Essentials of Neuro-ophthalmology

Declaration

Essentials of Neuro-ophthalmology

PK Mukherjee MS
Former Professor and Head
Upgraded Department of Ophthalmology
Pandit Jawaharlal Nehru Memorial Medical College
Raipur, Chhattisgarh, India

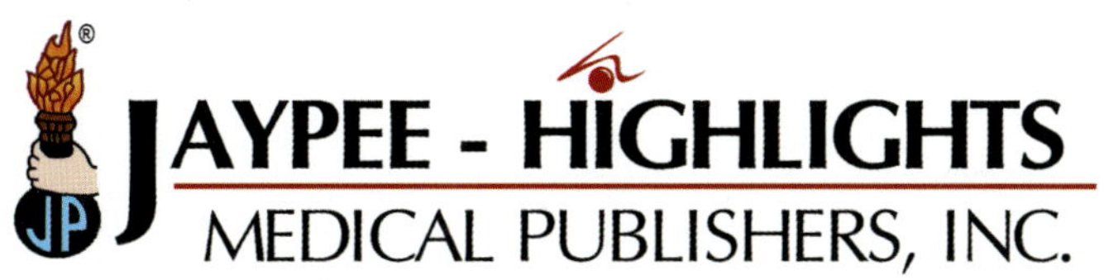

Published by

Jitendar P Vij

Jaypee Brothers Medical Publishers (P) Ltd

Corporate Office

4838/24 Ansari Road, Daryaganj, **New Delhi** - 110002, India

Phone: +91-11-43574357, Fax: +91-11-43574314

Registered Office

B-3 EMCA House, 23/23B Ansari Road, Daryaganj, **New Delhi** - 110 002, India

Phones: +91-11-23272143, +91-11-23272703, +91-11-23282021, +91-11-23245672

Rel: +91-11-32558559, Fax: +91-11-23276490, +91-11-23245683

e-mail: jaypee@jaypeebrothers.com, Website: www.jaypeebrothers.com

Offices in India

- **Ahmedabad**, Phone: Rel: +91-79-32988717, e-mail: ahmedabad@jaypeebrothers.com
- **Bengaluru**, Phone: Rel: +91-80-32714073, e-mail: bangalore@jaypeebrothers.com
- **Chennai**, Phone: Rel: +91-44-32972089, e-mail: chennai@jaypeebrothers.com
- **Hyderabad**, Phone: Rel:+91-40-32940929, e-mail: hyderabad@jaypeebrothers.com
- **Kochi**, Phone: +91-484-2395740, e-mail: kochi@jaypeebrothers.com
- **Kolkata**, Phone: +91-33-22276415, e-mail: kolkata@jaypeebrothers.com
- **Lucknow**, Phone: +91-522-3040554, e-mail: lucknow@jaypeebrothers.com
- **Mumbai**, Phone: Rel: +91-22-32926896, e-mail: mumbai@jaypeebrothers.com
- **Nagpur**, Phone: Rel: +91-712-3245220, e-mail: nagpur@jaypeebrothers.com

Overseas Offices

- **North America Office, USA,** Ph: 001-636-6279734, e-mail: jaypee@jaypeebrothers.com anjulav@jaypeebrothers.com
- **Central America Office, Panama City, Panama,** Ph: 001-507-317-0160, e-mail: cservice@jphmedical.com Website: www.jphmedical.com
- **Europe Office, UK,** Ph: +44 (0) 2031708910, e-mail: info@jpmedpub.com

Essentials of Neuro-ophthalmology

First Edition: **2010**

ISBN 978-81-8448-982-8

Typeset at JPBMP typesetting unit

Printed at Replika Press Pvt. Ltd.

To

My Wife and Soul Mate

Protima

Preface

The fascinating subject of neuro-ophthalmology is an enigma that frightens the undergraduates and the postgraduates are initially at ease with cases of neuro-ophthalmology and the general ophthalmologists find them too demanding hence are happy to handover them to neurophysicians or neurosurgeons at the earliest.

Neuro-ophthalmology is not an individual entity, it is very much ophthalmology. It has ramifications in other specialties like neuromedicine, neurosurgery, neuroimaging, oncology and otorhinology.

The riddle of neuro-ophthalmology is not difficult to crack provided the cases are examined by a fixed protocol, avoiding ordering investigations at random. The puzzles of neuro-ophthalmology are easier to solve if the clues in the form of history, clinical examination, etc. are given adequate attention to.

The number of books in neuro-ophthalmology are not too many. Most of those available are huge treatise which are almost classics by themselves. These books create awe in the beginners. The remaining books are too abridged to comprehend. The present book is a veritable "Neuro-ophthalmology Made Easy" meant for both undergraduates and postgraduates.

Management of a neuro-ophthalmic disorder is not always within the domain of ophthalmologists who should be aware of the significance of referring the case to consultants in other specialties. They should be able to decide when and to whom a case should be referred to.

The present book does not deal with systemic management in details, whenever needed only passing references have been given. The systemic management is better left to neurophysicians or neurosurgeons. The surgical procedures too have been left out. They may be read from specific books. Neuroimaging is proving to be a great boon in neuro-ophthalmic disorders. The students are advised to understand finer points of neuroimaging from books exclusively dealing with the subject.

PK Mukherjee

Acknowledgments

It was virtually impossible for me to write the book without the help from my friends, colleagues and family members.

On the top of the list of my peers, who extended unending help are the members of upgraded Department of Ophthalmology, Pandit Jawaharlal Nehru Memorial Medical College, Raipur, Chhattisgarh, India. They include Professor SL Adile, the present Director Medical Education, Government of Chhattisgarh, Professor and Head of the Department, Dr AK Chandrakar, Professor Dr ML Garg and Dr Nidhi Pandey, Associate Professor of Ophthalmology, all of whom have kept me supplied with unending stream of books and journals. Dr Santosh Patel has been generous enough to provide me maximum number of clinical pictures, who deserves special mention and thanks.

My niece, Dr Nupur Chakravarty, Professor of Ophthalmology, YD Patil Medical College, Mumbai, Dr OP Billore of Rotary Eye Hospital, Navsari, Dr Hetal Yagnik, Dr Sharad Sivasane and Dr Dishant Shant of the same institute as well, have sent me interesting photographs from their collection. Their contribution is acknowledged with gratitude. I am thankful to Dr Anand Saxena for the colored fundus photographs and fundus fluorescein angiography (FFA) used in the book.

I thank Dr Barun K Nayak, Editor of Indian Journal of Ophthalmology, to use some of the photographs published in the journal.

Dr Manik Chatterjee, Associate Professor of Anatomy, Pandit Jawaharlal Nehru Memorial Medical College, Raipur, Chhattisgarh, India was always available to solve my curiosity about intricacies of neuroanatomy. He was polite enough to point out the fallacies in my drawings. I am thankful to him.

I am highly obliged to Padamsri Professor AT Dabke PhD, former Director of Medical Education and Professor of Pediatric for permitting to use his personal library unfettered.

The book may not have seen the light of the day without the help from members of my family. My sons-in-law, Satayadeep Sahukar and Dr Abeer Bandyapadhya, took special interest in locating various references on Internet, drawing the diagrams and arranging them. I am thankful to my daughters, Dr Protibha Mukherjee Sahukar and Dr Preeti Bandyopadhya, for their unending help and suggestions from time to time in their respective specialties.

The real inspiration has been my wife, Protima, who awakened me often from the slumber in which I slipped occasionally.

Sri Maneesh Dandekar of Hypersoft Computers has taken great troubles in deciphering my handwritten manuscript and type them many a times. Sri Bhim Sona of Hypersoft also deserves appreciation for drawings used in the book.

Finally, I extend my thanks to Sri Jitendar P Vij (Chairman and Managing Director), Jaypee Brothers Medical Publishers (P) Ltd., New Delhi, India and members of his team for their constant interest in publishing my humble contribution towards continued medical education.

Contents

The ocular symptoms can broadly be divided into two groups:

1. Visual
2. Nonvisual.

Existence of both simultaneously in the same patient is very common. In less frequent cases one may follow the other.

The visual symptoms may be

1. Uniocular/binocular
2. Acute/gradual
3. May recover
4. Recover with relapse
5. May worsen.

The visual symptoms can be

A. Afferent
B. Efferent.

A. The afferent visual signs and symptoms are

1. Diminished vision:
   i. Distant
   ii. Near
   iii. Both.
2. Field defects:
   i. Central
   ii. Peripheral
3. Diminished color sense.
4. Diminished brightness.
5. Diminished night vision.
6. Amaurosis.
7. Obscuration.
8. Oscillopsia.
9. Visual hallucination.
10. Visual aura.
11. Photopsia.
12. Macropsia and metamorphopsia.

B. The efferent visual symptoms are mostly motility disorders.

They are:

1. Diplopia
2. Diminished near vision
3. Nystagmus
4. Squint and abnormal head posture
5. Abnormality of lid:
   i. Ptosis
   ii. Paradoxical lid movement

iii. Lagophthalmos
iv. Lid retraction
v. Blepharospasm
vi. Blepharoclonus
vii. Hemifacial spasms
viii. Myokymia
ix. Infrequent blinking
x. Proptosis and exophthalmos.

The nonocular symptoms of neuro-ophthalmic disorders are

1. Headache
2. Vomiting/nausea
3. Vertigo
4. Tinitus
5. Hearing defect
6. Regurgitation of fluid from nose
7. Myoclonus
8. Weakness in limbs
9. Paraplegia/hemiplegia
10. Neuralgia
11. Anesthesia
12. Tremors
13. Facial asymmetry.

Interpretation of afferent signs and of neuro-ophthalmic interest

(I) Visual disturbance

Diminished distant vision: It can be of **acute or gradual** onset, both of which can be **uniocular** or **binocular**. Binocular sudden loss of vision draws attention earlier than uniocular. It is necessary to find out that what the patient means is a real diminished vision. The patient with field loss with good central vision may complain of diminished vision. Patients with extraocular paresis may confuse mild diplopia as blurring. Persons with drooped lids may also complain of loss of vision (Flow chart 1.1).

While evaluating loss of vision the following points need to be looked into:

1. **Onset**
   i. *Sudden:* AION, papillitis, retrobulbar optic neuritis, compressive lesions of the optic nerve, central retinal artery and venous obstruction are the common causes of sudden loss of distant vision.
   ii. *Gradual:* The gradual causes of diminished distant vision are—papilledema, chronic retrobulbar optic neuritis, compressive lesions of the visual path.
2. **Progression**
   i. **Progressive:** Compressive lesion, chronic infection
   ii. **Fast deterioration:** Generally vascular or acute infection

Flow chart 1.1: To interpret diminished distant vision in relation to neuro-ophthalmic lesions

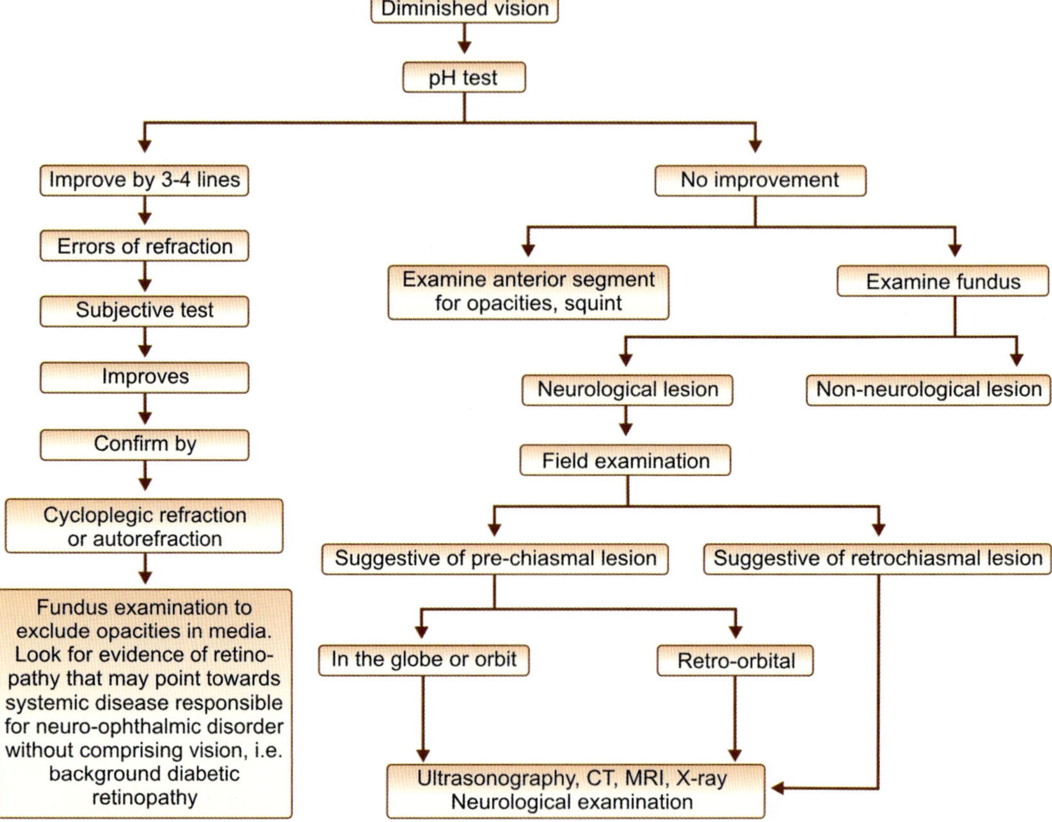

iii. **The progressive over days** followed by a state of low vision that improves over following weeks to months, i.e. optic neuritis.

3. *Deterioration:* Acute optic neuritis, there is fast deterioration over days followed by a state of stationary diminished vision and gradual improvement over weeks.
4. *Nonimprovement:* Anterior ischemic optic neuropathy, severe traumatic optic neuropathy.
5. **Duration of diminished vision**
   i. **Few seconds** – Raised intracranial pressure
   – Drusen of optic papilla
   ii. **Few minutes** – Amaurosis fugax (unilateral)
   – Occipital lobe ischemia (bilateral)
   – Postpartum, eclampsia
   iii. **20-30 minutes** with aura, scintillating scotoma—migraine.
6. **Associated with pain** – Optic neuritis.
7. **Associated with headache** – Raised intracranial tension
   – Diabetic neuropathy

- Intracranial aneurysms
- Benign intracranial hypertension
- Superior orbital fissure syndrome
- Giant cell arteritis.

8. Is the diminished vision due to neurological causes or is due to non-neurological cause?

   The non-neurological causes of diminished distant vision concurrent with neurological defects are:

   i. Errors of refraction: Error of refraction may coexist with neuro-ophthalmic conditions hence the best corrected vision should be recorded before further examination. Rest of the condition are found out on fundus examination.
   ii. Opacities in media
   iii. Retinopathies
   iv. Vitreous hemorrhage
   v. Amaurosis fugax: The loss of vision is unilateral of few second with recovery.

Causes of acute unilateral loss of vision

i. *Ischemic optic neuritis:* Both arteritic and nonarteritic ischemic neuritis have acute loss of vision. Acute profound loss of vision is seen in both anterior ischemic optic neuropathy and its posterior counterpart.
ii. *Acute papillitis:* This also gives acute loss of vision but the loss is not as dramatic as in acute ischemic optic atrophy.
iii. *Occlusion of central retinal vessels* both of artery and vein present as acute loss of vision but are not always associated with neuro-ophthalmic manifestation. The central retinal artery occlusion due to its pallor may be mistaken as optic atrophy and impending central vein thrombosis, may be confused as hyperemic disc or wrongly diagnosed as papilledema.
iv. Amaurosis fugax.

Causes of sudden bilateral loss of central vision

Bilateral sudden loss of central vision are **less common** than unilateral. For bilateral loss of vision the lesion has to be in such a location that involves **both the visual paths**.

i. Anterior ischemic optic neuritis due to temporal arteritis begins as unilateral but the other eye may be involved soon.
ii. Optic neuritis (bilateral simultaneous optic neuritis is rare)
iii. Acute chiasmitis
iv. Toxins and drugs
   - Methyl alcohol
   - Quinine
v. Vertebrobasilar artery insufficiency
vi. Cortical blindness
vii. Malignant hypertension
viii. Migraine

ix. Devic's neuromyelitis
x. Malingering.

Causes of gradual unilateral diminished vision

These are caused by chronic infection and inflammation, compressive neuropathy, heredofamilial degenerations and congenital anomalies. Many of the unilateral causes of diminished vision generally become bilateral with passage of time.

1. Congenital: Optic nerve hypoplasia, morning glory syndrome.
2. Heredofamilial optic neuropathy, generally bilateral but may start as unilateral.
3. Postinflammatory optic atrophy:
   i. Postneuritic atrophy
   ii. Consecutive optic atrophy
   iii. Primary optic atrophy
   iv. Postpapilledematous optic atrophy.
4. Compressive neuropathy.
5. Amblyopia (children).

Causes of gradual bilateral loss of vision are

1. Congenital: Bilateral optic nerve, hypoplasia.
2. Heredofamilial neuropathy:
   i. Lebers disease
   ii. Behr's neuropathy
   iii. Kjer's neuropathy.
3. Nutritional: Tobacco, alcohol amblyopia.
4. Drugs and toxins.
5. Raised intracranial tension.
6. Primary optic atrophy.
7. Consecutive optic atrophy.

(II) Diminished near vision

The commonest cause of diminished near vision, i.e. **presbyopia**, which is not of neurological origin. The next cause, i.e. **pharmacological** is also not of neurological origin. Pharmacological loss of vision can be brought about by local effect of cycloplegic or due to ingestion of parasympatholytic agents. Hence, in all cases of near vision defect in prepresbyopic age the two questions asked are regarding:

i. Use of parasympatholytic drugs, local/systemic
ii. History of trauma.

The Following points should be remembered:

i. All cycloplegic drugs are associated with mydriasis,
ii. All mydriatic are not cycloplegia,
iii. There is no drug that causes exclusive cycloplegia without mydriasis.

The neurological causes of diminished near vision are

Neurological diminished near vision is an efferent phenomenon.

(a) **Oculomotor palsy:**
- Total palsy
- Internal ophthalmoplegia only
- Third nerve palsy is generally associated with internal ophthalmoplegia
- Third nerve palsy without internal ophthalmoplegia is seen in vascular lesions, i.e. diabetes, hypertension
- Compressive lesions are mostly associated with internal ophthalmoplegia.

(b) **Infection of central nervous system:**
- Epidemic encephalitis: The lesion is nuclear and cycloplegia is bilateral.
- Poliomyelitis.
- Syphilis: In cerebral syphilitic the loss of accommodation may be independent of third nerve palsy, it is generally bilateral.

Tuberculosis: This generally cause unilateral paralysis of other extraocular muscles. The lesion involves the trunk.

Herpes zoster rarely cause diminished near vision.

(c) **Toxic causes:**

The two common bacterial toxins that cause loss of accommodation are:
- *Diphtheria:* It may be associated with diphtheria or may be a postdiphtheritic phenomenon.
- *Botulism:* It is associated with food poisoning due to *Clostridium botulinum*. The symptoms are acute and develop within first 24 hours of onset of food poisoning. It is bilateral, may be the only sign of botulism.
- *Tetanus:* Rarely cephalic tetanus may cause loss of accommodation.

(d) **Miscellaneous causes:**
- Progressive congenital ophthalmoplegia
- Adies syndrome
- Inverse Argyll Robertson pupil
- Parkinsonism.

Field defects

Field defects are always present in disorders of **visual pathway** from retina to occipital cortex. Field defects caused by retinal lesions are not of neuro-ophthalmic interest however they may be present with neuro-ophthalmic disorder and cause confusion (Fig. 1.1).

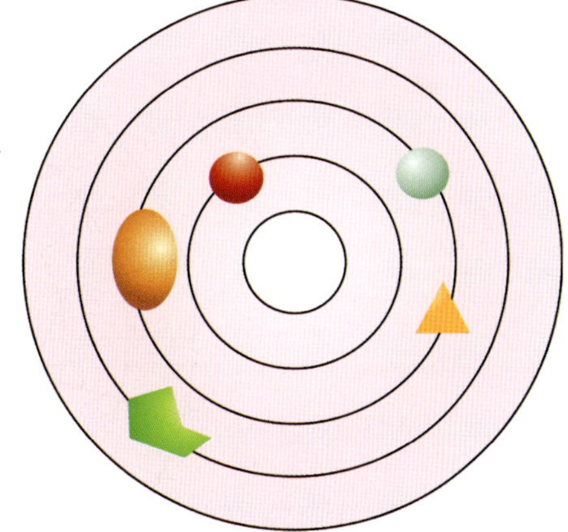

Fig. 1.1: Scotomas of chorioretinal lesion

Commonly used terms in relation to field defects are

- **Field of vision:** As per Traquair's definition, field of vision is an island of vision in a sea of blindness.
- **Central field:** Field within 30° of fixation (Fig. 1.2).
- **Peripheral field:** Field between 30° and 90° (Fig. 1.3).
- **Isopter** is the boundary of the scotoma. It joins points with same intensity.
- **Scotoma** is an area of blindness **total** or **partial** in field of vision. It is an area of depressed visual function surrounded by normal visual function.
- **Absolute scotoma:** No stimulus, i.e. bright or large is perceived any where in the scotoma.

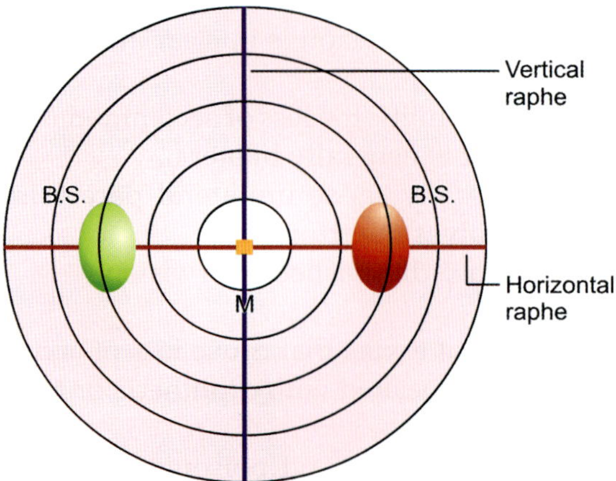

Fig. 1.2: Normal central field showing: M—Point of fixation; BS—Two blind spots

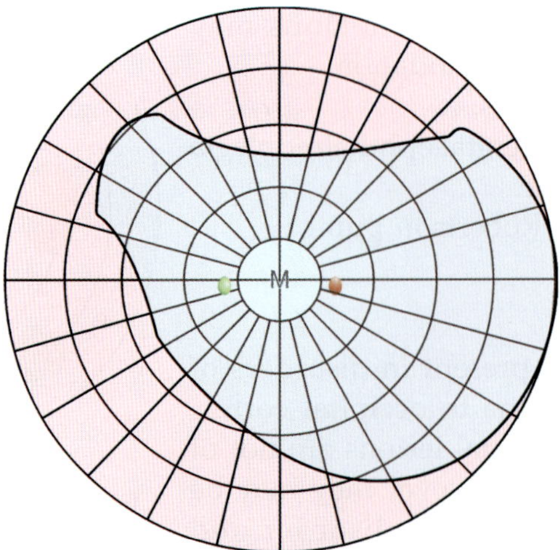

Fig. 1.3: Normal peripheral visual field right eye

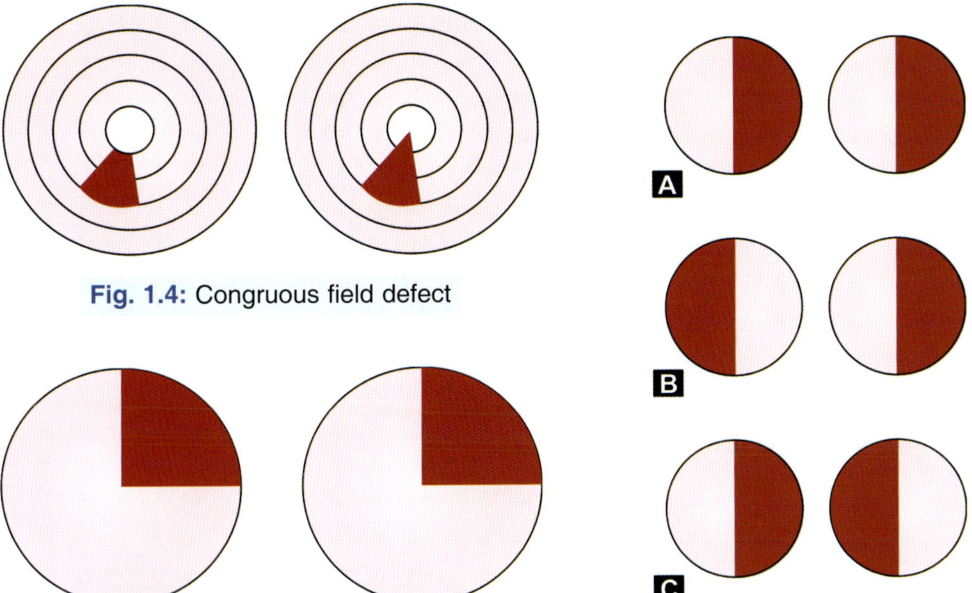

Fig. 1.4: Congruous field defect

Fig. 1.5: Quadrantanopia

Figs 1.6A to C: Various types of hemianopia

- **Relative scotoma:** The size, and depth of the scotoma changes with changes of stimulus. The size of scotoma is inversely proportionate to size of stimulus and intensity of stimulus.
- **Congruence:** A scotoma is said to be congruent when a scotoma coincides exactly with the scotoma in the other when superimposed. In simple terms both the scotomas are of the same size and shape. The term congruous is generally used for hemianopias or quadrantanopias (Fig. 1.4).
- **Quadrantanopia:** One-fourth or a quadrant of a field is affected (Fig. 1.5).
- **Hemianopia:** One-half of the field is affected.
- **Homonymous field defect:** Loss of field on the same side of both the eyes, i.e. loss of right temporal along with left nasal or vice versa (Fig. 1.6A).
- **Heteronymous field defect:** Loss of field on opposite sides in two eyes, i.e. right and left temporal or right and left nasal. They are known as bitemporal and binasal hemianopia (Figs 1.6B and C).
- **Sectoranopia:** The field defect is present in one sector, generally they start at the center and spread toward the periphery (Fig. 1.7).

Some examples of mono-ocular field defects (Fig. 1.8)

- **Enlargement of blind spot:** The blind sport enlarges both in vertical as well as horizontal direction.
- **Central scotoma:** Scotoma round the point of fixation, i.e. macula.

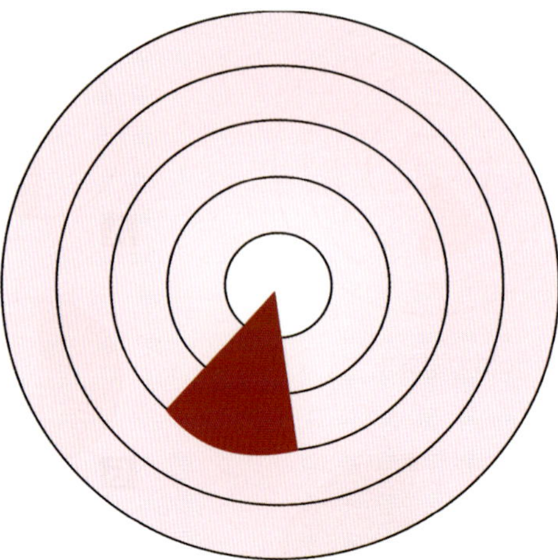

Fig. 1.7: Sectoranopia

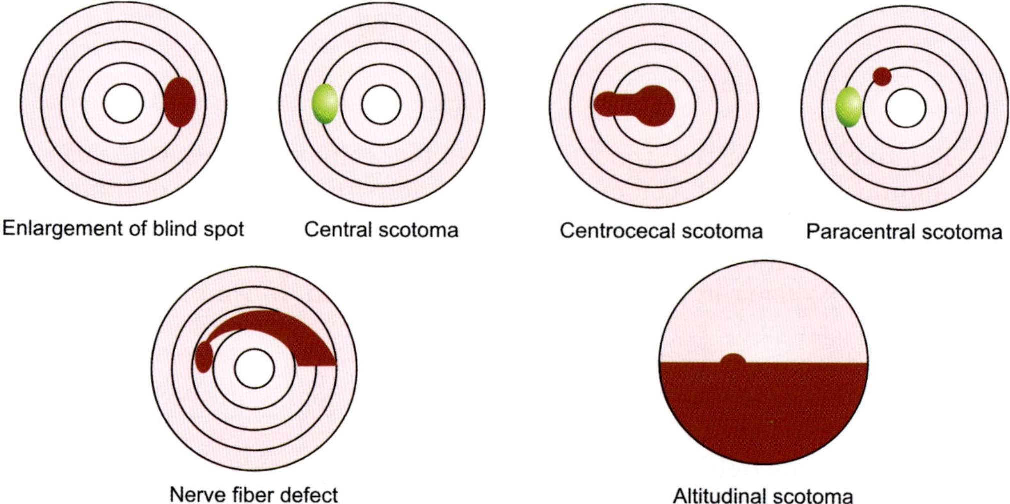

Fig. 1.8: Mono-ocular central field changes

- **Centrocecal:** Scotoma extending from point of fixation towards papilla, i.e. macula to optic nerve.
- **Paracentral scotoma:** They involve papillo-macular bundle little away from the macula but not involving the macula.
- **Arcuate scotomas** are the scotomas that start from the blind spot, arch over the macula and end on the horizontal raphe away from the macula. They are narrow at the blind spot and fan out as they arch over the point of fixation, they are caused due to **defects in nerve fiber bundles**. Rarely seen in neuro-ophthalmic lesion.

Altitude scotoma

Some examples of binocular field defects

- **Junctional scotomas:** They are bilateral scotomas. One eye has a central scotoma, the other has a sectoranopia they are caused due to lesion at the junction of optic nerve and the chiasma on the same side (Fig. 1.9).
- **Pie in the sky:** These are superior homonymous noncongruous scotomas in the mid periphery due to anterior temporal lobe lesion (Fig. 1.10).
- **Pie in the floor:** Inferior, homonymous incongruous field defects in the mid periphery due to lesion parietal lobe (Fig. 1.11).
- **Macular sparing** are bilateral field defects seen in homonymous hemianopia, leaving 5° of macular field intact. They are seen in occipital lobe lesions (Fig. 1.12).

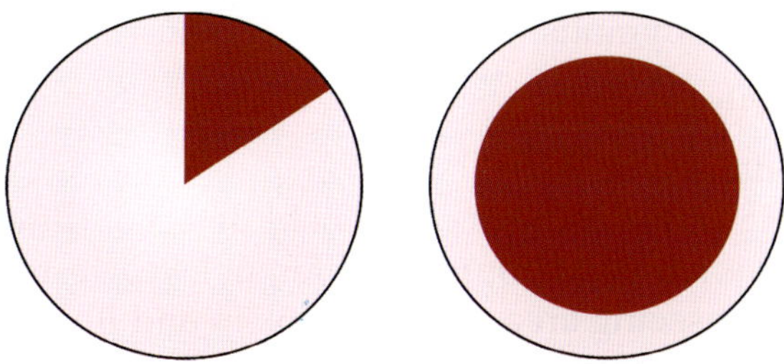

Fig. 1.9: Junctional scotoma

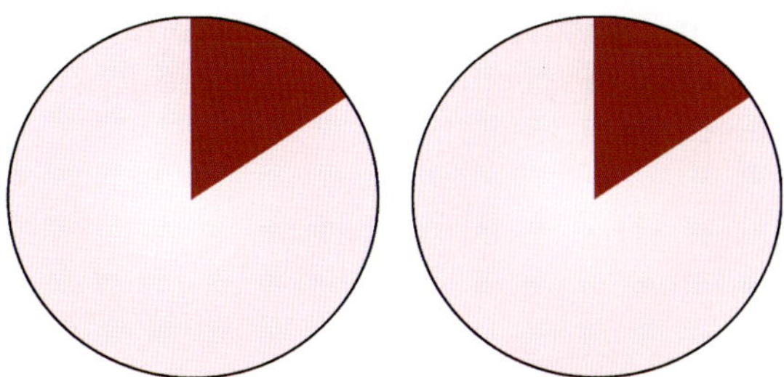

Fig. 1.10: Pie in the sky

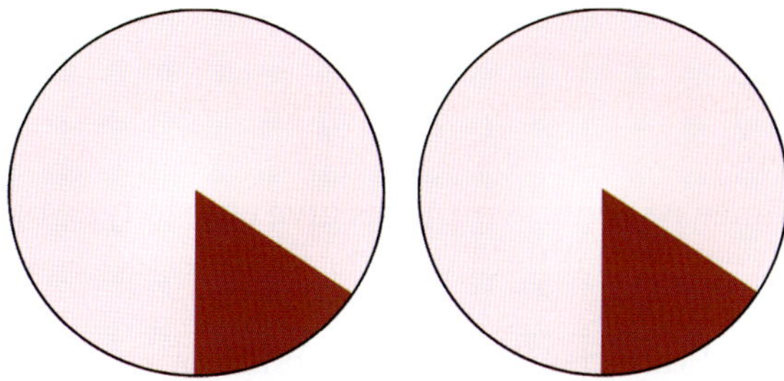

Fig. 1.11: Pie in the floor

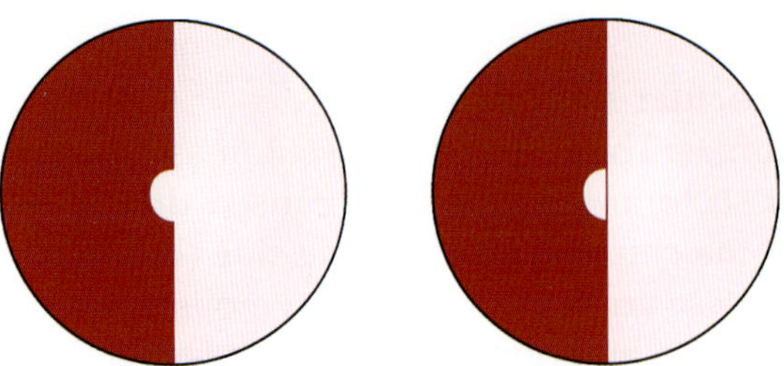

Fig. 1.12: Sparing of macula

- **Macular splitting** when the inner border of the homonymous hemianopia passes through the macula.
- **Sparing of the temporal crescent** is seen in lesions of visual cortex in presence of congruous homonymous hemianopia.

Methods of field charting

There are two methods:

1. **Kinetic:** This draws the contour of the field defect at different levels, isopter of each level tested is joined to isopter of different levels tested. The target is moved from seeing to nonseeing area. The size, colors and illumination of the target is variable. It produces horizontal section through the island of vision. The field testers can be **manual** or **automatic**. The examples are: **Bjerrum screen, Lister** and **Aimark** and **Goldmann perimeter** (Fig. 1.13).
2. **Static perimetery:** It measures each retinal receptors ability to perceive light. When the light is placed in specific location. It produces a vertical section through the island of vision (Fig. 1.13).

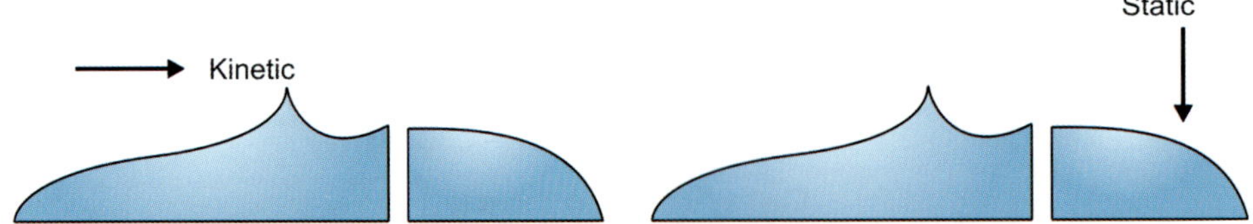

Fig. 1.13: Method of field charting movement of target in kinetic and static perimeter

Evaluation of field defects in neuro-ophthalmic cases

Points to remember:

1. **History:** Sometimes patients symptoms give clue to type of field defect expected:
   i. Central and centrocecal field defects are referred as loss of vision or black spot in front of the eye.
   ii. Bitemporal field defects: Patient with bitemopral defect complain that they bump into persons or objects on either side or cannot locate a vehicle coming from the side at a road junction.

iii. Unilateral outer field can be lost in ipsilateral homonymous homoanopia.
iv. Nasal hemianopia can be part of contralateral homonymous hemianopia.
v. Left homonymous field loss is reported as difficulty in seeing whole words or finding next line while reading.
vi. Right homonymous field loss is reported as difficulty in seeing the next word.
vii. Altitudenal field losses are felt as either lower field loss or upper field loss and are due to ischemic optic neuropathy.
viii. The nerve fiber defects in retina respect the horizontal raphe.
ix. The neurological defects respect the vertical raphe except in case of occipital lobe lesions which can respect the horizontal meridian.
x. The fields are drawn as the patient perceives them.
xi. The patient's best-corrected vision is recorded before the fields are being charted and patient uses his glasses or contact lenses during field charting.

Field changes in both eyes should be charted one at a time. A patient with symptoms in one eye may not be aware of peripheral field change in the other eye. Pre-existing field changes may influence and cause confusion in neuro-ophthalmic field defects.

Field changes in different locations in optic pathway

	Part involved	*Type of field defect*
1.	Optic nerve	Dense central scotoma, less common centrocecal scotoma and altitudinal scotoma. Arcuate scotoma rarely peripheral (see Fig. 1.8)
2.	Retrobulbar	Central scotoma (see Fig. 1.8)
3.	Junction of chiasma and optic nerve	Junctional scotoma consists of central scotoma on the side of optic nerve involved with sectoranopia, generally superior or central hemianopia (macular) on the other side (see Fig. 1.9)
4.	Chiasma:	
	i. Central	Bitemporal hemianopia begins as quadranopia (Fig. 1.14)
	ii. Posterior chiasma	Small central bitemporal scotomas—incongruous
	iii. Lateral	Binasal hemianopia requires two lesions
	All the above field defect respect vertical line	
5.	Optic track	Contralateral homonymous incongruous hemianopia (Fig. 1.15)
6.	Lateral geniculate body	Contralateral homonymous hemianopia small in size, incongruous, may be wedge shaped, wedge pointing towards point of fixation. They are rare (Fig. 1.15)

Confrontation methods of eliciting field defect in neuro-ophthalmic lesions

The methods used are helpful to elicit large central field defects, hemianopias and quadrantanopias. **They are not suitable for nerve fiber layer defects.**

It can be done in two ways:

a. **In adults:** To test the right field, the patient sits at arms length away from the examiner, closes the left eye and looks in the left eye of the examiner. The examiner closes his right eye. The examiner moves his index finger from the periphery towards the center slowly in jerks. The patient is asked to state when the finger is noticed for the first time. This is repeated all around the peripheral. This roughly delineates the outer border of the visible field. The method is good for peripheral contraction, tubular field, hemianopia and quadrantanopia.

b. **In children:** The child looks at the face of the examiner with both eyes open and a small object of interest is moved from the periphery to center. As soon as the object becomes visible the child moves the eyes to bring the object to the fovea.

c. **Ability to recognize and count fingers when kept at half a meter distance:**
   i. The ability of the patient to count the fingers placed in four quadrants. The patient looks into the eye of the examiner. One eye is tested at a time.
   ii. Simultaneous counting of fingers in each hemifield of one eye. The examiner presents fingers of different number, i.e. three of right hand and two of left hand. The patient is asked to tell the total number of fingers seen. This method is used to find out subtle hemianopia. The patient with hemifield change may not notice hemianopia when tested in individual field, which becomes apparent when tested simultaneously.
   iii. The patient is shown single finger in each quadrant and asked to state in which quadrant. The finger looks faint. The quadrant with faint image has a relative scotoma.

d. **Diminished color sense:** Acquired diminished color vision is an important feature of lesions of visual pathway from retina to retrochiasmal structures. The two common causes of diminished color sense involving the anterior pathway are:
   i. Optic neuropathy
   ii. Maculopathy.

   The two conditions should be differentiated. The maculopathies are not associated with neuro-ophthalmic signs. Before embarking upon examination of defective color sense of neuro-ophthalmic origin, it is mandatory to exclude possibility of color blindness especially in males by any of the standard screening procedures, i.e. using pseudoisochromatic plates.

Color blindness is an inherited disease seen almost exclusively in males with bilaterally symmetrical reduction of color sense and is a stationary condition. Color blindness per se, does not cause defective vision or field changes which are prominent feature of neuropathy and maculopathy.

The optic neuropathy and maculopathy are differentiated by following features

Comparison between optic neuropathy and maculopathy

Features	*Optic neuropathy*	*Maculopathy*
Distant vision	Diminished	Diminished
Field defect	Central/centrocecal	Central
Metamorphopsia	Absent	Present
Color vision	Diminished grossly	Dull
Pupillary reaction	Normal/RAPD	Normal
Brightness	Dull	Normal
Amsler grid	Central scotoma	Metamorphopsia
Photo stress test	Negative	Positive

For neuro-ophthalmic lesions colour vision is tested in

Two eyes separately and compared.

a. The effected eye has subnormal color vision.
b. The testing methods are gross. It consists of comparison of the brightness of the color of the same object in two eyes and followed by use of Ishihara color testing plates that can demonstrate presence of red-green defect and blue-yellow defect.
c. Color vision defect may return to normal with treatment in lesions of optic nerve.
d. Color vision defect is due to conduction defect in the optic nerve.
e. Color vision defect may precede diminished vision.
f. It may appear before ophthalmoscopic signs develop.
g. The color vision defect may not be proportionate to loss of vision. Loss of color sense is more profound than loss of vision.
h. Combination of loss of vision and diminished color sense goes in favor of optic neuropathy.
i. Compressive and demyelination cause more marked color defect than vascular lesions which produce more diminished vision than color vision.
j. Optic nerve diseases produce red-green defect except in chronic papilledema.
k. Glaucoma and macular diseases mostly produce blue-yellow defect.
l. The neurological causes of defective color vision are: Optic neuritis, retrobulbar neuritis, retrochiasmal lesion with defective field, lesion of inferior occipital lobe, heredofamilial optic atrophy, and many drugs.
m. **Achromatopsia** is total absence of color sense. The vision is monochromatic. It is a **rare congenital** condition associated with **pendular nystagmus**, **photophobia** and **diminished vision**.

3. **Diminished brightness:** An object looks dull both in optic neuropathy and maculopathy. Dimness is more pronounced in maculopathy than neuropathy.

4. **Diminished night vision** is not of much significance in neuro-ophthalmic disorders. In case of primary retinal and choroidal dystrophies, diminished night vision is a prominent feature which are associated with consecutive optic atrophy.
5. **Amaurosis** is defined as loss of sight without apparent lesion of in the eye. It is to be differentiated from amblyopia which is gradual in onset. Transient lowering of vision of neuro-ophthalmic importance can broadly be divided into:
   i. Monocular amaurosis:
      (a) Amaurosis fugax due to carotid insufficiency
      (b) Amaurosis due to vertebrobasilar insufficiency (less common)
   ii. Bilateral transient visual loss
   iii. Cortical blindness
   iv. Malingering.

I. **Amaurosis fugax** is—**transient, painless monocular** loss of vision that **lasts for few seconds to few minutes**. The loss of vision may involve whole of the visual field, may be hemianopic. The patient complains that a curtain has descended from above or ascended from below causing diminished vision that may be total or may be referred as lowering the intensity of ambient light. The dimness clears in the reverse direction, i.e. from below upward or vice versa. The vision generally returns to normal. Only in one percent of eyes, there may be permanent loss of field of vision.

Exact mechanism of the phenomenon is not clear. The common theories are:
i. Unilateral local vasospasm in ophthalmic retinal artery complex.
ii. Atheroma formation in internal or common carotid.
iii. Acute hypoperfusion in ophthalmic retinal system due to hemodynamic changes.

Other causes of transient visual loss are: Takayasu's disease, impending central retinal artery occlusion, giant cell arteritis, valvular heart disease, coagulopathy, and polycythemia.

II. **Bilateral transient loss of vision** is an indication of **vertebrobasilar insufficiency** is caused due to ischemic of the occipital cortex. The condition is painless, transient and reversible, may be associated with migraine. The attack lasts for one to five minutes.
The condition may be the only symptom of **vertebrobasilar insufficiency** or may be the beginning of more serious **brainstem lesion**.

III. **Cortical blindness** is a **bilateral amaurosis** that lasts for **weeks to months**. It is a **painless** condition where the **patient may deny blindness** in spite of obvious loss of vision. It is generally seen in **elderly** person who have other feature of vascular insufficiency resulting in bilateral occipital lesion. The **pupillary reactions are normal so are the fundi**. It may follow trauma or may be due to tumors.

IV. **Malingering:** The medical dictionary defines malingering as **wilful, deliberate and fraudulent feigning or exaggeration of the symptoms**. The ocular symptoms in malingering are mostly visual, i.e. loss of vision. Unilateral bilateral, partial or total less common are **diminished night or color vision**. The condition is not associated with any neuro-ophthalmic deficits. However before pronouncing a person to be malinger utmost care should be taken to rule out other causes.

6. **Obscuration** is similar to amaurosis but of shorter duration. The loss of vision lasts for only a few seconds with complete recovery. It is most commonly seen in **papilledema** due to ischemia of optic nerve secondary to raised intracranial tension. The episode lasts less than 30 seconds. It begins suddenly and passes of equally fast. It may be associated with flashes of light. Obscuration in **migraine** last for longer time, i.e. 25-30 minutes and is associated with scintillating scotomas.
7. **Oscillopsia** is a peculiar sensation where the patient feels that the stationary objects are moving. It is seen in **acquired nystagmus, superior oblique myokymia**, some disorders of **brain stem** and **vestibular system.**
8. **Visual aura** is seen in migraine. They may be scintillating with or without fortification.
9. **Visual hallucinations** are illusory feeling of presence of an external object in its absence.
   It can be:
   i. **Simple** (unformed): This mostly presents as flashes of light or change in color. The lesions of occipital lobe and anterior visual path generally cause unformed hallucination.
   ii. **Complex** (formed) result in seeing figures, persons, animals, etc. They are seen in temporal lobe lesions.

Hallucinations do not have any localizing value

They are also reported in **schizophrenia, mania, epilepsy, and Alzheimer's disease**. The list of drugs that cause visual hallucination is long.

1. Most of them are caused following administrations of the drug.
2. Less common are the drugs that cause hallucination on withdrawal, i.e. alcohol and baclofen.

Besides therapeutic substances, there are some toxins and poisons that also cause hallucination.

The commonly used therapeutic drugs are: Atropine, home atropine, cyclopentolate are known to cause hallucination when used locally. Other substance are: Marijuana (Marihuana), LSD, ecstasy (MDMA).

10. **Photopsia** is sensation of light in various forms of **flashes, sparks and illuminous points** in the field of vision. Sometimes the patient may complain of sparking or streaks light inside the eye. They are generally due to **irritation of the retina** that may be precursor of retinal detachment and should not be dismissed as trivial. All such cases should be examination by indirect

ophthalmoscope. Photopsia of any origin do not have any localizing value. They may be caused by lesions extending from **visual cortex to optic nerve**.

11. **Micro, macro and metamorphopsia:** These are the visual sensations where the shape of the object is changed. In micropsia the object look smaller, in macropsia larger and metamorphopsia distorted. The common cause is **macular lesion**. The neurological lesions casing them are **deep-seated cerebral lesion** sometimes felt in **epilepsy**. They do not have any localizing value. In all eases of distorted shape of object the first line of investigations should be directed towards a macular lesions.
12. **Dyslexia** is a common neurological disorder with widespread psychogenic and social ramification. The condition is first noticed in **childhood** when an apparently normal child fails to cope up with lessons and is generally thought to be dull. The term is generally referred to **word blindness**. The child has good corrected vision. The child fails to appreciate the meanings of written word, signs and symbols.
    The **Alexia** is complete inability to understand written words and symbols. Causes are cortical or subcortical lesions.
13. **Visual agnosia** is inability to recognize objects by sight but may be recognized by touch or sound.
14. **Palinopsia:** Patients with hemianopic field defect complains that the image of an object lingers even when it has been removed. They are seen in lesions of occipital or partial lobe.
15. **Apraxia** is diminished, voluntary, horizontal movement with retained voluntary vertical movement. It can be **congenital** or **acquired** and is caused due to parieto-occipital lesions. It may be localized in lid as well.
16. **Agraphia** is in ability to write in absence of motor paralysis.

Efferent visual symptoms in neuro-ophthalmic disorders

1. Diplopia (Flow chart 1.2)

Diplopia is a **subjective feeling** of seeing every object two. Most common type of diplopia is binocular diplopia (Fig. 1.18).

Binocular diplopia is that diplopia where closing any of the eyes causes disappearance of diplopia, irrespective of the eye involved. In neurological disorder, i.e. a person has diplopia due to paralysis of one of the extraocular muscle in right eye. The diplopia will disappear even when the left eye is closed. To have diplopia both the eyes should have fairly good and almost equal vision. The pupillary area should not be obscured by lid. The image formed on the retina should be central. Binocular diplopia is of great importance in neuro-ophthalmic lesion.

Uniocular diplopia is that diplopia which disappears when the diseased eye is covered; diplopia persists on covering the contralateral eye. **Uniocular diplopia has no neuro-ophthalmic significance**. It is **less common** than binocular diplopia and

Flow chart 1.2: Behaviors of diplopia

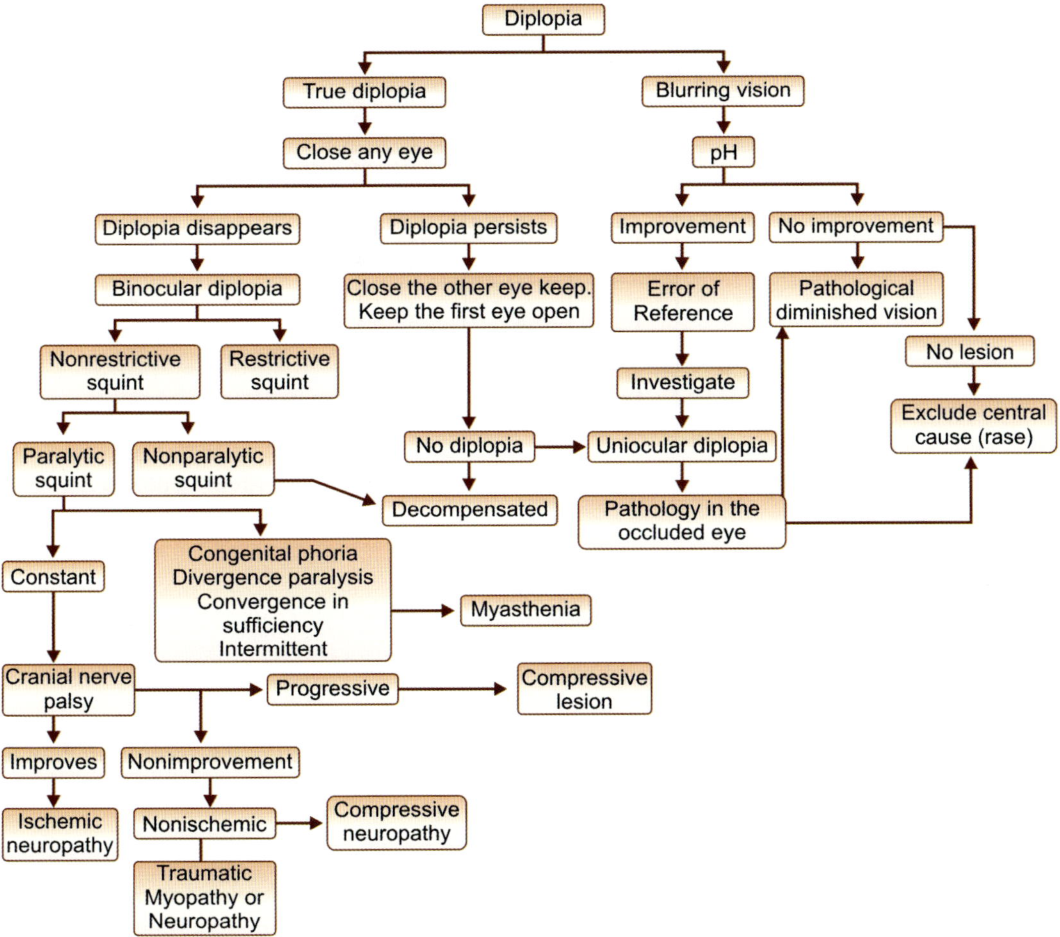

caused by lesions in the eyeball. The extraocular muscles are normal the amount of diplopia does not change with change in gaze. The common causes of uniocular diplopia are: Recent corneal opacity, astigmatism, iridodialysis, subluxated lens, subluxated 10 L recent retinal detachment, air in AC or vitreous. Rarely uniocular diplopia can be of central origin.

Polyopia is sensation of seeing multiple. This can either be **uniocular** or **binocular**. The uniocular polyopia disappears when one closes the effected eye but in binocular polyopia the multiple images persist. In rare cases there may be super imposition of binocular diplopia on uniocular diplopia, i.e. person with uniocular diplopia goes into paralysis of extraocular muscles. This patients will also get polyopia.

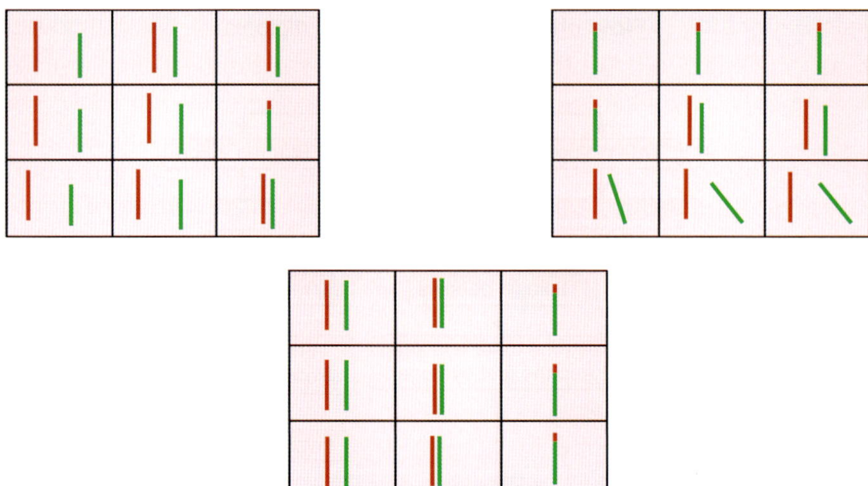

Fig. 1.18: Various types of binocular diplopia tested with red-green glasses

Evaluation of diplopia

a. The first thing to be determined is if the complain is:
   i. Binocular diplopia
   ii. Uniocular diplopia
   iii. Polyopia.

b. Once it has been ascertained that the diplopia is binocular the examiner has to decide if the diplopia is:
   i. **Neurologic:** Cranial nerve
   ii. **Myogenic:** Myasthenia
   iii. **Restrictive:** Thyroid ocular disease, traumatic, orbital pseudotumor, orbital tumors.

c. The neurological lesion are either constant, improve gradually over days or worsens. Improvement is seen in **ischemic neuropathy**, i.e. diabetes and hypertension. The paralysis in **multiple sclerosis** have frequent recurrence following apparent improvement. Worsening of diplopia is seen in **compressive lesions** of cranial nerves, and **thyroid ophthalmopathy**. Intermittent diplopia and change in the side is seen in **myasthenia**. Diplopia in myasthenia worsens with increased activity. Congenital lesions generally do not cause diplopia they are frequently associated with head tilt and amblyopia.

d. Find out if the separation of the image are:
   i. Horizontal: Third nerve palsy, sixth nerve palsy.
   ii. Vertical: Isolated superior oblique palsy, partial third nerves palsy, thyroid ophthalmopathy and myasthenia.
   iii. Tilting: Cyclovertical muscle palsy. Commonest is superior oblique palsy.

e. Is the diplopia crossed (heteronymous) or uncrossed (homonymous): The principle involved in crossed/uncrossed diplopia lies in projection of false image in relation to the position of the globe. The false image is projected in a direction opposite to the displacement of the eye hence in esotropia the diplopia is uncrossed and in exotropia it is crossed. Paralysis of adductors will cause crossed diplopia and abductors will cause uncrossed diplopia.
f. Is diplopia equal in all fields of gazes, if so it is due to nonparalytic squint? If it worsens in the field of action of the muscle involved, the squint is paralytic.
g. Onset of diplopia: Acute onset is seen in noncompressive cranial nerve palsy and trauma.
h. Diplopia with horizontal separation which is worse for distance is due to lateral rectus palsy while diplopia which is worse for near work and climbing stairs with vertical separation is due to fourth nerve palsy. Total third nerve palsy does not cause vertical diplopia. Patients with third nerve palsy may have initial diplopia that disappears if the lid comes down to cover the pupil only to reappear as the paralysis improves exposing the pupil.
i. Diplopia associated with proptosis is generally caused due to thyroid oculopathy, tumors in the orbit, pseudotumor of orbit, cavernous sinus thrombosis, and cavernous sinus fistula.
j. Diplopia with multiple muscle involvement in both eye without proptosis is seen in myasthenia, progressive ocular myopathy, and botulin toxin.
k. Diplopia with adduction defect and abducting nystagmus is seen in intranuclear ophthalmoplegia.
l. In evaluating vertical diplopia only vertical separation is taken into consideration. Horizontal separation is ignored.
m. In vertical diplopia find out which vertically acting muscles are involved—elevators/depressors.
n. In case of vertical diplopia if the eye is abducted the rectus are at fault and if the eye is adducted oblique are at fault.
o. In red-green glass test for diplopia the red image belongs to the right eye.
p. The more peripheral image belongs to the paretic eye.

2. Diminished near vision (see page 8)

3. Nystagmus (see Chapter 16)

4. Squint and abnormal head posture

Squint of recent origin is an obvious sign of neuro-ophthalmic importance that brings the patient for examination. This is associated with diplopia and in ability to move the eye equally in all direction. A patient with slowly developing ocular deviation may not be aware of its presence. The squints of recent origin are mostly paralytic in nature less common are: Phorias breaking into tropia, divergence in sufficiency and convergence paralysis. This makes it imperative to differentiate between:

- Paralytic
- Nonparalytic squint.

Paralytic squint itself can be due to any of the following causes:

- Neurogenic
- Myogenic
- Restrictive.

The following chart shows the differentiating features of paralytic and nonparalytic squint:

Features of paralytic and nonparalytic squint

Features	*Paralytic squint*	*Nonparalytic squint*
Symptoms	1. Cosmetic deviation may be associated with ptosis or lagophthalmos.	1. Cosmetic deviation. No lid changes.
	2. Diplopia common.	2. Absent, except in congenital phoria getting converted to tropia. Convergence paralysis or divergence insufficiency.
	3. Abnormal head posture common.	3. No abnormal head posture.
	4. Giddiness may be present.	4. Giddiness absent.
Heredity	Absent	Has strong hereditary tendency.
Vision	Variable diminished vision not related to squint except in involvement of optic nerve.	Variable, diminished vision may be the cause or effect of the squint.
Error or refraction	Not contributory.	May be the cause of squint.
Onset	Sudden	Generally gradual may be periodic or intermittent.
Movement	Restricted in the field of action of effected muscle.	Equal and full in all fields of gaze.
Primary deviation	Secondary deviation is more than primary deviation.	Primary and secondary deviation are equal.
Secondary changes in the muscles	Common	Rare
Spontaneous recovery	Possible	Nil
Amblyopia	Common in children	Common in children.

The following features differentiate paralytic squint from restrictive squint

Differences between paralytic squint and restrictive squint

Feature	*Paralytic squint*	*Restrictive squint*
Onset	Sudden	Gradual
Laterality	Mostly unilateral	May be bilateral
Movements	Restricted in the direction of action of involved muscle	Restricted in the opposite direction
Duction and version	Duction is more than version	Both equal
Forced duction test	Negative	Generally positive

Abnormal head posture

Abnormal head posture is not only a prominent symptom of paralytic squint but are also important signs.

The abnormal head posture is mostly seen in paralytic squint but can be seen in some nonparalytic conditions like:

i. Loss of field
ii. A esodeviation
iii. V exodeviation
iv. Astigmatism
v. High degree of ametropia
vi. Congenital ptosis
vii. Nystagmus.

Some of the nonocular condition are:

i. Torticolis
ii. Unilateral deafness
iii. Habitual.

Abnormal head posture due to nonocular causes are not rectified by patching one of the eyes.

The pathophysiology behind the abnormal head posture of neurological causes are:

The head turns when the eye cannot move:

- To increase the field of the under acting muscle.
- To avoid diplopia.
- Improve vision.
- To get binocular single vision as far as possible.

The abnormal head posture can be

i. Elevation/depression of the chin.
ii. Turning the head left/right (face turn)
iii. Tilting the head towards left or right shoulders.
iv. Combination.

Neuro-ophthalmic causes of various abnormal head posture

1. Chin	I. Elevation	i. Ptosis
		ii. Paralysis of elevators
		iii. Over action of depressors
		iv. Entrapment of inferior rectus
		v. Double levator palsy
		vi. General fibrosis syndrome.
	II. Depression	i. Paralysis in depressors
		ii. Over action of elevators
		iii. Supranuclear lesion.
2. Head	I. Turn right	i. Paralysis of right abductor RLR, oblique
		ii. Paralysis of left adductor, right SR, right IR and left inferior oblique
		Right supranuclear gaze paresis
		iii. Contracture of right MR
		iv. Left supranuclear gaze paresis.
	II. Turn left	i. Paralysis of left abductor, left LR and obliques
		ii. Paralysis of right adductors, RMR, right SO, right IO, left IR
		iii. Contracture of left MR
		iv. Left supranuclear gaze paresis.
	III. Tilt right	Left superior oblique, right inferior oblique, left superior rectus. Right inferior rectus.
	IV. Tilt left	Right superior oblique, left inferior oblique. Right superior rectus, left inferior oblique
	V. Either side	Infantile esotropia nystagmus. DVD (sometimes). Superior oblique sheath syndrome, blow out fracture.

Clinical features of paralysis of individual muscle

Muscle	*Deviation*	*Compensatory head position*	*Ocular movement*	*Diplopia*
MR	Temporal	Head turned towards sound side	Diminished adduction	Horizontal crossed increase in adduction
SR	Down and slightly temporal upper pole rotated temporally	Face up toward paralysed side, chin elevated tilt towards the healthy side	Diminished up movement on paralysed side. Up shoot of the sound eye when looking toward paralysed side	Vertical crossed
IR	Up and out toward the paretic side intortion toward sound side	Face rotated toward affected side c hin down	Diminished movement down and out	Vertical
IO	Down towards sound side intorsion	Face turned toward sound chin raised	Limited up towards the sound side	Homonymous
SO	Up and towards the sound side	Face turned towards sound side Chin depressed tilting of head towards same shoulder	All downward mount of paralysed eye are sub-normal except in extreme abduction	Homonymous vertical seperation more on looking down and to sound side
LR	Adduction	Face turned towards the affected side	Limitation of abduction	Uncrossed attempt abduct

Characteristics of nuclear palsies

- Muscles of both eyes are involved
- May be symmetric or asymmetric
- Loss of parallelism
- Diplopia
- Generally pupil are spared.

Nuclear lesion of IV cannot be differentiate from trunk lesion.
Nuclear lesion VI: Signs of ipsilateral horizontal gaze palsy.

5. Ptosis

(a) The neurological ptosis due to third nerve involvement is generally acute in onset (Fig. 1.19). Congenital ptosis may be unilateral or bilateral (Fig. 1.20A).

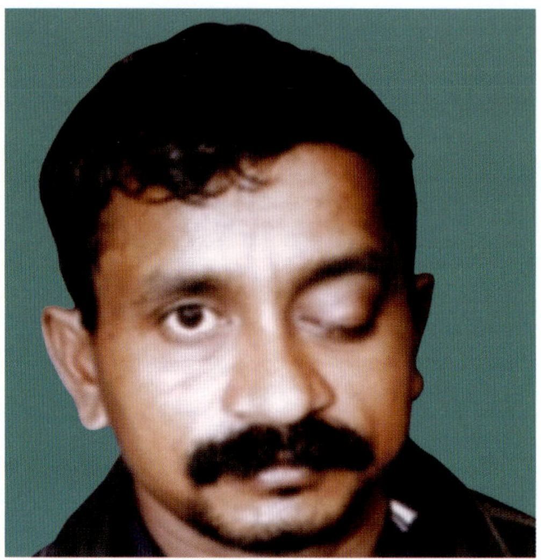

Fig. 1.19: Neurological ptosis

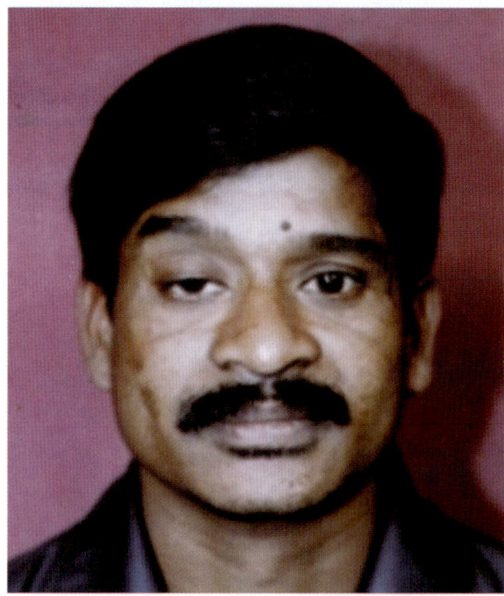

Fig. 1.20A: Congenital ptosis

(b) Neurological ptosis can also be unilateral or bilateral.
(c) When bilateral is generally unequal.
(d) It may be isolated without any other extraocular muscles involvement. Such incidences are infrequent, commonest cause is trauma either to the nerve to levator or to the muscle itself.
(e) Associated involvement of superior rectus is more common because the levator and superior rectus of the same eye are supplied by the upper division of the third cranial nerve.
(f) Ptosis with involvement of other cranial nerves is possible when the pathology is either in the cavernous sinus or anterior to it.
(g) In case of multiple muscle palsy especially in oculomotor involvement onset of ptosis is invariably preceded by extraocular muscle palsy.
(h) In case of central cause of ptosis the extraocular muscle palsies follow onset of ptosis.
(i) Ptosis due to third nerve lesion is not always associated with paralysis of intrinsic muscle.
(j) **In Horner's syndrome** no other extraocular muscle except levator is involved because of under action of **Muller's muscles** only. The ptosis is unilateral and associated with **miosis**, **enophthalmos** and **anhydrosis**. The lesion can be anywhere between hypothalamus to ascending sympathetic chain.
(k) **In supranuclear lesions** the ptosis is mild and generally unilateral, involvement of contralateral lid is also possible. There is defective up gaze and mydriasis.
(l) Ptosis of **nuclear lesion** have the following feature:
   i. Bilateral
   ii. Relatively symmetric
   iii. Ptosis sets in earlier than other oculomotor palsy
   iv. Bilateral superior rectus involvement is common
   v. The part of the oculomotor nucleus that serves the levator is caudal to other nuclei and near the fourth nerve nucleus, involvement of the fourth nerve is also possible.
(m) Variable, asymmetric ptosis that may change sides and worsen with activity, is due to **myasthenia**. This is confirmed by Tensilon test.
(n) Bilateral, progressive, ptosis with ophthalmoplegia is due to myopathy.

6. *Paradoxical lid movements* are either drooping (ptosis) of the lid or elevation of the lid (retraction) due to movements either of the eye or muscles of the jaw. It may be associated **with ptosis** or **without ptosis**. The paradoxical movements are **generally unilateral**. It is commonly a **congenital phenomenon** but can be acquired too. The mechanism is thought to be **lack of lid oculomotor synergies** or **lid jaw synergies**. The commonest paradoxical lid movement is **Marcus Gunn jaw winking**. Others are its inverse form and aberrant regeneration of third nerve—cyclic oculomotor spasm.

7. *Lid retraction:* Normal upper lid covers the upper 2 mm of the cornea and the lower lid just touches the limbus at six o' clock of the cornea without any visible sclera above

or below. Lid retraction is said to be present when the upper lid is elevated sufficiently to make some sclera visible above or the lower lid is depressed to expose the sclera below or both. The lower lid is depressed. This gives a startled look to the eyes. It can be unilateral or bilateral, may be symmetric or unequal.

The neurological causes of lid retraction can be

a. **Stimulation of the cervical sympathetic:** This produces clinical feature diagonally opposite to Horner's syndrome, i.e. the interpalpebral aperture is widened. The eye looks exophthalmic, the pupil is dilated and there is excessive sweating on the forehead and lids. This is commonly seen in **thyrotoxicosis**. Some patients may develop mild to moderate lid retraction following instillation of **10% phenylpherine** in the conjunctival sac and intravenous injection of **Tensilon** or **prostigmine** in myasthenia (Fig. 1.20B).
b. **Spastic lid retraction** is due to lesion in the corticonuclear pathway of mesencephalon.

8. Lagophthalmos

Lagophthalmos is **inability to close the eyes**. It is due to involvement of **facial nerve**. It is commonly **unilateral** and acute due to lesion in the peripheral trunk (Fig. 1.21).

Bell's palsy: Symptoms vary according to severity of the lesion the commonest symptom is inability to close the lid on the effected side with watering, which is both lacrimation and epiphora. The interpalpebral fissures is wide. The creases of the forehead are flattened.

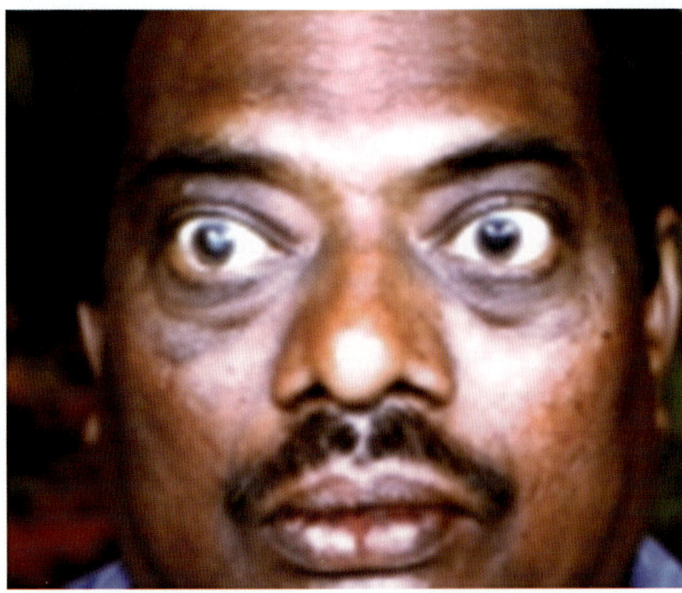

Fig. 1.20B: Lid retract due to drugs mydriasis

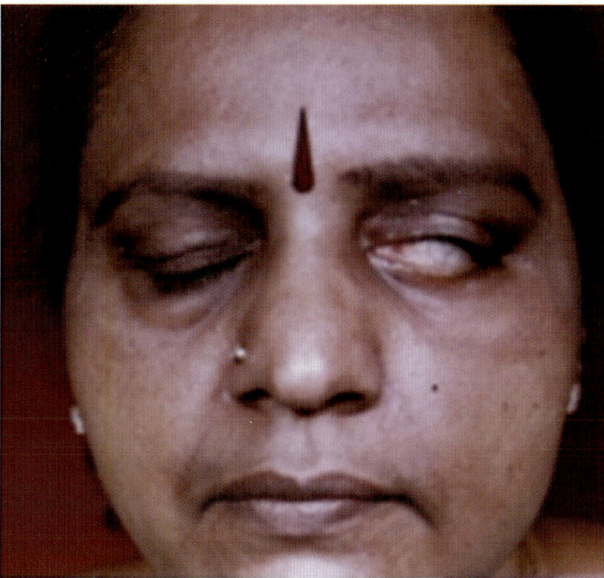

Fig. 1.21: Lagophthalmos

Bilateral involvement of orbicularis is far less common than unilateral lagophthalmos. The lagophthalmos can be isolated, i.e. only the orbicularis is involved.

Other combinations are

- Ipsilateral sixth nerve palsy with loss of conjugate gaze and contralateral hemiplegia. The syndrome is known as **Millard Gubler syndrome**.
- Lagophthalmos with ipsilateral loss of hearing, loss of taste and diminished lacrimation—cerebellopontine angle pathology and **Ramsay Hunt syndrome**.
- Lagophthalmos with hyperacusis. The nerve to the stapedius muscles involved.
- Lagophthalmos with multiple cranial nerve palsy, i.e. fifth to eighth nerve, Horner's syndrome, gaze palsy, cerebellar symptoms, nystagmus (cerebello-pontine angle tumor)
- Lagophthalmos with hearing loss and vestibular symptoms: The seventh nerve can be involved at various sites which range from its supranuclear connections, the nucleus, lesion in the pons and in the trunk.

The causes of bilateral facial palsy can be

a. Infection: Leprosy, polio, lyme disease, AIDS
b. Demyelination: Gullian Barr's syndrome
c. Myasthenia
d. Mobius syndrome
e. Melkersson Rosenthal syndrome
f. Myotonic dystrophy
g. Others: Leukemia, sarcoid.

Causes of isolated seventh nerve palsy are: Lesion in the nerve trunk either in stylomastoid grove or more peripheral part.

The causes are: Bell's palsy, trauma to mastoid or zygomatic bone, facial trauma, parotid surgery, parotid tumor.

9. *Blepharospasm* is defined as forceful involuntary closure of lids. It can be due to peripheral cause referred to as **reflex blepharospasm**. This is very common especially in children, has no neuro-ophthalmic significance. The lesions are in cornea, or anterior uvea. Rarely such blepharospasm can be seen in meningitis.

The blepharospasm of neuro-ophthalmic importance is due to irritation of seventh nerve, central connection or basal ganglion.

The commonest among the causes of blepharospasm is known as **essential blepharospasm** which is a repetitive, bilateral, progressive condition of adults.

The other causes of blepharospasm are

- Focal seizure
- Drug induced
- Meig's syndrome (the essential blepharospasm involving the whole of the face)
- Infection of herpes zoster of geniculate ganglion
- Parkinson's disease
- Huntington's disease
- Brainstem stroke
- Demyelinating disease
- Tetany
- Tetanus
- Postencephalitic.

10. *Blepharoclonus* is milder than blepharospasm. Blepharoclonus is increased frequency of blinking either reflex, central or psychogenic.

11. *Hemifacial spasm* is contracture of facial muscles on half of the face without weakness of other half of the face without weakness of the muscles. Contracture, with weakness of facial muscles is known as **facial myokymia.** This is caused due to lesion of the pons i.e. demyelination, haemorrhage, tumours. Other causes are cerebello pontine angle tumor, Gullian-Barre syndrome and some times Bell's palsy.

12. *Infrequent blinking* is seen in progressive supranuclear palsy.

Proptosis and exophthalmos is seen in thyroid oculopathy, and total ophthalmoplegia.

BIBLIOGRAPHY

1. Deniston, AKO, Murry PI. Oxford handbook of Ophthalmology, 1st edn, Oxford University Press, 2006.
2. Duke Elder S. System of ophthalmology, Vol. 12.
3. Gami NK. Bed sight approach to clinical neurology, 1st edn, Current Book International, 1985.
4. Glasser JS. Neuro-ophthalmology, Harper and Row, London, 1978.

5. Karna S. Neuro-ophthalmology: Clinical examination and diagnosis. 1st edn, Jaypee Brothers Medical Publishers, New Delhi, 2006.
6. Kline LB, Bajandas FJ. Neuro-ophthalmology, 5th edn, Jaypee Brothers Medical Publishers, New Delhi, 2004.
7. Kumar SM. Neuro-ophthalmology, 4th edn, Arvind Eye Hospital, Madurai, 2007.
8. Mason, S, Swash M. Hutchinson's clinical methods, 17th edn, ELBS and Bailliere Tindal, London, 1980.
9. Mukherjee PK. Clinical examination in ophthalmology, 1st edn, Elsevir, New Delhi, 2006.
10. Mukherjee PK. Pediatric Ophthalmology, 1st edn, New Age International, New Delhi, 2005.
11. Mukherjee PK, Dongre RC. A case of acquired facial diplegia, macular edema and lingua plicate. Ind Jr Oph 1971;21:36-39.
12. Natchiar G. Neuro-ophthalmology, 1st edn, Arvind Eye Hospital Madurai, 1987.
13. Swaiman KF. Pediatric Neurology, Vol. 2, 2nd edn, Mosby, St Louis, 1994.
14. Vijayalakshi P. Paediatric Ophthalmology, Arvind Eye Hospital, 2007.

2 Applied Anatomy of the Cranial Nerves of Neuro-ophthalmic Interest

Out of the twelve cranial nerves only following are of neuro-ophthalmic importance:

- The optic nerve
- The oculomotor nerve
- The trochlear nerve
- The trigeminal nerve
- The abducent nerve (abducens)
- The facial nerve
- The vestibulo-cochlear ocular nerve.

The **vestibulo-cochlear** nerve is not involved directly with the eye. It is associated with supranuclear horizontal movements. Its lesions produce nystagmus which has otherwise far reaching neurological significance.

The **optic nerve** is a sensory nerve, in fact it is not a true nerve. It is best considered to be a neural tract. It does not have a formed nucleus.

The **trigeminal nerve** is sensory nerve for ocular structures. Its motor function is not related to ocular structure.

The **facial nerve** has limited motor function related to eyes, i.e. it supplies only the orbicularis. Its secreto motor fibers supply the lacrimal gland.

The **oculomotor**, **trochlear** and **abducent** are the cranial nerves that serve the extraocular muscles. The oculomotor also supplies the intraocular smooth muscles through its parasympathetic component and sensory supply through ciliary ganglion.

The fascicules of these cranial nerves come in close relation with different nuclei and tracts.

In the base of the skull, the nerves come in close contact with blood vessels and other cranial nerves.

All the above three cranial nerves also carry **propioceptive impulses** from extraocular muscle.

The cranial nerves involved with movement of the eyes can have **supranuclear, nuclear and infranuclear defect.**

The supranuclear path

1. The supranuclear motor path descends from the **cerebral hemisphere** to end in **pontine horizontal gaze complex**.
2. In between these two ends, the fibers **decussate in the midbrain** (Figs 2.1 and 2.2).
3. Besides the supranuclear connections the cranial nerve nuclei are connected to the contralateral precentral gyri via corticonuclear paths.

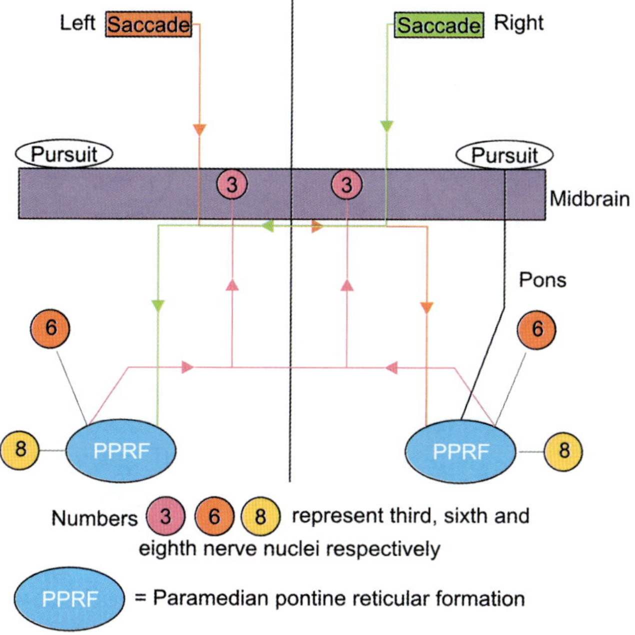

Fig. 2.1: Supranuclear connection of eye movement

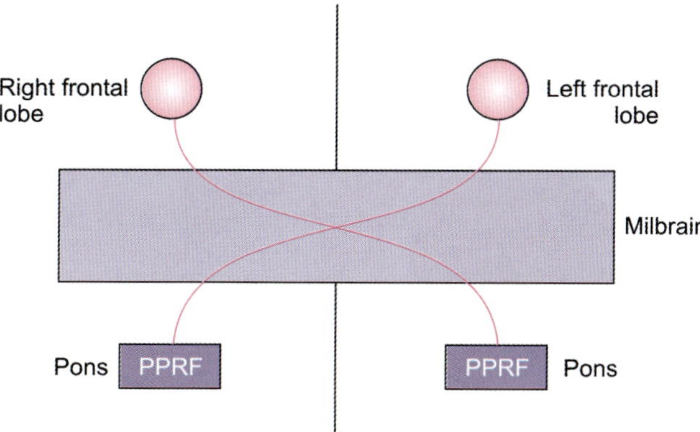

Fig. 2.2: Path of horizontal saccade

Supranuclear connections of the eye movement

The movements of the head, the body and the objects are constant threat to clear vision. To overcome these, eyes have to be constantly aligned in a position to have a sharp macular image, most of which is reflex and partly voluntary. This is brought about by supranuclear mechanism, the exact anatomy of which is not well understood. It is presumed to be extending from **cerebral cortex to pontine horizontal gaze centers** (Fig. 2.1).

The supranuclear eye movements are:

1. Saccadic
2. Smooth pursuit
3. Vergence
4. Vestibular (nonoptical reflex).

The **saccadic movements** can either be **voluntary** or **reflex** (Fig. 2.2). The purpose of this movement is to move the eye from one object to another, to project it on the fovea. The movement is jerky in nature. It could be horizontal or vertical. The path of horizontal saccade starts in premotor cortex. The fibers pass to the pontine paramedian reticular formation (PPRF) to reach the horizontal gaze center. The left saccade is under influence of right frontal cortex and vice versa.

Irrigative lesions of any of the frontal lobes cause a deviation of the eye to the other side.

Smooth pursuit

The purpose of this movement is to **keep the fixation** on the object of interest after it has been located by saccade.

The movement is a slow eye movement (SEM). The path extends from occipital motor cortex to horizontal gaze center in PPRF.

The area initiating the movement is situated in the parieto-occipito-temporal junction. The path undergoes a double decussation before reaching the nuclei of third, fourth and sixth nerves. **The path has ipsilateral control**. The right lobe controls the right pursuit and the left lobe the left pursuit.

Vergences

The purpose of this movement is to keep convergence under control. It is associated with accommodation, pupillary constriction and fusion. It keeps the image on the fovea irrespective of the distance. The stimulus originates in the retina.

The vestibular reflex

This maintains the eyes in required position in spite the change in the head and body position. The path gets the impulse from the changed position of the head and propioceptors in the muscles of the neck. The fibers relay in the vestibular nucleus and pass in the horizontal gaze center in PPRF and then to nuclei of third and sixth.

Vertical gaze

The vertical gaze too have saccadic pursuit and vestibular reflexes. The center for vertical gaze lies in the pretectal mid brain. The impulses start in nuclei of the vertically acting extraocular muscles (Fig. 2.3).

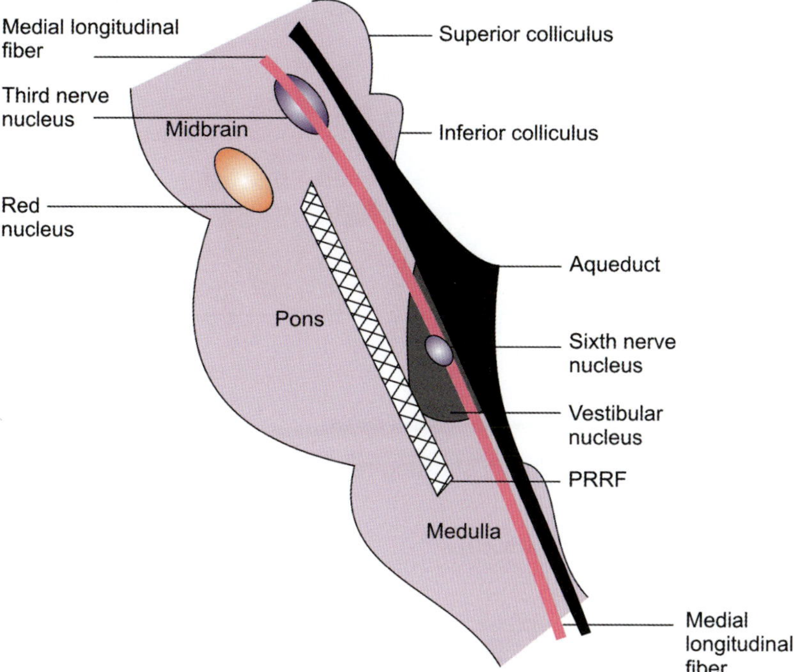

Fig. 2.3: Structures related to vertical and horizontal gazes

APPLIED ANATOMY OF OCULOMOTOR NERVE

The **oculomotor nerve** is the **third cranial nerve** concerned with movements of maximum number of extraocular muscles and intraocular plain muscles.

The nucleus is longitudinal column of cells in the midbrain at the level of superior colliculus (Flow chart 2.1). The nucleus extends from floor of third ventricle above to upper part of the nucleus of fourth nerve below (see Fig. 2.22). The nucleus lies in front of the pre-aqueductal gray matter on each side of the midline. The medial longitudinal bundle is still more ventral and lateral to the nucleus (Fig. 2.4).

The third nerve **does not have a single nucleus**. The nucleus is a conglomeration of many subnuclei situated either in the midline or on either side of the midline. The nuclei are subdivided into two broad groups:

1. The principle nucleus complex (Fig. 2.5)
2. Edinger-Westphal nucleus.

The presence of a separate nucleus for convergence, i.e. the nucleus of Perlia is no more considered valid.

The principle nuclear complex is again divided into two groups:

i. Unpaired single nucleus that is situated in the midline, is also called caudal central nucleus. It innervates levator palpebral superior on both the sides.

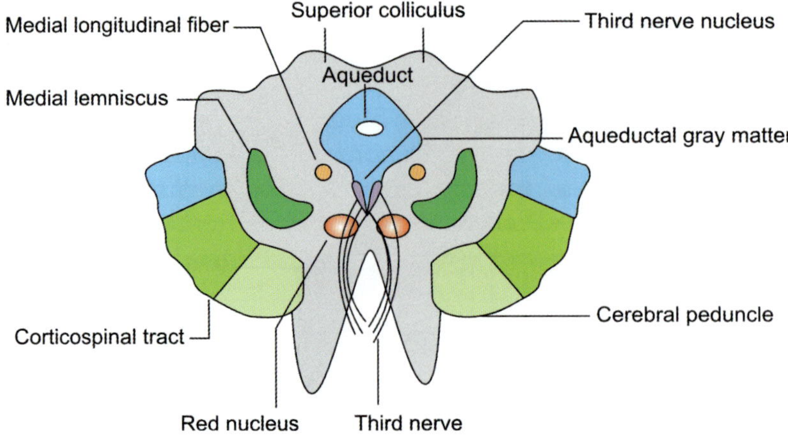

Fig. 2.4: Section through midbrain showing relation of third nerve to other structures

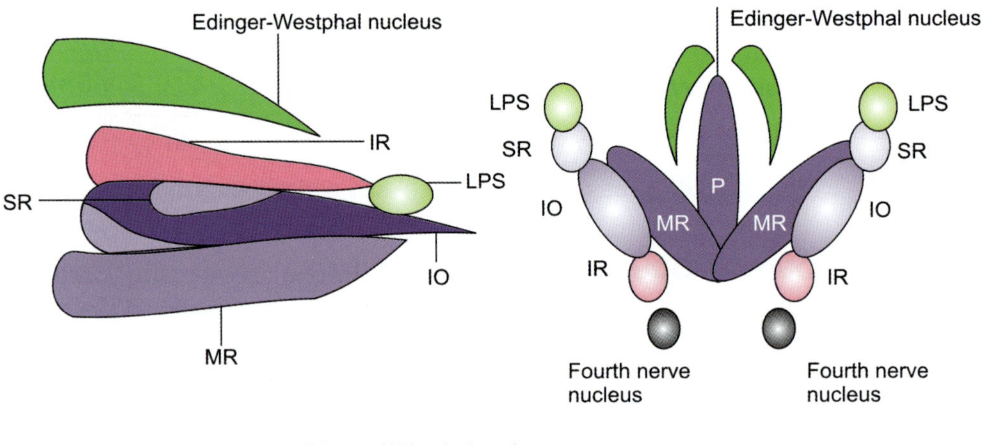

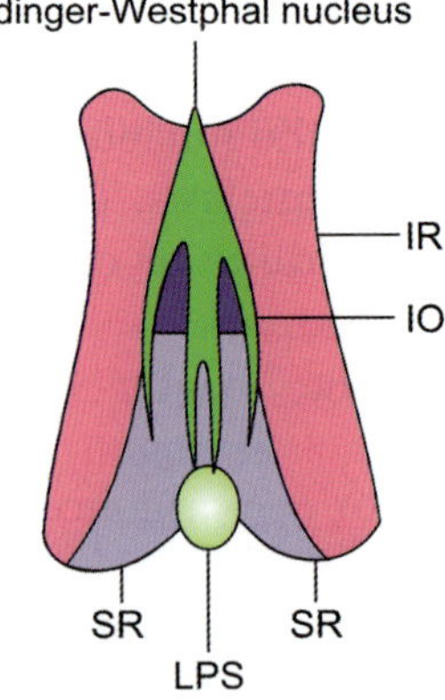

Fig. 2.5: Three views of arrangement of subnuclei of third nerve: SR—Superior rectus, MR—Medial rectus, IR—Inferior rectus, IO—Inferior oblique, LPS—Levator palpebral superior, P—Perlas nucleus

Flow chart 2.1: Scheme of oculomotor nucleus

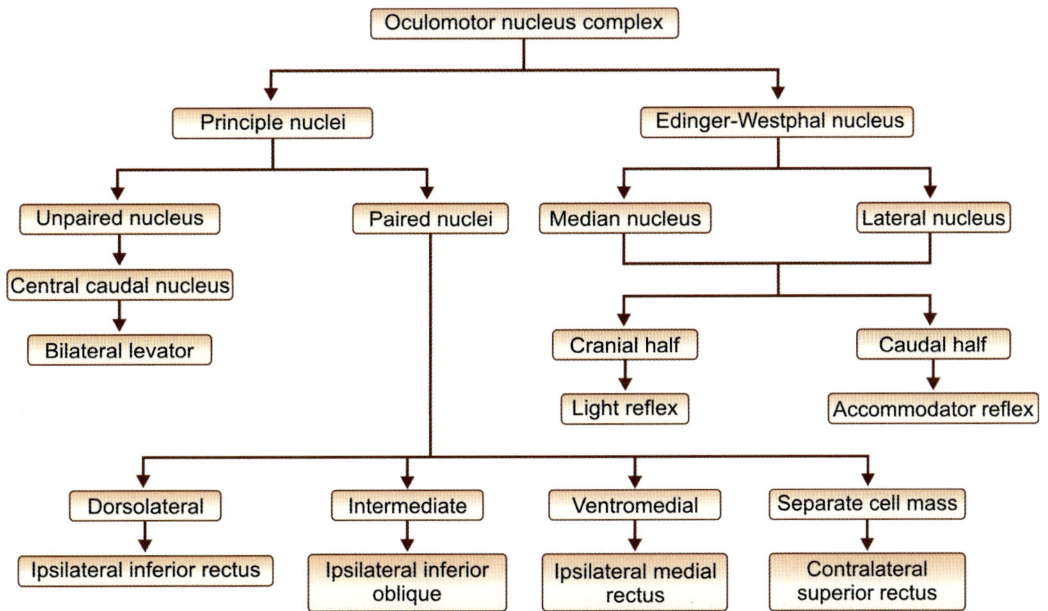

ii. The paired nuclei. They are:

Nucleus	*Muscle supplied*
1. Dorsolateral nucleus	Ipsilateral inferior rectus
2. Intermediate nucleus	Ipsilateral inferior oblique
3. Ventromedial nucleus	Ipsilateral medial rectus
4. Nucleus mass of superior rectus	Contralateral superior rectus

The paired nuclei supply superior rectus, medial rectus, inferior rectus and inferior oblique. The superior rectus is supplied by contralateral subnuclei which is a combination of large multiple polar cells.

Nuclear third nerve palsy should have paralysis of superior rectus, medial rectus, inferior rectus and inferior oblique of one side and superior rectus of other side.

The **Edinger-Westphal nucleus** contains **parasympathetic fibers**. The cranial half is concerned with light reflex and caudal half is concerned with accommodation.

Connections of third nerve nucleus

The third nerve is connected to the following structure

Connection	Purpose
Pyramidal tract	Supranuclear connection
Pretectal nuclei	Light reflex
Medial longitudinal fibers.	Connects 4th, 6th and 8th nerve for coordination of eye movement.

The course of the third nerve

The course of the third nerve can be divided into two parts:

1. Central (midbrain, fascicular)
2. Peripheral:
   i. Basilar
   ii. Cavernous
   iii. Orbital.

The fascicular part

The portion of the third nerve between its nuclei and exit from the midbrain constitutes the fascicular part. **The fibers are efferent** in nature.

During its course in the midbrain, the fibers pass through red nucleus. The medial lemniscuses and substantia nigra are lateral to the fibers.

Before exit in the oculomotor sulcus, the fibers pass through the medial part of the corticospinal tract (pyramidal tract) in the cerebral peduncle (Fig. 2.6).

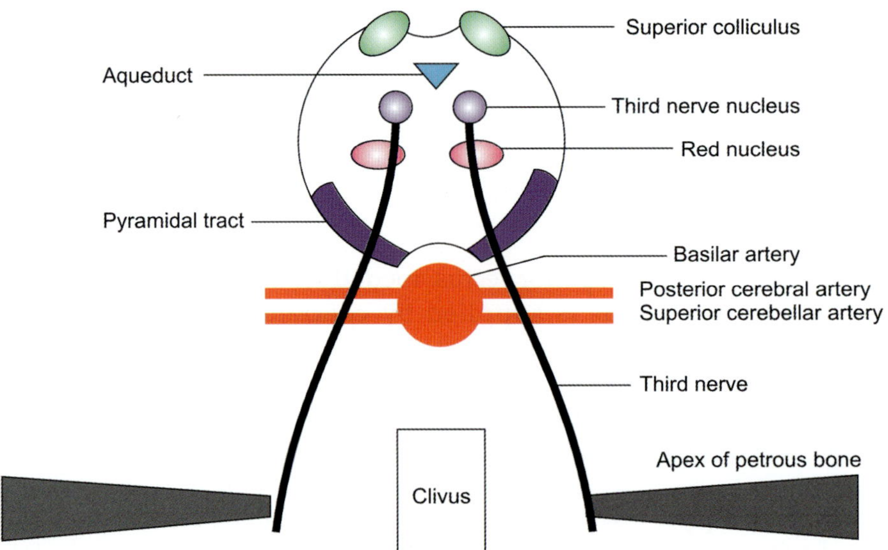

Fig. 2.6: Relation of fascicular and basilar part of third nerve to various structures

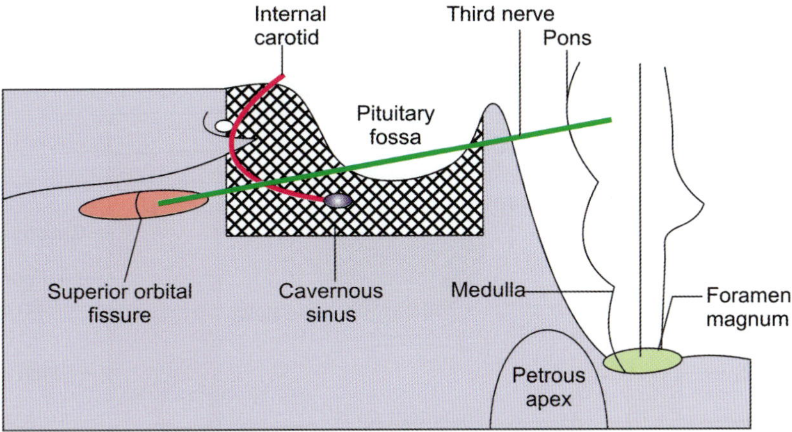

Fig. 2.7: Basilar part of third nerve

The basilar part

The oculomotor nerve leaves the midbrain along the oculomotor sulcus (medial sulcus) as 15-20 rootlets that join to make the trunk of the nerve in the interpeduncular fossa. The main trunk of the third nerve is formed by confluence of two large roots, i.e. the medial and lateral roots. The former is larger than the latter. The big roots are formed by combination of smaller rootlets. The trunk is initially flat in shape but becomes rounded cord latter. The cord of the oculomotor nerve passes between the **posterior cerebral** and **superior cerebellar arteries** near the basilar artery. Then the cord traverses parallel and almost snug with the posterior communicating artery on its lateral side to enter the cavernous sinus without coming in direct relation to any neural tract.

Lesions of third nerve in the basilar part produces isolated third nerve palsy.

During its course between the posterior cerebral and superior cerebellar arteries, the fourth nerve is lateral to the nerve, away and slightly below. The optic tract, is superior to the oculomotor nerve (Fig. 2.7).

The cavernous part

The nerve after it has passed between the free edge of tentorium and posterior clinoid process pierces the dura and reaches the superior aspect of the cavernous sinus on its medial side. The nerve travels towards the lateral wall to become the superior most nerve in the cavernous sinus. In the anterior cavernous sinus the trochlear nerve moves upwards to reach the lateral part of the superior orbital fissure.

In the anterior cavernous sinus the **third nerve divides into two divisions**, **a small superior division** and **a large lower division**. The two divisions enter the orbit through the middle part of the superior orbital fissure with nasociliary nerve and sympathetic twig in between them. The abducent nerve is below and medial to the two divisions (Fig. 2.8).

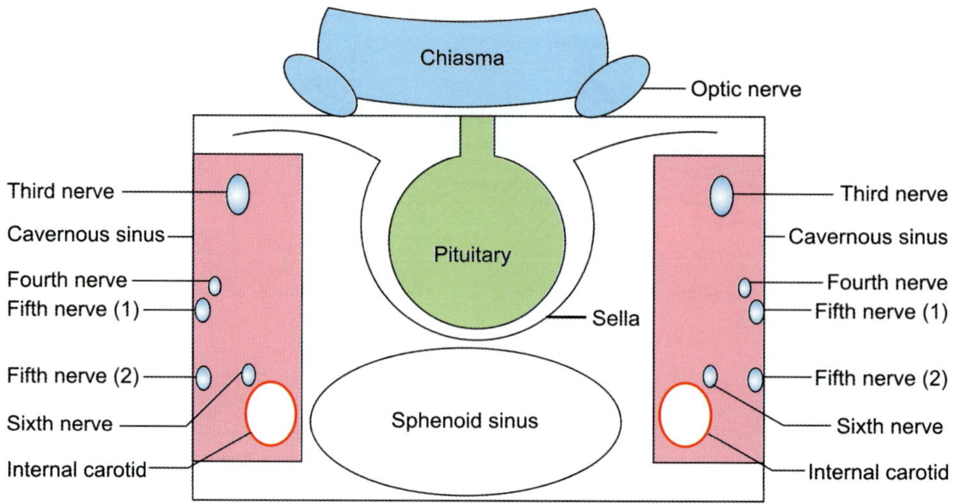

Fig. 2.8: Relation of third, fourth and fifth nerves in cavernous sinus

The orbital part

1. The superior division runs through the central surgical space and enters the superior rectus from the ocular surface. Thereafter, it pierces the substance of the superior rectus to reach the levator palpebral superior (Fig. 2.9).
2. The inferior division also runs through the central surgical space to supply the medial rectus, inferior rectus and inferior oblique from their ocular surfaces. The branch to inferior oblique also gives a twig to the ciliary ganglion that carries the parasympathetic fibers.

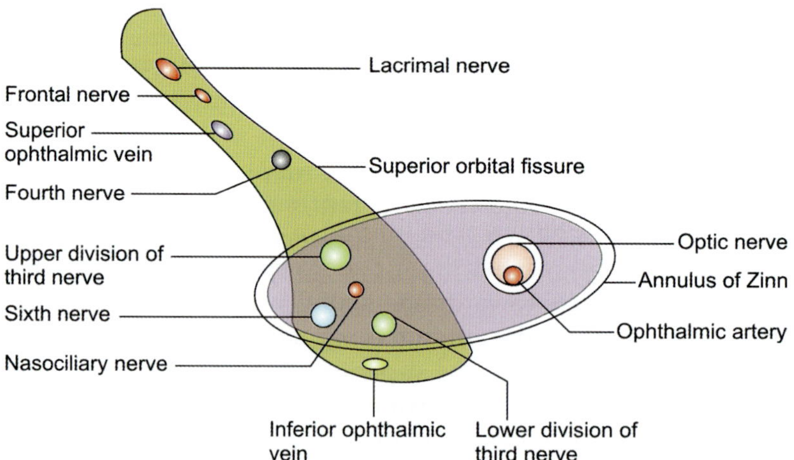

Fig. 2.9: Relation of structures at apex of orbit

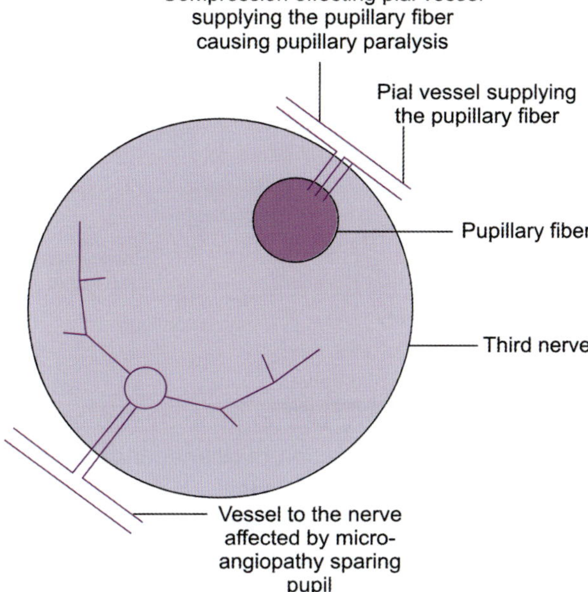

Fig. 2.10: Blood supply to the third nerve trunk

Position of fibers of different functions

1. The fibers of different functions are arranged in an order that does not change once the third nerve has assumed a cord like appearance.
2. The pupillary fibers are most medial, the fibers of inferior oblique are most lateral, in between these two are the fibers for inferior, medial and superior recti along with fibers for levator.
3. The position of parasympathetic pupillary fibers, which are superficial as well as medial have great clinical significance due to their position in the nerve and their blood supply between brainstem and cavernous sinus. The pupillary fibers are supplied by pial branches. The rest of the fibers are supplied by vasa nervosum. Hence, a compressive lesion produces total third nerve palsy that include pupil (Fig. 2.10). A microvasculopathy involves only the vasa nervosum but not the pial vessels. Thus, they produces various degrees of third nerve palsy without involving the pupil. This is called **pupillary sparing oculomotor palsy**. The commonest cause being diabetes. In contrast to this, the common compressing lesions are various aneurysms. The other causes are tumors.

Aberrant regeneration of the third nerve fibers

There are two types of aberrant regenerations:

1. The primary: This is less common of the two, seen mostly in compressive lesion in cavernous sinus, i.e. aneurysms and meningiomas.

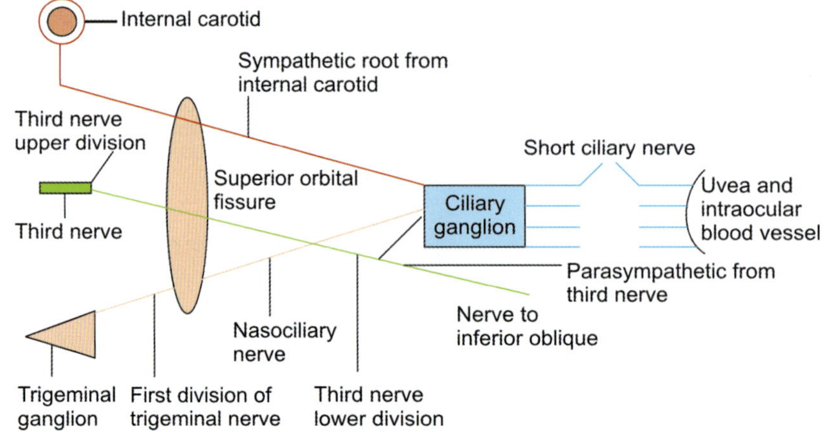

Fig. 2.11: Connection of ciliary ganglion

2. The secondary: This is more frequent, seen following acute clinical features of trauma or aneurysm and not seen in microvasculopathy.

Ciliary ganglion

Ciliary ganglion is one of the small ganglions with important neuro-ophthalmic significance. **It is considered as peripheral sympathetic ganglion for eyes**. However, it contains parasympathetic, sympathetic and sensory fibers as well. Only parasympathetic fibers relay in the ganglion. The ganglion is situated deep in the orbit about 1.5 to 2 cm behind the globe and 1 cm in front of the apex of the orbit. It is rectangular in shape 2 mm × 1 mm. It lies in the loose fatty tissue between the optic nerve and the lateral rectus. The orbital part of the ophthalmic artery is on medial side of the ganglion (Fig. 2.11).

The ganglion has three roots

1. The parasympathetic
2. The sympathetic
3. The sensory

The parasympathetic is derived from the third nerve, the sensory is derived from the fifth nerve. Thus, the function of the ganglion can be jeopardised in lesion of either.

1. **The parasympathetic root** is small stout that originates from the nerve to inferior oblique. It contains preganglion fibers from Edinger-Westphal nucleus. Theses fibers synapse with the postganglion, i.e. fibers in the ciliary nerve that supply constrictor pupillae and ciliary body. It is also known as motor root. Paralysis of this leads to mydriasis and cycloplegia. The root joins the nerve to inferior oblique to the ganglion on the inferoposterior angle.
2. **Sensory root** is relatively long and slender; it arises from the nasociliary nerve. It enters the ganglion on the posterosuperior angle. The sensations from the eyes are transmitted through this root. It carries pain sensation from the cornea

and uvea. Paralysis of this leads to loss of sensation from the cornea and the uvea. This phenomenon is utilized in retrobulbar anesthesia.

3. **The sympathetic root** is variable. It originates from the wall of the internal carotid in the cavernous sinus, enters the orbit through the superior orbital fissure either as an independent root or along the parasympathetic root. It contains postganglionic fibers from the cervical sympathetic. It supplies the dilator pupillae and intraocular blood vessels. The fibers do not relay in the ciliary ganglion.

The branches of the ciliary ganglion are the short ciliary nerves which are about 12 to 20 in numbers. They contain sensory, motor and sympathetic fibers.

Applied anatomy of the trochlear nerve

The trochlear nerve is the fourth cranial nerve. It is an unique cranial nerve that differs from both third and sixth nerve. It has more similarity with sixth nerve than with the third nerve. Some of the features of the fourth nerve are:

1. It is the most slender cranial nerve.
2. It has longest intracranial course.
3. It is the only cranial nerve that decussates completely. The sixth nerve does not decussate; the third nerve decussates partially.
4. It is the only cranial nerve that emerges on the dorsal surface of the midbrain.
5. Its nucleus supplies the superior oblique of the opposite side.
6. Its fascicular part is so small that it is impossible to differentiate between the nuclear and fascicular lesion (Fig. 2.12).
7. Its basilar part does not come in relation to other nerve trunks (Fig. 2.13).
8. It enters the orbit through the superior orbital fissure outside the tendinous ring of Zinn.
9. It is the only nerve that supplies the extraocular muscle from the orbital surface.
10. It is generally not paralysed by moderate amount of retrobulbar anesthesia.

Note: The points 1 and 2 make it vulnerable to trauma and 8 and 9 prevents it from retrobulbar anesthesia.

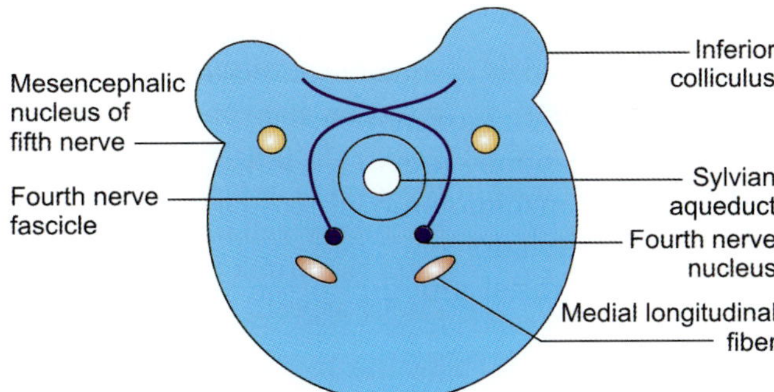

Fig. 2.12: Section of midbrain through inferior colliculus showing dorsal decussation of fourth nerve

Comparison between salient features of third, fourth and sixth cranial nerve (Figs 2.14, 2.15 and 2.21)

Features	*Third nerve*	*Fourth nerve*	*Sixth nerve*
1. **Nucleus**			
I. Position	At the level of superior colliculus inferior to aqueduct of sylvius extending from floor of third ventricle to upper border of fourth nerve nucleus.	Ventrolateral to the cerebral aqueduct at the level of upper part of inferior colliculus in midbrain.	Lower pons anterior to the upper part of fourth ventricle beneath the facial colliculus.
II. **Number**	Group of subnuclei that may be paired/ unpaired or single, e.g. Edinger-Westphal nucleus.	Single, the right nucleus supplies the left superior oblique, the left supplying the right.	Single, supplies ipsilateral, lateral rectus.
III. **Relation**	Preductal gray matter is posterior to the nucleus, the medial longitudinal bundle, red nucleus. Medial lemniscuses and substantia nigra are anterolateral to the nucleus. The medial longitudinal bundle is nearest to the nucleus and the substantia nigra most anterior.	The medial longitudinal bundle is antero-lateral.	The MLF lies medial to the nucleus, the fifth nerve nucleus complex is ventrolateral, the vestibular nucleus in dorsolateral. The fascicle of seventh nerve wind round the nucleus.
2. **Fasciculus**	The fascicular part passes successively through red nucleus medial lemniscuses substantia nigra and the corticospinal tract. The fibers partly decussate.	The fascicular part winds round the aqueduct in posterior direction and completely decussates at the level of anterior medullary vellum to form two trunk on the dorsal aspect.	The fascicular part passes successively lateral to MLF, PPRE and through the pyramid.

Contd...

Contd...

Features	*Third nerve*	*Fourth nerve*	*Sixth nerve*
3. **The basilar (Figs 2.14 and 2.15)**	a. The trunk passes between the posterior cerebral and superior cerebellar arteries. b. The fourth nerve is lateral to third nerve between the above two arteries. c. The posterior communicating artery is medial to the trunk.	The basilar part passes between the posterior cerebral and superior cerebellar arteries lateral to third nerve.	1. The vertical part is crossed by antero-inferior cerebellar artery. 2. The basilar artery lies between the two trunks. 3. It passes over the petrous apex. 4. Under the Grubber's ligament.
4. **Cavernous sinus**			
I. Posterior	a. In the lateral wall. b. The fourth nerve of the ophthalmic and maxillary nerves are below.	In the lateral wall. In the posterior part below the third nerve.	It lies in the cavity of the sinus below the level of third and fourth nerve. The internal carotid is superomedial.
II. Anterior	a. The nerve divides in two division. b. The fourth nerve move upwards. c. The sixth nerve is below and medial.	In the anterior part it move up to enter the superior orbital fissure.	It is joined by oculo-sympathetic.
5. **Superior orbital fissure**	The nerve passes with in the: a. Common tendenous ring. b. The superior division along with nasociliary and sympathetic pass through the middle part, superior to the lower division and the sixth nerve.	Enters the superior orbital fissure outside the annulus of Zinn. The upper division of third nerve is medial to it and inside the annulus.	Enters inside the common ring below and lateral to third nerve and nasociliary nerve.
6. **Orbit**	The nerve supplies the levator, superior rectus, inferior rectus, medial rectus and inferior oblique from ocular surface.	It supplies single nerve, i.e. superior oblique from the orbital surface.	It supplies single muscle, i.e. lateral rectus from ocular surface.

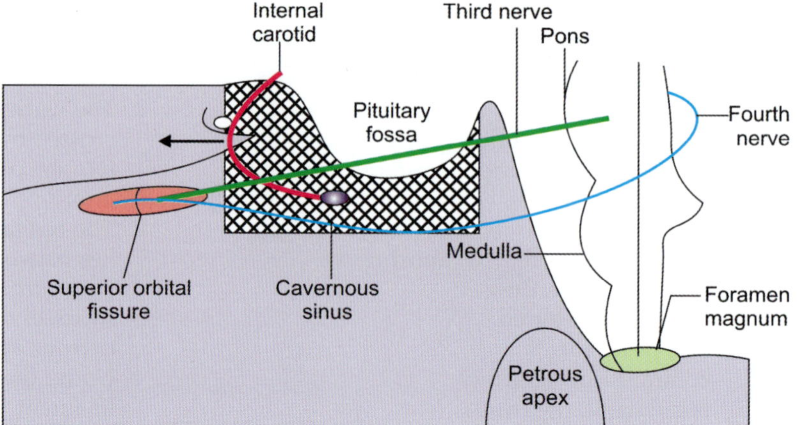

Note:
1. Dorsal origin of the fourth nerve
2. The fourth nerve enters the orbit outside the common tendinous ring
3. It is longer than third and sixth nerve

Fig. 2.13: Basilar part of fourth nerve

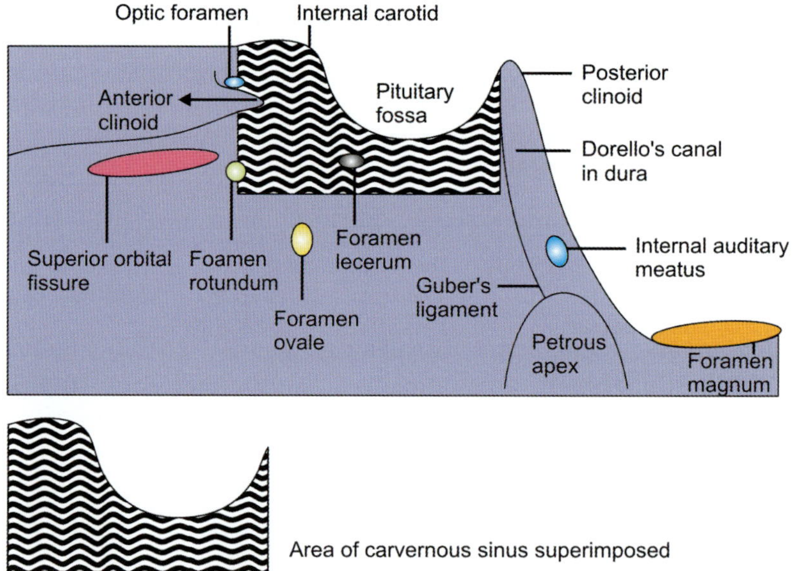

Fig. 2.14: Bony and vascular landmarks of neuro-ophthalmic interest (lateral views)

The nucleus of the trochlear nerve lies in the vertical line of the oculomotor nucleus above and abducent nucleus below. The caudal end of the third nerve may reach up to the upper limit of the fourth nucleus. The fourth nerve nucleus is oval mass of multipolar neurons situated anterolateral to the cerebral aqueduct. The medial longitudinal bundle

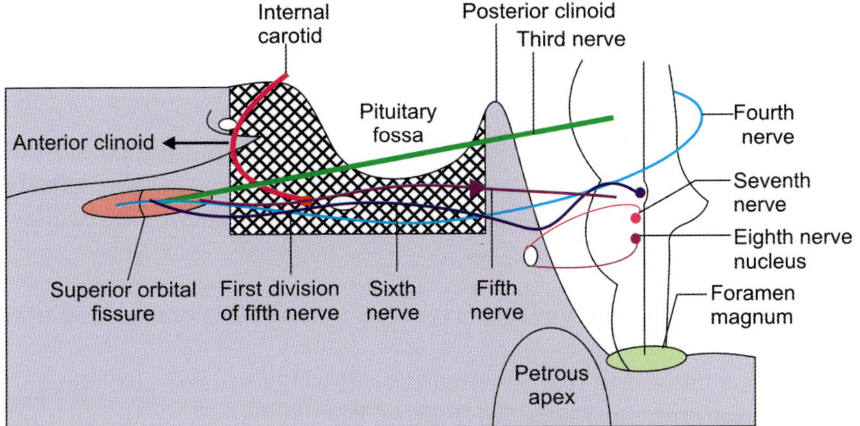

Note: All nerve enters the orbit inside common tendinous ring except the fourth nerve

Fig. 2.15: Cranial nerves of neuro-ophthalmic interest and their course between pons and orbit

is anterior and lateral. The nucleus is situated slightly lateral to the midline in the midbrain at the level of upper part of inferior colliculus. There may be a **smaller subsidiary nucleus** inferior to the main nucleus.

The connection of the fourth nerve nucleus

The nucleus is connected to

i. The medial longitudinal fasciculus joins the fourth nerve nuclei to nuclei of third above and nuclei of sixth and eight below on either side of the midline.
ii. The tectobulbar tract and superior colliculus join the fourth nerve nucleus with visual cortex.
iii. Cerebral cortex is joined by corticonuclear tract on either side.

The course of the fourth nerve

The course of the nerve is divided into fascicular, basilar, cavernous and orbital portion like third and sixth nerve.

The fascicular part

The fascicular part of the fourth nerve is **smallest** among all the cranial nerves serving the eyes. The fibers of the nerve **curve round the Sylvian aqueduct** to reach the dorsal part of it where the **fiber decussate completely** to cross the midline, i.e. the axons of the right nucleus cross over to the left side to form the left trochlear nerve and vice versa. The decussation takes place in the **anterior medullary velum**. Before decussation, the axons pass medial to the **mesencephalic root of the trigeminal**. The **oculosympathetic path** passes through the dorsolateral tagmentum in the vicinity of the fascicular part. The fascicles of the fourth nerve emerge from the midbrain below the inferior colliculi, medial to the superior cerebellar peduncle, close to the upper border of pons in between the temporal lobe and pons.

The basilar part

The basilar part passes **under the free edge of the tentorium**, then passes between the **posterior cerebral artery** and **superior cerebellar artery** lateral to the third nerve. The posterior cerebral artery is superior to the nerve and the superior cerebellar below.

The Cavernous part

The nerve pierces the dura to enter the cavernous sinus and is **embedded in the lateral wall** of the sinus.

In the cavernous sinus the relations between the third nerve and fourth nerve are different in the posterior and anterior part of the cavernous sinus. In the posterior cavernous sinus the fourth nerve is below the third nerve. In the anterior part it moves upwards to reach the superior orbital fissure. **In the cavernous sinus the nerve communicates with ophthalmic nerve**. It enters the superior orbital fissure **outside the annulus of Zinn** lateral to the superior division of third nerve, the frontal nerve is superior to it.

The orbital part

After entering the orbit the nerve runs anteromedially without entering the muscle cone. It gives three to four twigs to innervate the superior oblique. The twigs pierce the belly of the muscle from its orbital surface (see Fig. 2.9).

Applied anatomy of the abducent nerve

The abducent nerve is the **sixth cranial nerve**. It differs from the third and the fourth in the sense that **it does not decussate anywhere in its course**. Like fourth nerve it **supplies only one extraocular muscle**. The similarity between fourth and sixth ends here because the fourth nucleus supplies the contralateral superior oblique while the sixth nerve nucleus is designated for **ipsilateral lateral rectus only**.

The nucleus

The nucleus of the sixth cranial nerve is a **small oval nucleus** that is situated in the **lower pons** anterior to the upper part of the fourth ventricle at the level of facial colliculus. The nuclei of two sides are placed on either side of the midline. **Most of the axons innervate the ipsilateral lateral rectus. The contralateral medial rectus sub-nucleus also gets some fibers** through the medial longitudinal bundle which is situated medial to the nucleus (Fig. 2.16). The fifth nucleus complex is ventrolateral while the vestibular nucleus is dorsolateral to the nucleus (Fig. 2.17).

The nucleus of the seventh nerve is placed more anteriorly and nearer to midline as compared to the fifth nucleus complex. The faciculus from the seventh nerve, travel posteriorly to encircle the sixth nucleus from all sides except anterior lateral aspect. This anatomical relation explains frequent involvement of both the nerves in lesion at this level.

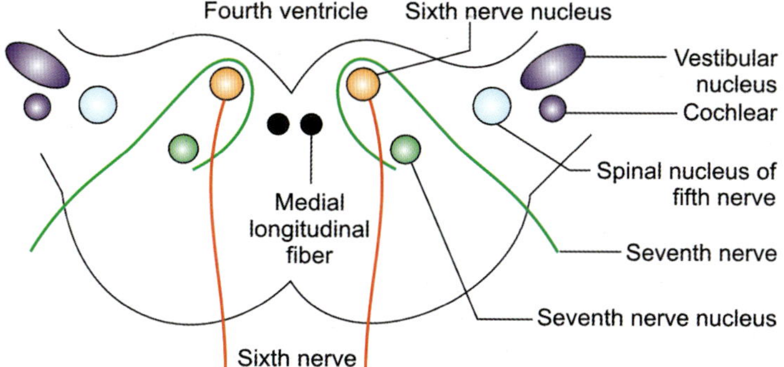

Fig. 2.16: Various cranial nerve nuclei in pons

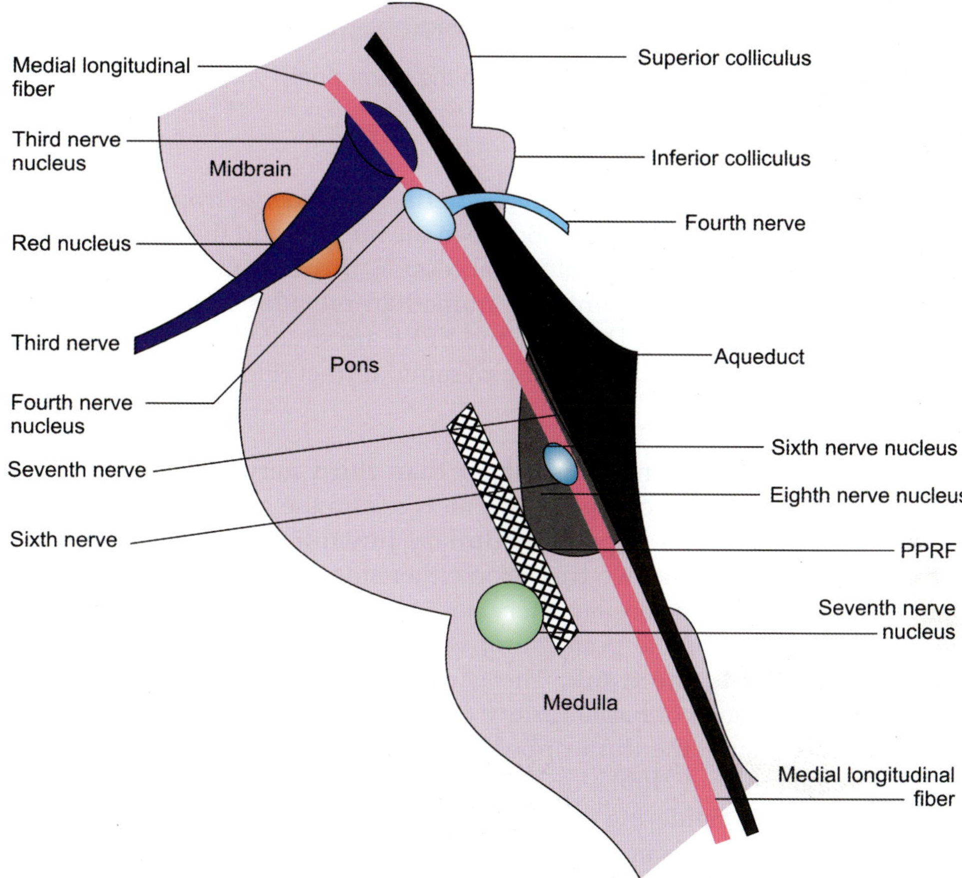

Fig. 2.17: Vertical section of brainstem showing thrid, fourth, sixth and seventh nerves

Connection of the sixth nerve nucleus

The nucleus of abducent nerve is connected to third, fourth and eighth nerve via medial, longitudinal, fasciculus and the cortex via corticonuclear tract of the other side.

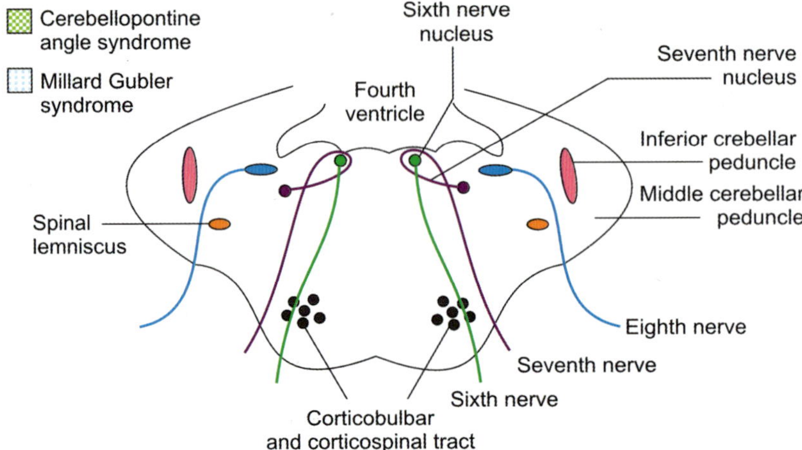

Fig. 2.18: Lesions in the lower pons

The fascicular part

The efferent fibers of the sixth nerve travel anteriorly to emerge from the brainstem **at the junction of pons and the medulla**. Between the nucleus and the exit of the fascicles from the midbrain the fibers travel in succession through the vicinity of medial longitudinal fasciculus (MLF), pontine paramedian reticular formation (PPRF) and pyramidal (corticospinal) tract. The MLF and PPRF are situated medial to the fibers of the third nerve which travels through the pyramidal tract (Fig. 2.18).

The basilar part

The basilar part of the sixth nerve is **longer than third nerve but shorter than the fourth nerve**. The two trunks of the nerves emerge from the midbrain on either side of midline by multiple rootlets at **pontomedullary junction**. The rootlets join to form single trunk on each side. The two trunks on either side are separated from each other by about one centimeter. The basilar artery lies in between the two. The nerve ascends on the anterior surface of the pons, snug with the surface for about 15 mm. **The pyramids are medial to the trunk**. The trunk is crossed by the **anterior inferior cerebellar artery**, a branch of basilar artery (Fig. 2.19).

The sixth nerve pierce the dura opposite the dorsum sella and bends round the inferior petrosal sinus and climbs up on the posterior surface of petrous bone then turns forwards sharply rendering it vulnerable to be impinged against **the apex of the petrous bone**. Then it passes under the **Grubber's ligament** and the superior petrosal sinus. Before entering the cavernous sinus, it passes through the **Dorello's canal** (Fig. 2.20).

The cavernous part

In contrast to the third and fourth nerve, which are embedded in the lateral wall of the cavernous sinus, the sixth nerve lies free in the cavity of the cavernous sinus in close

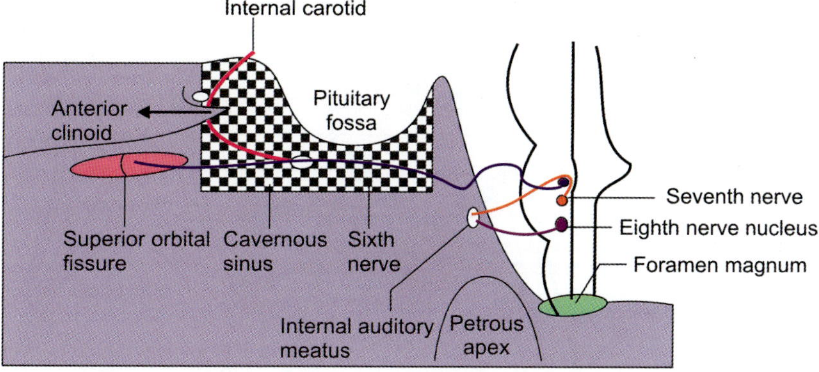

Note:
1. Upward showing of sixth nerve on the anterior face of pons
2. Fascicules of seventh nerve round the sixth nucleus
3. Common entry of the seventh and eighth nerve through auditory meatus

Fig. 2.19: Course of the sixth nerve in the prepontine space and cavernous sinus

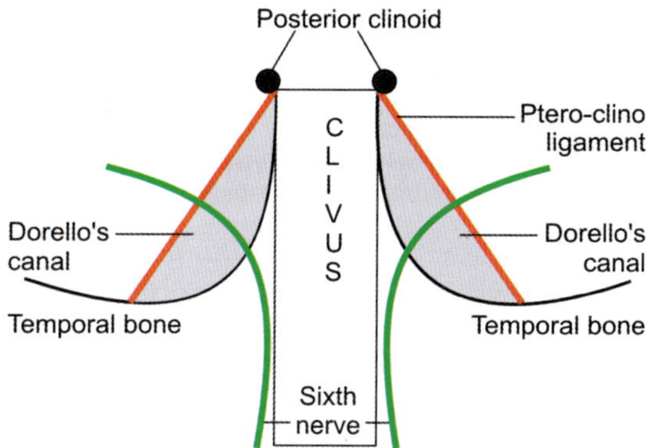

Fig. 2.20: Position of sixth nerve in relation to Dorello's canal

relation to the internal carotid inferior to both the nerves. It lies superomedial to the artery. In the cavernous sinus, it is joined by oculosympathetic (Figs 2.21 and 2.8).

The orbital part

The sixth nerve enters the orbit through the superior orbital fissure inside the common tendinous ring below and lateral to the third nerve and the nasociliary nerve. In the orbit, it travels in the muscle cone and pierces the lateral rectus from the ocular surface (see Fig. 2.9).

Applied anatomy of the trigeminal nerve

The trigeminal is the **fifth cranial nerve**. It is the largest cranial nerve of neuro-ophthalmic interest. It is a **mixed nerve** that has both **sensory and motor component**

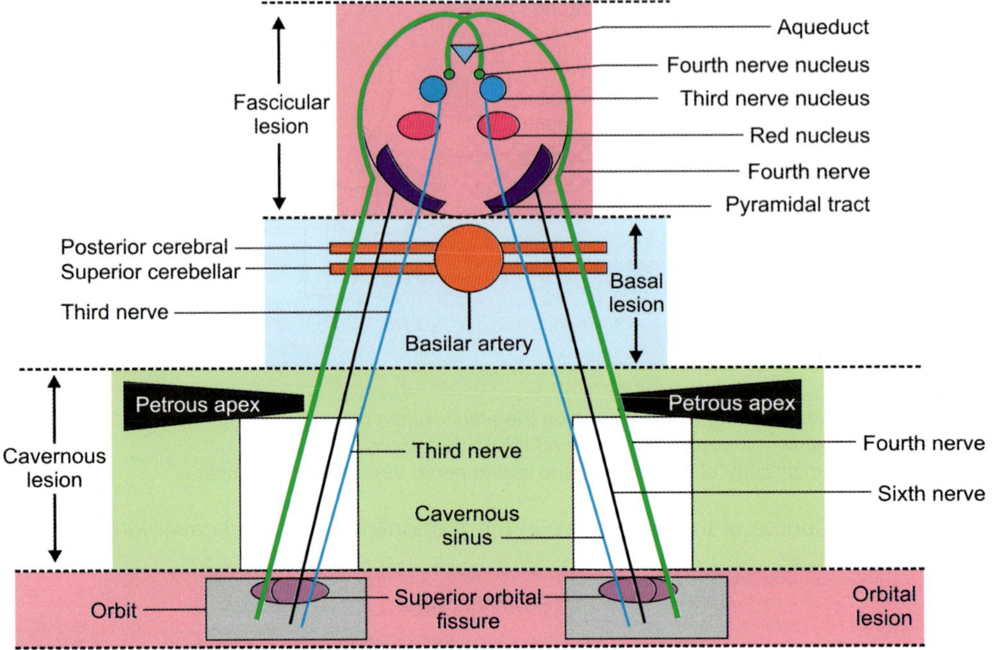

Note:
1. Only fascicular lesions involve neural tracts
2. The third nerve and fourth nerve pass between posterior cerebral and superior cerebellar arteries
3. The sixth nerve passes under the anteroposterior cerebellar artery below the third and fourth in the plane of them

Fig. 2.21: Various possible levels of infranuclear lesion of third, fourth and sixth nerves

besides it supplies postganglionic secretomotor fibers to the lacrimal gland. The motor component lacks neuro-ophthalmic features and is smaller than the sensory part. The motor part supplies the striated muscles developing from first branchial mesoderm. It is efferent in nature.

The sensory part of the trigeminal is **afferent somatic** that carries sensation from **anterior half of skull, face, eyeball, all ocular adnexa, nasal cavity, paranasal sinuses, external ear** and **mouth**. The fifth nerve also carries **sympathetic fibers** from the internal carotid and **parasympathetic** from facial and glossopharyngeal nerve.

Nuclei of trigeminal (Figs 2.22 and 2.23)

The trigeminal does not have a single nucleus. The nuclei complex consists of **four nuclei** which functionally are divided into two broad groups (Fig. 2.22):

1. Sensory
2. Motor

1. Sensory comprising of:
   i. Mesencephalic nucleus
   ii. Principle sensory nucleus
   iii. Spinal nucleus

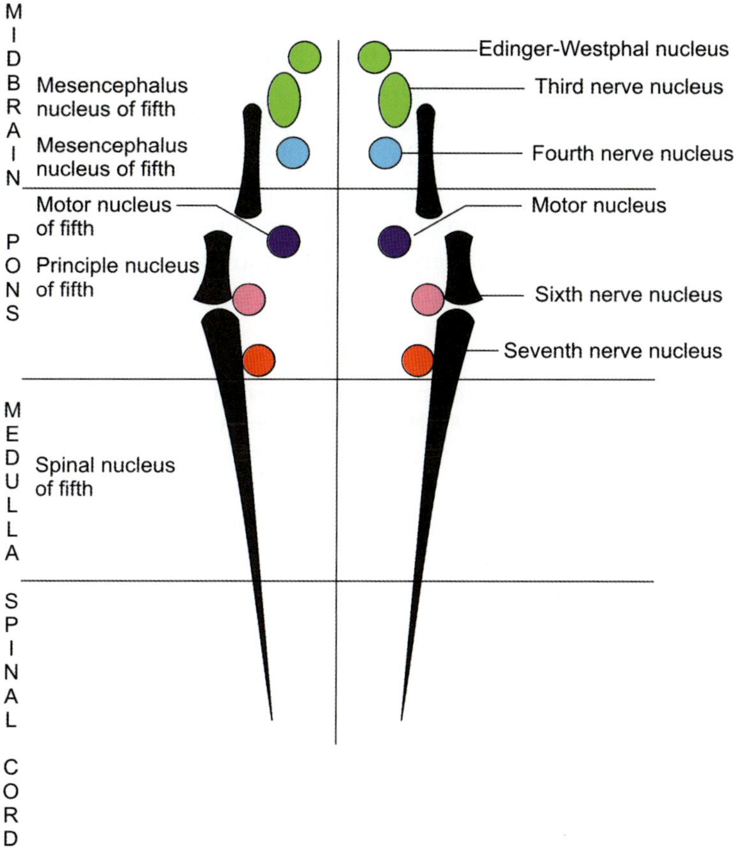

Fig. 2.22: Arrangement of nuclei of third, fourth, fifth and sixth cranial nerves

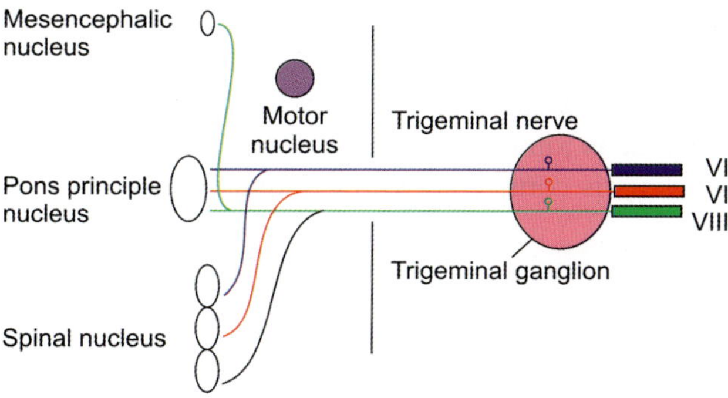

Fig. 2.23: Connection of nuclei of fifth nerve

2. Motor: The sensory nuclei are **spread over a long area** vertically on either side of the midline extending from the **lower pons to the dorsal horn of the spinal cord** up to second cervical vertebra.

The mesencephalic nucleus is most superiorly placed sensory nucleus of trigeminal. It is situated on either side of the aqueduct dorsolateral to it and ventral to the lateral lemniscuses and inferior colliculus. The third nerve nucleus is superomedial to it. It extends upwards from the cranial end of the principle sensory nucleus into the midbrain. It gets the **propioceptive sensation** from the muscles supplied by not only the trigeminal but also by third, fourth, sixth, seventh and twelfth cranial nerves.

The principle sensory nucleus

It lies in the **pons** lateral to the motor nucleus **below the mesencephalic nucleus**. The sixth nerve nucleus is on the inferomedial to it. It is an oval structure **ment for tactile sensation**.

The spinal nucleus of the trigeminal

It is **longest** among all the nuclei of the fifth nerve. It begins at the lower end of the principle nucleus and descends up to second cervical segment of the spinal cord. It gets sensory fibers from all the areas supplied by the fifth nerve. It is also connected to sensory fibers of facial, glossopharyngeal and vagus.

The motor root

The motor root does not have any neuro-ophthalmic significance. It is situated medial to the principle sensory nucleus in the tagmentum of the pons above the nucleus of the sixth nerve and motor nucleus of the seventh nerve.

The connections of the fifth nerve nucleus

1. The axons of various nuclei of the trigeminal join the main trunk of the fifth nerve.
2. The axons of the motor nucleus travel separately to exit as motor root of fifth nerve.
3. The trigeminal sensory nucleus is joined to cerebral cortex via thalamus.
4. The motor nucleus is joined to the cortex via corticonuclear tract.
5. The spinal nucleus is connected to the sensory fibers of glossopharyngeal and vagus nerve.
6. The mesencephalic nucleus is connected to third, fourth, sixth, seventh and twelfth by propioceptive fibers.

The course of the trigeminal can be divided into two parts

1. The afferent
2. The efferent

The afferent part is **sensory** that supply various tissues **ocular** as well as **nonocular**, i.e. the skin, mucous membrane, meninges, uvea, blood vessels. They extends between the gasserian ganglion and the target tissues via cavernous sinus.

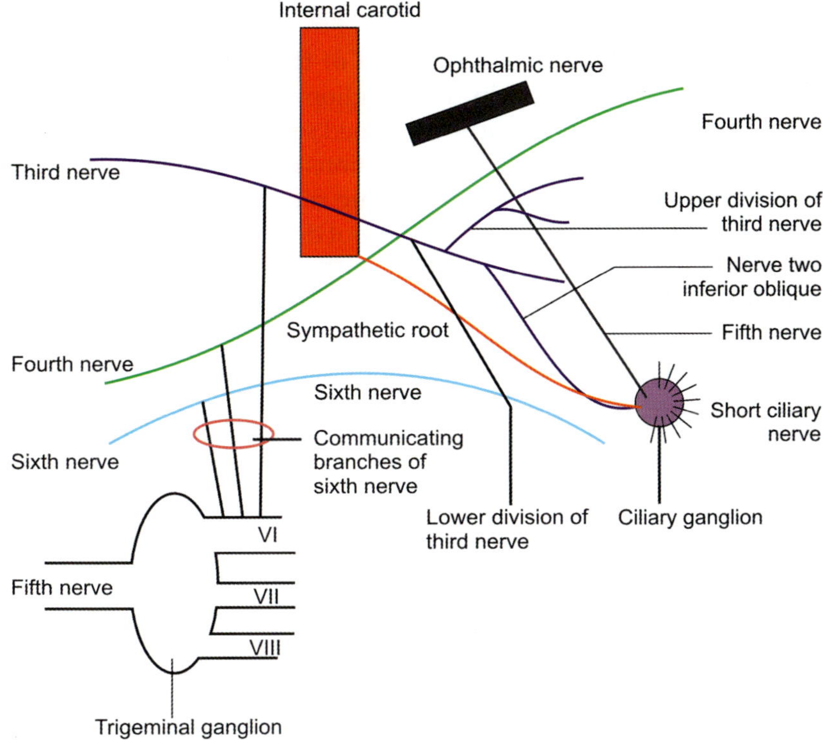

Fig. 2.24: Connection of trigeminal ganglion and ciliary ganglion

The fibers from the principle nucleus in the pons pass straight into the sensory root. It carries three sets of fibers destined to be **ophthalmic, maxillary** and **mandibular** division after passing through the **gasserian ganglion**.

The fibers from the spinal nucleus ascend upwards in the pons to join the sensory fibers of the principle sensory root and pass in the sensory root. The fibers arising from the upper part form the ophthalmic, the fibers form the middle part form the maxillary and those arising from lower part form the mandibular division (Fig. 2.24).

The mesencephalic nucleus sends two sets of fibers; one that joins the sensory part in the pons and exits from the pons to become sensory root. It also supplies fibers to the motor nucleus.

The fibers form motor nucleus do not mingle with sensory fibers in brain they form a separate part that emerge from the pons as motor root.

The trigeminal nerve exists from the pons as two roots, i.e. a large sensory root and a small motor root. The two roots travel anteriorly in a superolateral direction in the cisterna pontis to reach the gasserian ganglion. The two roots are below the fourth nerve, above the seventh and eighths nerve. Here the root passes above the apex of the petrous bone and lies below the superior petrosal sinus.

The gasserian ganglion

The gasserian ganglion is the **sensory ganglion of the trigeminal nerve**. The sensory nerves are relayed and re-arranged in the ganglion. It lies in the **Meckel's cave** near the apex of the petrous bone, which is a bean shaped structure with concavity backwards in which the sensory roots merge. The three divisions of the trigeminal join the gasserian ganglion at its anterior border. The ophthalmic most superiorly; mandibular most inferiorly; the maxillary in between. The motor root does not join the gasserian ganglion. It bypasses it to join the mandibular nerve.

The temporal lobe of cerebrum is above. The foramen lacerum, the greater superficial petrosal nerve and the motor root of trigeminal are below the ganglion. The middle meningial artery is lateral to it while cavernous sinus with its content and pituitary gland is medial to it.

The branches of the trigeminal nerve

The trigeminal has three division

- The ophthalmic or the first division V1
- The maxillary or the second division V2
- The mandibular or the third division V3

Out of these whole of V1 and part of V2 are of neuro-ophthalmic value.

The ophthalmic division

It is the smallest division of the fifth nerve. It arises from the anteromedial part of the gasserian ganglion and after a short course enters the cavernous sinus and is embedded in the lateral wall of the cavernous sinus. The third and the fourth nerve are superior to it. In the lateral wall just before entering the orbit, it divides into three branches—the **lacrimal**, **frontal** and **nasociliary**. The lacrimal nerve is the lateral most structure to enter the superior orbital fissure. In the orbit, it is joined by zygomaticotemporal nerve, a branch of maxillary division. The combination carries the postganglionic parasympathetic secretomotor fibers to the lacrimal gland. The frontal nerve also enters the superior orbital fissure outside the common tendinous ring between the lacrimal and trochlear nerve. The nasociliary nerve enters the orbit inside the tendinous ring below the upper division of the third nerve and above the lower division and the sixth nerve. It gives sensory root to the ciliary ganglion (Fig. 2.25).

Applied anatomy of the facial nerve

The facial nerve is the **seventh cranial nerve**. Its lesions have lesser number of neuro-ophthalmic manifestation than cranial nerves—third, fourth, sixth and fifth. The only neuro-ophthalmic manifestation is **facial palsy and its variations**.

The facial nerve is a **mixed nerve**, it has a **motor**, **a sensory** and a **secretomotor component**. It is also called nerve of the **second branchial arch**. The motor component is **efferent** while the somatic and visceral sensations are **afferent** (Flow chart 2.2).

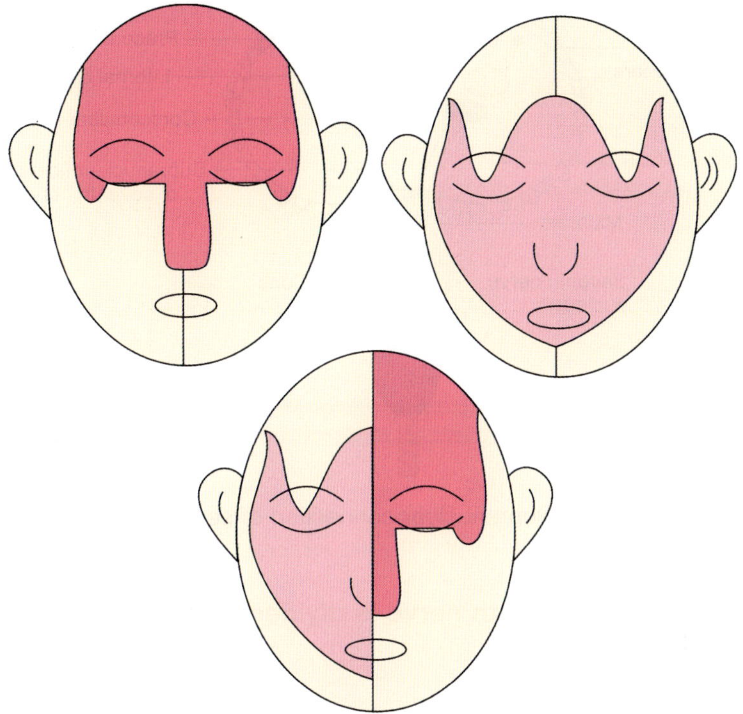

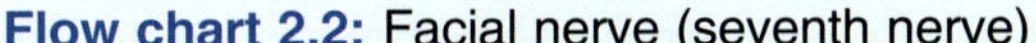

Fig. 2.25: Sensory distribution of V1 and V2 showing areas of overlap

Flow chart 2.2: Facial nerve (seventh nerve)

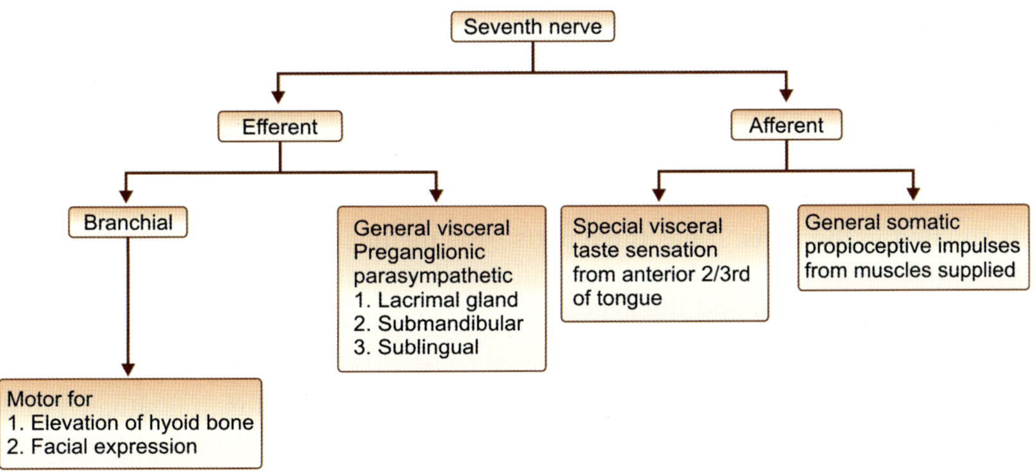

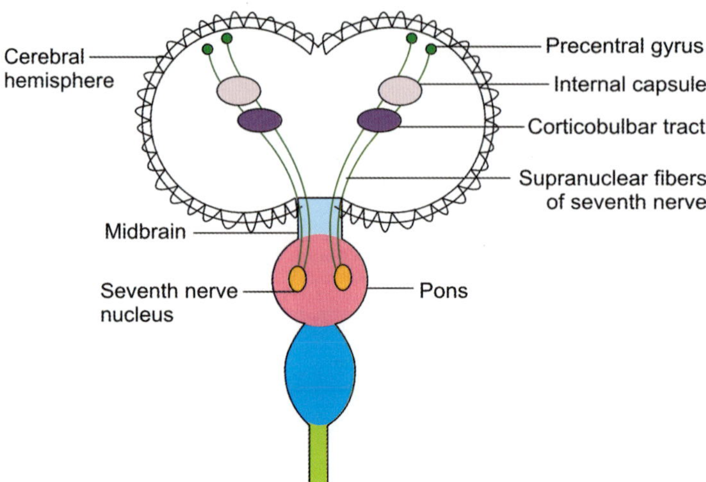

Fig. 2.26: Supranuclear connection of seventh nerve

For clinical purpose the seventh nerve is divided into

1. Supranuclear part
2. Nucleus
3. Infranuclear part

The supranuclear fibers start in the cerebral hemisphere in lower third of precentral gyrus, pass through the **internal capsule**, **corticobulbar tract** and come down to **midbrain** and **pons**. At this level some the fibers cross the midline to reach the opposite nucleus of the facial nerve the remaining terminate in nucleus of same side (Fig. 2.26).

The nuclei of seventh nerve

The seventh nerve too dose not have a single nucleus. It has **four nuclei**, i.e. **one sensory**, **one motor** and **two secretomotor**. The nuclei are situated in the lower part of the pons. The sensory component is called the **nervus intermedius** (Figs 2.27 and 2.28).

The motor nucleus

It is situated in the **pons**. It has three parts—the medial, intermediate and the lateral. The medial nucleus sends fibers to auricular and cervical nerves. The intermediate is cornered with temporal and the zygomatic nerves.

The sensory nucleus

The sensory nucleus is also known as nucleus of **tractus solitarius**. It is situated in the upper part of the medulla. It receives fibers from anterior two third of tongue and auricle.

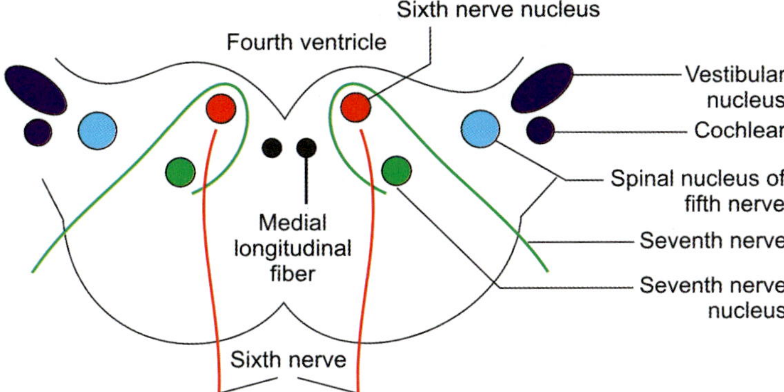

Fig. 2.27: Position of seventh nerve in relation to fifth, sixth and eighth nerve

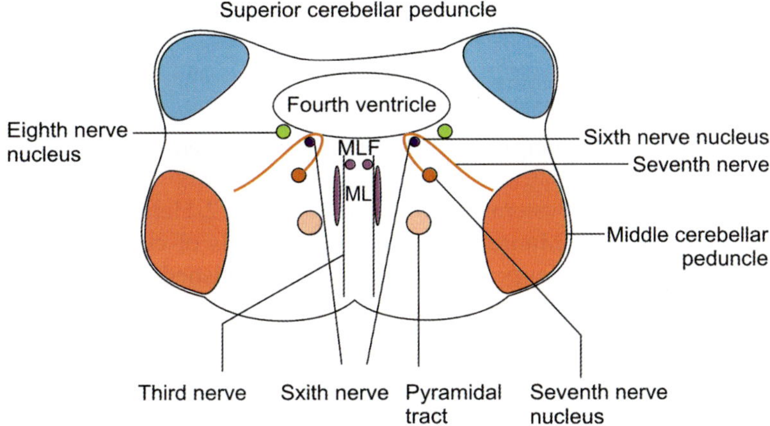

Fig. 2.28: Position of seventh nerve in relation to other neural tract

The secretomotor nuclei

The superior salivatory nucleus: It is situated in the pons dorsolateral and inferior to the motor nucleus. It sends parasympathetic fibers to the submandibular and sub-lingual glands.

The lacrimal nucleus is situated in the lower pons. It sends preganglion fibers to lacrimal gland.

The course of the facial nerve

The interpontine course of the seventh nerve consists of two roots, i.e. the motor root and the sensory root. They are independent structure up to the **internal acoustic meatus** thereafter they fuse to form a common trunk. In the intracranial course they are lateral to the eight nerve. Once the two roots fuse the eight nerve moves away. The common trunk enter the **facial canal** and then traverse the boney facial canal. The bony canal is not a straight canal, it has **two bends** that divide the canal in **three parts** which are again not in a same plane.

The first part is directed laterally, the second part backward and the third part is longest and vertical. The **geniculate ganglion** is situated at the junction of first and second part. As the nerve is intracanalicular in this part its course is identical to the boney canal. The nerve leaves the canal at the **stylomastoid foramen**. Thereafter it crossed the styloid process and enters the parotid gland after it has crossed the external carotid. Near the neck of the mandible it divides in **five branches:** The temporal, zygomatic, buccal, mandibular and cervical. Out of which the **temporal and zygomatic** branches are of neuro-ophthalmic interest. The zygomatic supplies the orbicularis oculi the muscle that closes the lid. The temporal supplies the **frontalis**, the corrugators superior.

BIBLIOGRAPHY

1. Banumathy SP, Natchair G. Anatomy of the eye, 2nd edn, Arvind Eye Hospital, Maduari, 1998.
2. Chaurasia BD. Human anatomy, Vol. 3, 3rd edn, CBS Publishers and Distributors, New Delhi, 2000.
3. Datta AK. Essentials of human anatomy: Neuroanatomy. 1st edn, Current Book International Calcutta, 1995.
4. Duke Elder S, Wyber KC. System of Ophthalmology, Vol. 2, Henry Kimpton London, 1961.
5. Gilman S, Newman SW. Manters and Gatz's Essentials of clinical neuroanatomy and neurophysiology, 7th edn, Jaypee Brothers Medical Publishers, New Delhi, 1990.
6. Nema HV. Anatomy of the eye and its adnexa. 2nd edn, Jaypee Brothers Medical Publishers, New Delhi, 1991.
7. Poddar Bhagat A. Anatomy of central nervous system, 8th edn, Scientific Book Company, Patna 2004.
8. Romanes GJ. Cunninghamis manual of practical anatomy, 15th edition, ELBS Oxford University, 1993.
9. Singh I. Textbook of human neuroanatomy, 6th edn, Jaypee Brothers Medical Publishers, New Delhi, 2002.
10. Wolff F. The anatomy of the eye and orbit, 7th edn, HK Lewis, London, 1976.

3 Disorders of the Visual Pathway

The **visual path** extends from the **retina** to the **visual cortex**. It is responsible for transmitting visual impulses from the retina to the visual cortex, besides visual fibers, the fibers responsible for **light reflex**, **near reflex** and **convergence reflexes** also traverse part of this path. The lesions of visual pathway cause disorders that may be **visual—pupillary** or **field changes** in various combinations. The visual deficiencies depend mostly on involvement of macular fibers. Pupillary changes are seen only in pregeniculate lesions while the field changes are produced by lesions any where between optic nerve and visual cortex (Table 3.1).

For clinical purposes, the visual path which is known as the **retinocalcarine** path also, can be divided into:

1. Anterior visual path extending from retina to chiasma, i.e. optic nerve and chiasma.
2. Middle visual path extending from posterior end of the chiasma to the lateral geniculate body, the optic tract.

Table 3.1: Field changes in relation to location in visual pathway

Location of the lesion	*Field changes*
Retina	Unilateral, ipsilateral, may be single or scattered, central or peripheral, do not respect vertical meridian
Optic nerve	Unilateral, ipsilateral, central/centrocecal, arcuate, junctional, generalized constriction.
Chiasma	Bilateral, heteronymous, bitemporal or binasal, congruous, respect the vertical line, may start in a quadrant, may cause junctional scotoma.
Optic tract—anterior	Bilateral, homonymous, incongruous, have variable density with sloping margins, macular splitting.
Posterior	Complete homonymous hemianopia.
Lateral geniculate body	Rare, difficult to chart, when present are a combination of field changes of optic tract and optic radiation. When detected they are highly incongruous, and cause homonymous hemianopia.
Optic radiation	Congruous, hemianopia, bilateral, homonymous, hemianopic or quadranopic, macular sparing, peripheral crescent, contralateral altitudinal scotoma.
Visual cortex	Homonymous, central hemianopia congruous.

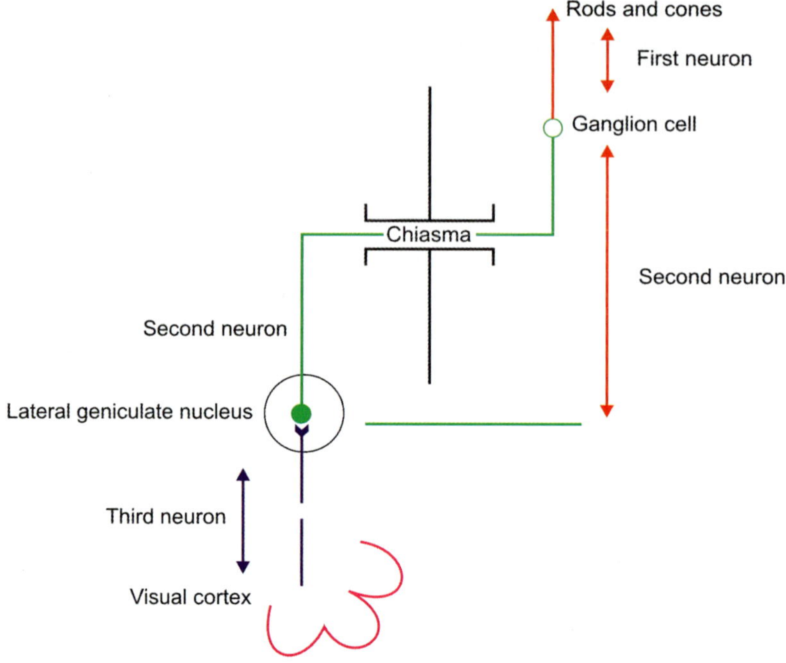

Fig. 3.1: Representation of three neurons of visual path

3. Posterior visual path extending from lateral geniculate body to the visual cortex called optic radiation or geniculocalcarine tract.
4. The lateral geniculate body and the area around it lie in the twilight zone of second and third part.
5. Each part has its distinct clinical features in the form of: (i) Field changes, (ii) Vision, (iii) Color vision, (iv) Pupillary changes, (v) Fundus changes, (vi) Dark adaptation, (vii) Opto-kinetic nystagmus.

The visual path has **three neurons** (Fig. 3.1)

(i) The first neuron extends from rods and comes to ganglion cells.
(ii) The second neuron joins the ganglion cells to the lateral geniculate body.
(iii) The third neuron extends from lateral geniculate body to visual cortex.

There are **two synapses** in the visual path:

(i) Between the bipolar cells and the ganglion cells of the retina.
(ii) Between the second neuron and the third neuron at lateral geniculate body.

The visual pathway is intimately related to many vessels but does not come in direct proximity of neural tracts like corticospinal tract and other cranial nerves, hence lesion of visual pathway alone are not associated with sensory and motor loss.

Some peculiarities of optic nerve

1. Though the optic nerve is listed among the cranial nerves, it is not a true nerve but a neural tract.

2. It does not have a nucleus like other cranial nerves, i.e. third nerve onwards.
3. It starts in the ganglion cell of the retina.
4. In its intraorbital part it shares the **covering of the brain,** i.e. **dura**, **arachnoid** and **pia** with corresponding spaces, i.e. **subdural** and **subarachnoid spaces** that are continuous with the corresponding spaces of the brain. The **CSF** bathes the optic nerve from all sides and plays an important part in production of **papilledema**.
5. It has very specialized blood supply
6. The optic nerve is a pure sensory nerve without any motor function.

Disorders of the optic nerve

1. The sensory function is visual that comprises of:
   (i) Vision
   (ii) Color vision
   (iii) Field of vision
   (iv) Pupillary changes
2. In disorders of the optic nerve, any of the functions singly or in combination become subnormal.
3. Disorders of the visual pathway can be:
   (i) Part of central nervous system disease
   (ii) Part of intraocular disease.
4. Disorders of the optic nerve, like any other part of the central nervous system can be:

Congenital	Dystrophic
Traumatic	Nutritional
Infectious	Vascular
Inflammatory	Demyelinating
Neoplastic	
Degenerative	

Clinical features of disorders of visual path

1. **Vision:** Most of the lesions of visual path cause diminished distant vision depending on location and severity of the lesion.
2. **Color vision:** Color vision defects are seen only in lesions of optic nerve.
3. **Field changes** depend on the arrangement of nerve fibers in retinocalcarine path, i.e. visual path. Shape, size, laterality and similarity of the visual field depend on the position of the fibers involved:
   (i) Central/peripheral
   (ii) Nasal/temporal
   (iii) Superior/inferior
   (iv) Crossed/uncrossed

The visual fields are outward projection of the retinal fibers in the space. The position of the visual fibers in the retina differ from that of in the visual path. The relation between the retina and the visual field have an inverted relationship, i.e. inferior retinal fibers are responsible for upper field defect and vice versa. They also have reversal of sites, i.e. temporal retina is responsible for nasal field defects and nasal retina is representing temporal field.

The retinal fibers within central 30° cause a disproportionately large field defect.

The temporal fibers of the ipsilateral retina remains uncrossed as the fibers proceeds towards the chiasma. The nasal fibers cross in the chiasma to join the uncrossed fibers of the other side.

The relative position of the fibers are shown in Figures 3.2A to G.

The relative position of fibers in visual pathway

The arrangement of the nerve fibers in the **distal part of the optic nerve** is shown in Figure 3.2A.

The macular fibers occupy a large temporal part in the form of a wedge with wider surface outwards. The macular fibers are sandwiched between upper and lower wedge of temporal fibers. The remaining part is occupied by nasal fibers. The horizontal raphe represents the line of demarcation between the upper and lower fibers.

As the fibers proceeds towards the chiasma the macular fibers shifts medially to become central (Fig. 3.2B). The area occupied by macular fibers shrink as compared to area in the distal part. The area occupied by the nasal fibers also gets reduced. Most of the remaining part is occupied by temporal fibers. The horizontal raphe still remains the line of demarcation between the superior and inferior fibers.

In the chiasma, the macular fibers remain central (Fig. 3.2C). Chiasma is the structure in which both central and peripheral fibers decussate partially (Fig. 3.3). The fibers lateral to the macula go straight in the optic tract without crossing the chiasma (Fig. 3.4).

The inferior fibers become lateral in the optic tract. The superior and crossed fibers occupy the medial part of the optic tract. The nasal fibers traverse the chiasma to reach the medial part of the optic tract on the other side. The inferior peripheral nasal fibers cross low and anteriorly. The superior nasal fibers cross posteriorly. The inferior peripheral nasal fibers form a loop in the opposite optic nerve and the loop is called anterior knee of **Willebrand's** (Fig. 3.5).

Similarly the superior peripheral nasal fibers form a loop in the optic tract and is called posterior knee of Willebrand.

In the optic tract the macular fibers are central and superior. The inferior lateral fibers both crossed and un crossed are situated medially (Fig. 3.2D).

The arrangement of the fibers in the lateral geniculate body (Fig. 3.2E).

In the optic radiation fibers sweep laterally and inferiorly round the temporal horn of the lateral and ventrical. The anterior most fibers of the optic radiation form **Meyer's loop** in the temporal lobe.

Visual cortex— (see Figs 3.2F and G)

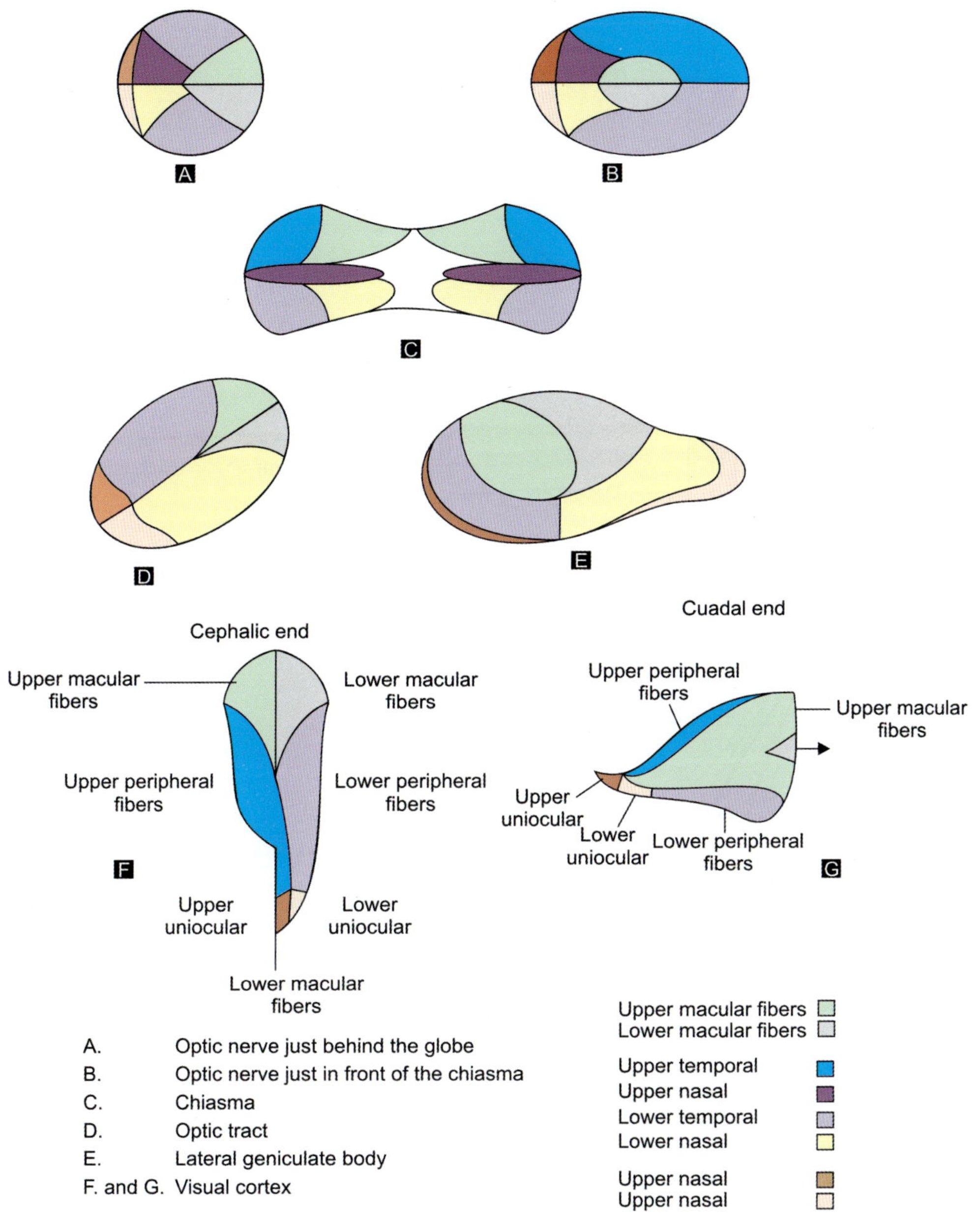

Figs 3.2A to G: Arrangement of visual fibers in visual path

4. **Field changes (see Figs 1.1 to 1.14)**
   The position, shape and congruence of the field defect depends upon the location of the lesion and the fibers involved.
   i. The lesions of retina and optic nerve produce uniocular ipsilateral field defects.
   ii. Lesion of chiasma cause heteronymous field defects.

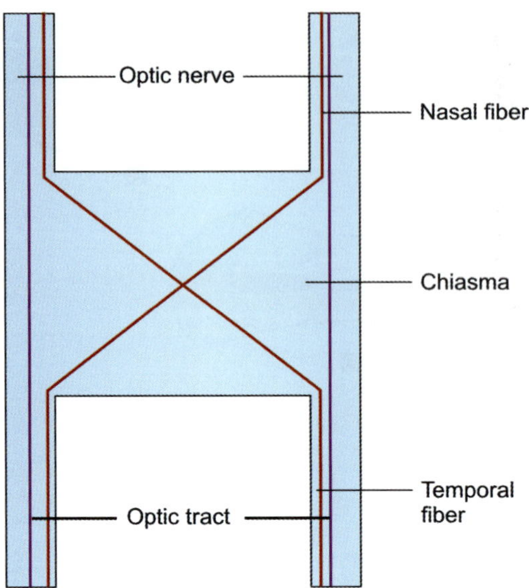

Fig. 3.3: Crossing of nasal fiber in chiasma

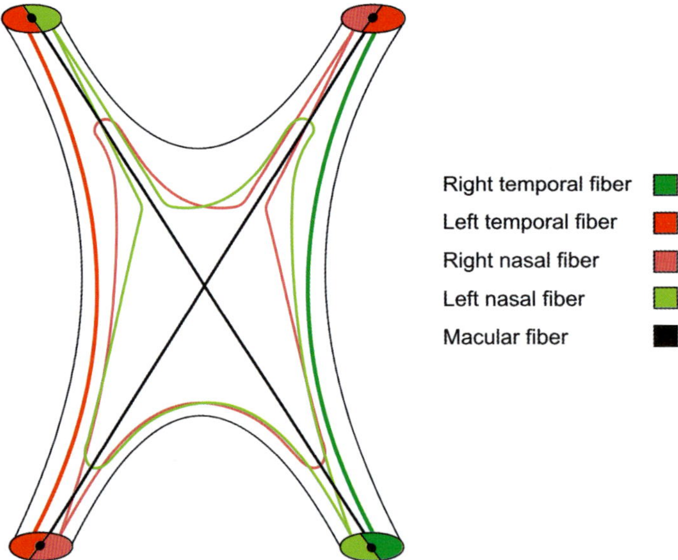

Fig. 3.4: Arrangement of fibers in chiasma showing crossed fibers and their rotation

iii. Those beyond chiasma produce bilateral homonymous field defects, may be sectorial, quadranopic or hemianopic that may be congruous or non-congruous, may be with macular sparring or without macular sparring.
iv. The lesions in chiasma and beyond produce bilateral field defects.

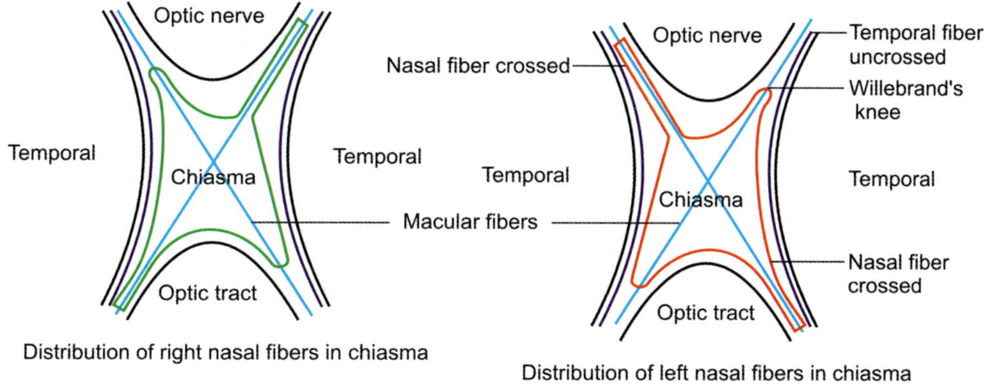

Fig. 3.5: Decussation of fibers in the chiasma

Lesions of **chiasma** and **beyond** generally respect the vertical meridian, i.e. they are either temporal or nasal field defects and rarely superior or inferior field defects.

5. **Pupillary changes** are brought about by lesions anterior to lateral geniculate body (see Chapter 4).

An eye may be blind but may retain pupillary reaction, i.e. cortical blindness.

6. **Fundus changes:** Swelling and vascular changes in optic nerve head is visible in papillitis and papilledema. Atrophy can occur with lesions from disk to lateral geniculate body and is visible on fundus examination.

   Lesions beyond geniculate body do not cause change in the fundus.
7. **Dark adaptation** is poor in lesion of the optic tract in the hemianopic scotoma.
8. **Optokinetic nystagmus** is of importance in lesions of middle and posterior part of the radiation.

DISORDERS OF OPTIC NERVE

Congenital anomalies of optic nerve of neuro-ophthalmic interest are

Most of the congenital anomalies of optic nerve do not have any neuro-ophthalmic features yet they are often mistaken as neuro-ophthalmic disorders.

1. Pseudoneuritis (pseudopapillitis)
2. Drusen of optic disk
3. Tilted disk
4. Hypoplasia and dysplasia of the disk
5. Pits of optic nerve.

1. Pseudoneuritis

Pseudoneuritis is the **commonest congenital anomaly of the disk**. The condition is self-limiting, does not have any neuro-ophthalmic manifestation. However, it is the commonest dilemma faced by a clinician while differentiating other causes of disk elevation, i.e. **early papilledema, papillitis or disk drusen**. The condition is **bilateral**, mostly seen in **hypermetropic eyes** which are otherwise normal. It may occasionally be seen in emmetropic eyes.

The condition is **asymptomatic** and found on routine fundus examination. The difficulty arises when the patient has symptoms suggestive of raised intracranial pressure, i.e. headache, diminished vision, etc. It is commonly mistaken as early papilledema or papillitis.

Bilateral involvement without loss of vision, good color vision, absence of central or centrocecal field changes exclude optic neuritis.

Papilledema is more difficult to exclude, it may require FFA, CT and MRI to clinch the diagnosis of early papilledema.

On fundus examination**, the disk is small**, the **cup is obliterated**. The margins are blurred without any peripapillary edema, exudates or hemorrhage. There is no venous dilatation, normal venous pulsation. The disk itself is not hyperemic. There may be abnormal branching of the retinal vessels. The elevation of disk is between one-dimensional to two-dimensional. Field examination may show normal or enlarged blind spot. Possibility of **drusen of optic nerve** may require exclusion by CT and fundus fluorescein angiography. No treatment is required except associated error of refraction.

2. Drusen of optic nerve

It is yet another condition that causes panic even in experienced clinicians too because it is one of the foremost causes of pseudopapilledema. The exact cause of the condition is not clear. The lesion is thought to be accumulation of immature neuroglia with degenerative changes and calcium deposition.

The condition is thought to be **congenital** but **does not manifest unless the child is about ten years old**. When its presence is felt as pseudopapilledema. By second or third decade they are fully developed and may protrude on the surface of the disk without any knowledge of the person. In 75% of the cases, they are bilateral. The parents may have ophthalmoscopic picture suggestive of disk drusen.

Presence of drusen like pictures in one of the parents, spares the child from costly investigation.

Ophthalmoscopic picture in adult is almost diagnostic. A fully developed drusen in adult looks like a small mulberry on the disk surface obliterating the normal cup, the disk margins are blurred and irregular. The growth glows in green filter. On fundus fluorescein angiography the drusen shows **autofluorescence, ultrasonograhy** delineates the outline of drusen even before it has reached the surface.

The condition is **asymptomatic** with good vision unless there is **spontaneous hemorrhage** on the disk surface that may spill over the retina or may become sub-hyaloid. Occasionally there may be transient obscuration of vision that may be mistaken as amaurosis fugax.

The fields changes

In spite of benign nature of the condition, the disk drusen has variable field changes that includes:

1. Enlargement of blind spot
2. Nerve fiber defect
3. Irregular peripheral constriction. Loss of lower nasal peripheral field is thought to be characteristic.

The condition progresses slowly and not known to cause blindness, does not require any treatment.

3. Tilted disk

It is a **bilateral condition** where the disk is **small and tilted**, generally seen in **myopic astigmatism**, the axis of astigmatism is generally oblique. It is often associated with congenital conus of the disk.

The vision is generally sub normal due to myopic astigmatism. The commonly seen field defects are bitemporal reduced sensitivity. The field defect does not respect the vertical meridian. Sometimes there may be altitudinal field defect. No specific treatment except correction of myopic astigmatism is required.

Hypoplasia and dysplasia of the disk

Hypoplasia of the disk is more common than dysplasia. The former is a small disk while the latter is a large disk and are known as micropapilla and megalopapilla respectively.

The hypoplasia of the disk may be **unilateral** or **bilateral**. The size varies between just below average diameter to very small disk. **The vision is directly related to the size of the disk**, smaller the disk poorer is the vision. Associated of forebrain deformity is not rare. It may be associated with short stature and nystagmus. Nystagmus is common in cases with normal stature also.

There is no known treatment. Subnormal vision is managed by low vision aids.

Morning glory syndrome is unilateral. It is a form of **dysplastic coloboma** of the disk, may be associated with retinochoroidal coloboma or peripapillary staphyloma. **The vision is very poor**. The disk is large and **excavated like advanced glaucoma** without much pallor. The vessels emerge from the disk in a spoke like fashion. The disk is surrounded by an elevated oval ring of hypopigmentation. Retinal detachment is frequent.

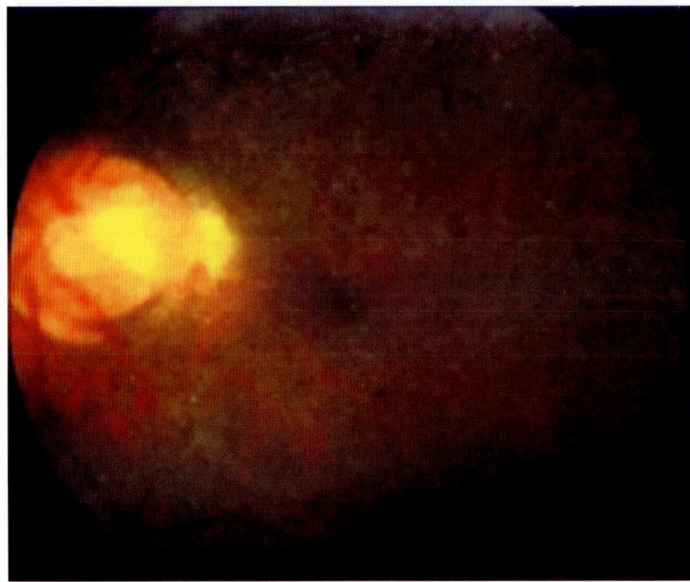

Fig. 3.6: Fundus photograph of congenital pit of optic nerve (*Courtesy:* Dr Anand Saxena)

Many cases are associated with congenital anomalies of forebrain which includes encephalocele, pulsating exophthalmos, nasopharyngeal and frontonasal mass.

Congenital pits of the optic nerve (Fig. 3.6)

This condition is not very rare. In the past it was listed as dysplastic change of optic disk. Exact cause of the condition is not known. The condition is not known to cause any neuro-ophthalmic manifestation except some field defects, i.e. arcuate scotoma and central scotoma. Serous detachment of macula is very common.

In all cases of serous detachment of the macula, the disk should be examined for evidence of congenital pits.

Differential diagnosis consists of primary optic atrophy and glaucoma.

Acquired swelling of the optic nerve head

All acquired swelling of the optic nerve head have neuro ophthalmic manifestation.

For clinical purposes the optic nerve swelling can be broadly divided into two categories:

1. Papilledema
2. Nonpapilledematous swelling.

Papilledema

The term should strictly be confined to **passive optic disk swelling secondary to elevation of intracranial** (cerebrospinal fluid pressure). The swelling is generally bilateral which need not be symmetric without visual loss until the condition passes into a stage of optic atrophy which is an irreversible state, may terminate in blindness. The condition is **rapid to develop and slow to subside** that too when the intracranial CSF tension has been brought down.

The exact mechanism of papilledema is not well understood.

Some of the accepted factors in producing papilledema are

1. The CSF pressure is critical for the mechanism.
2. The raised CSF pressure is transmitted to the optic nerve head through the subarachnoid space.
3. The tension in the subarachnoid spaces rises enough to compress the nerve fibers in the intraorbital part.
4. There is intra-axonal swelling and accumulation of axoplasmic fluid.
5. The axoplasmic flow slows down.
6. There is leak of axoplasmic fluid in the extracellular space at the prelamilar part of the disk.
7. The venous flow is obstructed.
8. There is hypoxia of the nerve fibers.
9. There is dilatation of capillaries on the nerve head.
10. There is venous dilatation with peripapillary edema leading to superficial hemorrhages and exudates on the disk and surrounding retina.

Clinical presentation

Papilledema can be seen at **any age** after closure of the cranial sutures. **In children subtentotial lesions are more common causes of papilledema than supratentorial lesions.** Generally papilledema is a slow progressive disorder that takes about a week to manifest following onset of raised intracranial pressure. Slow rise of CSF pressure causes gradual onset of papilledema. **Acute papilledema** develops within two to four hours following subarachnoid hemorrhage or intracerebral hemorrhage.

The symptoms of papilledema are

1. Systemic
2. Ocular

The systemic manifestations are secondary to raised intracranial tension. Sometimes even well developed papilledema may be asymptomatic or may have very little symptoms.

The common symptoms are: Headache, worse on waking in the morning, nausea, vomiting, diplopia, grey out or black outs, well developed papilledema may have hemiparesis, specific ocular motility disorders. Acute papilledema may be associated with lowered levels of consciousness.

The visual symptoms

Visual disturbances are **late** features of papilledema.

Vision

Good central vision is retained unless exudates or hemorrhages develop on the macula. However **black outs** and **grey outs** are common following sudden change of posture. Gradual loss of vision is a sign of onset of postpapilledematous optic atrophy that may terminate in blindness unless the cause of raised intracranial tension is removed.

Diplopia

Diplopia depends on involvement of cranial nerves. Commonest and first nerve to be affected is **sixth nerve** that has no localizing significance. However there may be other cranial nerve involvement with corresponding diplopia and tract involvement. These generally have localizing significance.

Extraocular muscle palsy may be associated with paralytic squint.

Field changes

The earliest detectable field change is enlargement of blind spot. Loss of peripheral field of vision is a sign of onset of postpapilledematous optic atrophy.

Fundus changes

Most significant ocular changes are seen in fundus. The fundus picture in turn depends on duration and severity of condition.

The fundus changes can be:

1. Early papilledema,
2. Fully developed papilledema,
3. Chronic papilledema

1. **Early papilledema:** Diagnosis of early papilledema is tricky, however some of the points that go in its favor are:
   - Good central vision
   - Bilaterality
   - Preservation of central part of the optic cup
   - Absence of spontaneous venous pulsation
   - Absence of centrocecal field changes.

Presence of signs and symptoms of raised intracranial pressure

Early changes (Fig. 3.7)

i. The earliest sign is obscuration of the retinal vessel at the disk margin.
ii. This is followed by development of prominent striation in nerve fibers near the disk margin.
iii. Blurring of the disk margin for which no rule of thumb is available, develops more frequently in the upper pole followed by lower pole, the nasal margin is last to be blurred.

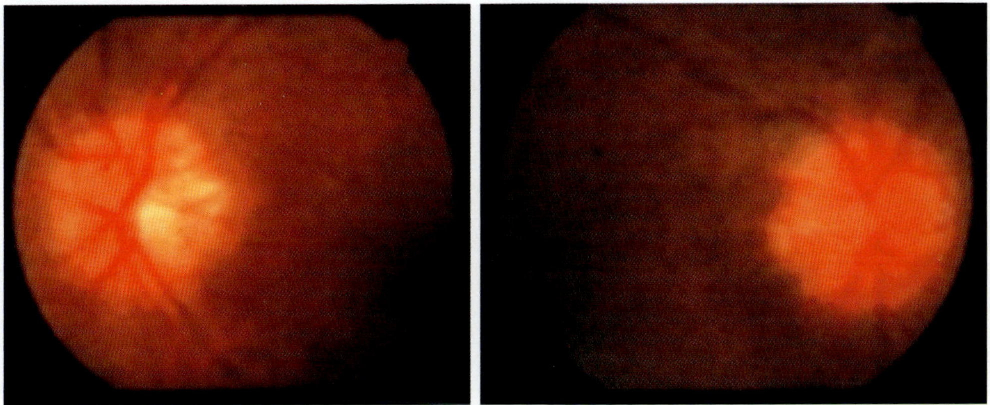

Fig. 3.7: Early disk changes in papilledema

iv. Hyperemia of the disk is due to capillary engorgement.
v. The central cup is visible.
vi. Spontaneous venous pulsation may be absent.
At this stage the central vision is good and there are no field changes. Fluorescein angiography alone is not very reliable investigation at this stage, it should be matched with other feature.

2. **Fundus changes in fully developed papilledema (Figs 3.8 and 3.9)**
   i. The whole circumference of the disk margin is blurred.
   ii. The whole of the disk is hyperemic.
   iii. The cup is no more visible.
   iv. The top of cup is elevated more than 1 mm which is equal to three-dimensional above the peripapillary retina. The edema may be more.
   v. Superficial hemorrhages on or near the disk are common.
   vi. Cotton wool spots on the retina represent infarction in the nerve fiber.
   vii. The venous pulsation is absent (this is not very reliable sign).
   viii. Retinal edema:
      a. Macular star or half star formation
      b. Development of Paton's line. These are stress lines which are concentric with the disk margin.

The vision is still maintained.

The field changes consists of enlargement of blind spot.

Fluorescein angiography at this stage differentiates **pseudopapilledema** and **drusen** from papilledema. However FFA does not always differentiate papilledema from papillitis which should be confirmed by other clinical signs and investigations.

The fluorescein picture consists of (Fig. 3.10)

i. Leak of fluorescein from disk capillaries.
ii. Extensive leak from disk capillaries and venous channels.
iii. Diffuse spread of dye in nerve fiber layer.

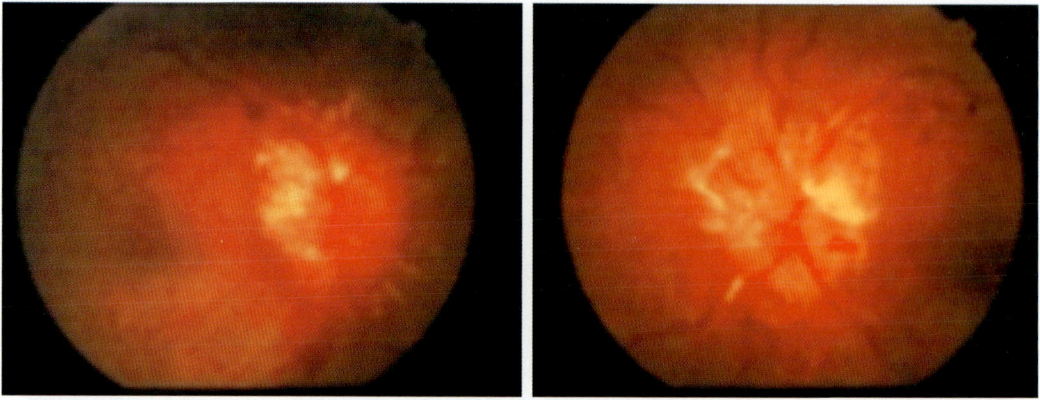

Fig. 3.8: Disk changes in fully developed papilledema (*Courtesy:* Dr Anand Saxena)

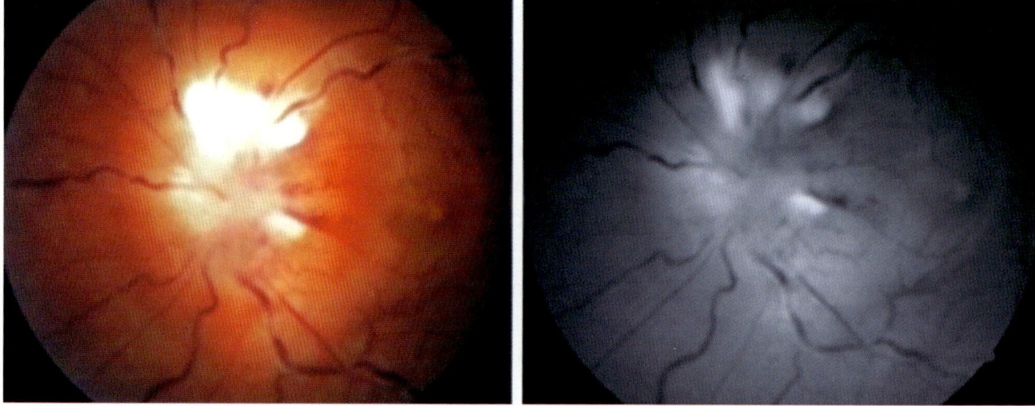

Fig. 3.9: Disk changes in fully developed papilledema—color and red free photograph (*Courtesy:* Dr OP Billoe, Dr Praveen and Dr Roopam Janak Desai)

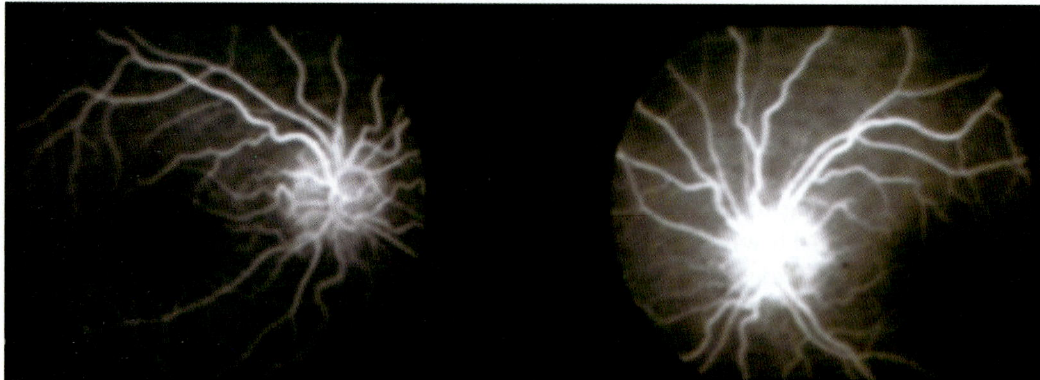

Fig. 3.10: Fundus fluorescein picture of papilledema (*Courtesy:* Dr Anand Saxena)

Neuroimaging

X-ray at this stage may not be of much help. Better results are obtained by thin section contrast enhancement CT and MRI. Ultrasonography in primary gaze and 30° eccentric gaze. In case of papilledema, the optic nerve diameter is more in primary gaze than at 30° eccentric gaze.

3. **Changes in chronic papilledema**
   i. The swelling of the disk starts subsiding with development of glial tissue.
   ii. The color of the disk changes from pink to dirty yellow.
   iii. The hemorrhages fade away.
   iv. The exudates still persists.
   v. The cup is permanently obliterated.
   vi. The vessels are sheathed.
   vii. The macular star is replaced by scar and mottled pigment.
   viii. The vision is diminished ranging from moderately low to total loss of vision.
   ix. Peripheral constriction of field is added to already existing enlarged blind spot.

Diagnosis

Diagnosis of well established papilledema is not difficult which is characterized by bilaterality, vision preserved for long, no pupillary changes, preserved cup for considerable time, obliteration of cup is signs of raised intracranial pressure go in favor of papilledema (Table 3.2).

Differential diagnosis consists of pseudopapilledema, drusen of optic disk, papillitis, anterior ischemic optic neuropathy, optic nerve tumor, infiltration of optic nerve, hypertensive and diabetic optic neuropathy, neuroretinitis, hypotony, central retinal vein and branch vein occlusion (Figs 3.11 to 3.13).

The pseudopapilledema, drusen of optic disk and anterior ischemic optic neuropathy and hypertension are generally bilateral.

Hypotony, papillitis and neuroretinitis are generally unilateral but may be bilateral and cause difficulty in differential diagnosis. Papillitis and neuroretinitis are associated with diminished vision.

Common causes of papilledema

1. *Congenital:* Oxycephaly, Crouzon's syndrome, Apert's syndrome, syringomyelia.
2. *Infection:* Meningitis, encephalitis, lateral venous thrombosis, subacute bacterial endocarditis, Guillain-Barre syndrome, chiasmatic arachnoiditis.
3. *Cardiovascular diseases:* Hypertensive encephalopathy, congenital heart disease.
4. *Intracranial:* Intracranial space occupying lesions
   i. Tumors
   ii. Brain abscess
   iii. Subdural hematoma
   iv. Subarachnoid hemorrhage

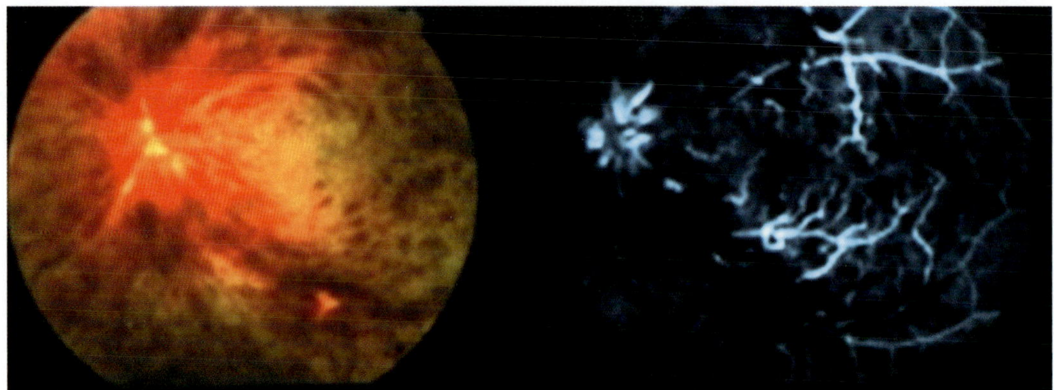

Fig. 3.11: Fundus photograph of central retinal vein thrombosis (*Courtesy:* Dr Anand Saxena)

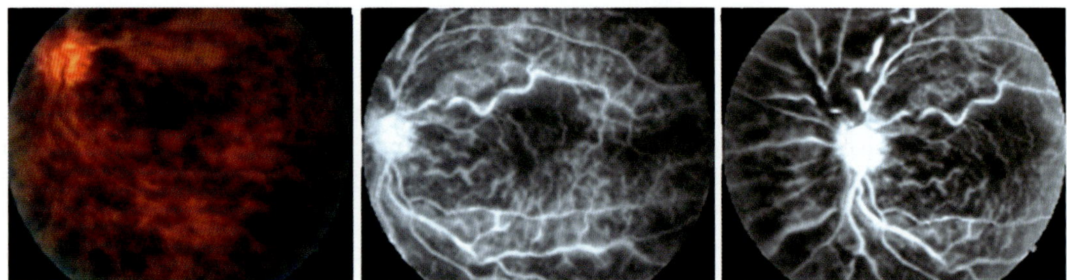

Fig. 3.12: Fundus photograph and FFA of central retinal vein thrombosis (*Courtesy:* Dr OP Billore)

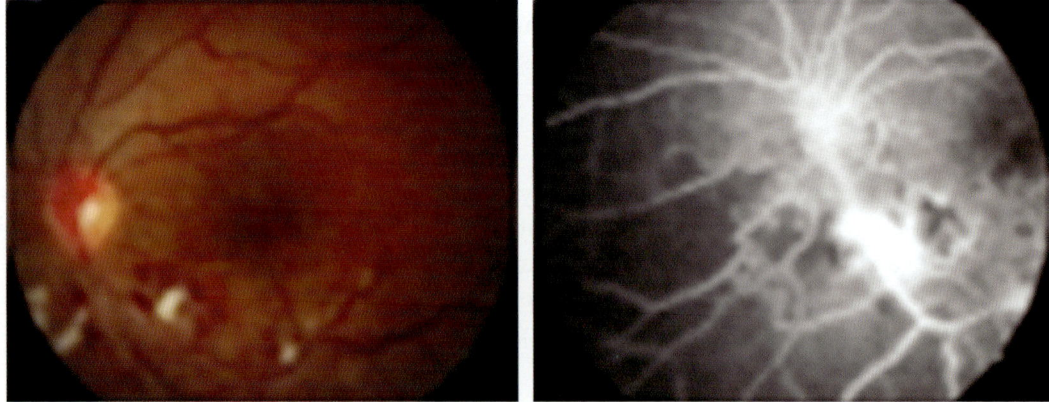

Fig. 3.13: Fundus photograph and FFA of central retinal branch vein thrombosis (*Courtesy:* Dr Praveen and Dr Roopam Janak Desai)

Table 3.2: Clinical features of common condition that form differential diagnosis of papilledema

Clinical features	*Pseudo-neuritis*	*Papilledema*	*Papillitis*	*AION*
Age	Discovered in childhood	Any age after the sutures have closed	10 to 40 years	After 60 years
Laterality	Bilateral	Bilateral	Unilateral/ bilateral	Unilateral, other eye may follow
Pain	Absent	Absent	On movement of eyeball	Tenderness on temple
Vision	Normal	Normal for long time	Poor	Gross loss
Field of vision	Normal	Enlarged blind spot, constricted peripheral field	Central or centrocecal	Altitudinal field loss
Pupillary change	Nil	Nil unless atrophy sets-in	Afferent pupil defect	Afferent pupil defect
Neurological signs	Absent	Invariably present	Absent	Absent
Other feature	Non-significant	Signs of raised intracranial pressure	Not significant	Raised ESR
Treatment	Not required	Lowering of intracranial pressure surgically or medically	May be self-limiting, role of steroid variable	Steroids may be required

v. Intracerebral hemorrhage
vi. Aqueductal stenosis
vii. Benign intracranial hypertension

5. Drugs and toxins: Vitamin A, oral contraceptives, tetracycline, steroid, withdrawal of steroid, nalidixic acid, heavy metals.
6. Others: Eclampsia, Addison's disease, Schilder's disease, lupus erythematosus, anemia, leukemia, spinal cord tumors, pulmonary emphysema.

Unilateral causes of swollen disk

It is better not to use term papilledema for unilateral swelling of the optic nerve head because they do not fulfil the criteria of papilledema, i.e. raised intracranial tension, bilaterality, slow loss of vision, delayed field loss, unilateral disk swellings are not associated with neurological defects.

The causes are either **ocular** or **orbital**.

The ocular causes of swollen disk are

1. Hypotony:
   - i. Postinflammatory
   - ii. Trauma
     - (a) Accidental
     - (b) Surgical
2. Acute congestive glaucoma
3. Intraocular inflammation: Chronic cyclitis, retinal vasculitis, granuloma of optic nerve head.
4. Intraocular tumors: Glioma of optic nerve, neurofibromatosis, hemangioma.

The orbital causes of unilateral swelling of optic disk are

Space occupying lesion

- i. Orbital tumors:
  - (a) Primary
    - – Benign
    - – Malignant
  - (b) Secondary
- ii. Inflammatory – Sinusitis, cavernous sinus thrombosis, orbital abscess
- iii. Vascular – Aneurysm of ophthalmic artery
- iv. Metabolic – Thyroid orbitopathy
- v. Trauma to optic nerve.

The disks that are not likely to develop papilledema are:
Myopia, optic atrophy, coloboma of disk, glaucomatous cup.

Management of papilledema

The management of papilledema is basically management of the cause of raised intracranial tension.

1. General: Acetazolamide, IV mannitol, large dose of steroid, they reduce the pressure for short period.
2. Specific: Management of infection by specific antibiotic.
3. Surgical:
   - i. Removal of expanding mass when possible.
   - ii. Fenestration of optic nerve.

It takes six to eight weeks for the papilledema to subside after the intracranial pressure has been brought down. Once secondary optic atrophy has set in, chances of improvement of vision is always remote.

Optic neuritis

Optic neuritis is an inflammatory condition of the optic nerve from papilla to chiasma due to infection, demyelination, autoimmune reaction, degeneration, rarely trauma or infiltration.

Topographically optic neuritis is divided into

1. **Papillitis**: When the ophthalmoscopic changes are visible on the disk head.
2. **Retrobulbar neuritis:** When there is no visible change in the fundus in spite of clinical features of the neuritis.
3. **Optic neuroretinitis:** When both the retina and neural elements of the optic nerve are involved. The changes are visible on fundus examination.
4. Both papillitis and retrobulbar neuritis can be topographically divided in following categories.
   i. **Axial neuritis** denotes predominant involvement of papillomacular bundle.
   ii. **Periaxial neuritis** means that the papillomacular bundle is less involved or not involved in the process.
   iii. **Perineuritis** denotes involvement of sheath of the neuritis.
   iv. **Transverse neuritis** means that the inflammatory process cuts across the whole diameter of the optic nerve, generally associated with myeilitis.

Infection may reach the optic nerve through

1. **Blood-borne infection**
   Blood-borne infections of the optic nerve are secondary to systemic infections which are mostly endogenous, rarely it may be exogenous brought about by trauma.
2. **Extension from**
   a. Paranasal sinuses
   b. Orbital contents
   c. Meninges
   d. Intraocular structures—retina, choroid.

Papillitis

This is inflammation of **visible part of the optic nerve**. The commonest age group to develop optic neuritis is **25 years to 50 years**.

It is more common in **females**. In **75% of cases**, it is **unilateral**. In most of the instances it is of abrupt nature, lasting for few weeks to few months and gradually improving to almost normal level. Recurrence is common.

The symptoms are

1. Ocular
   i. Visual
   ii. Nonvisual
   iii. Neurological

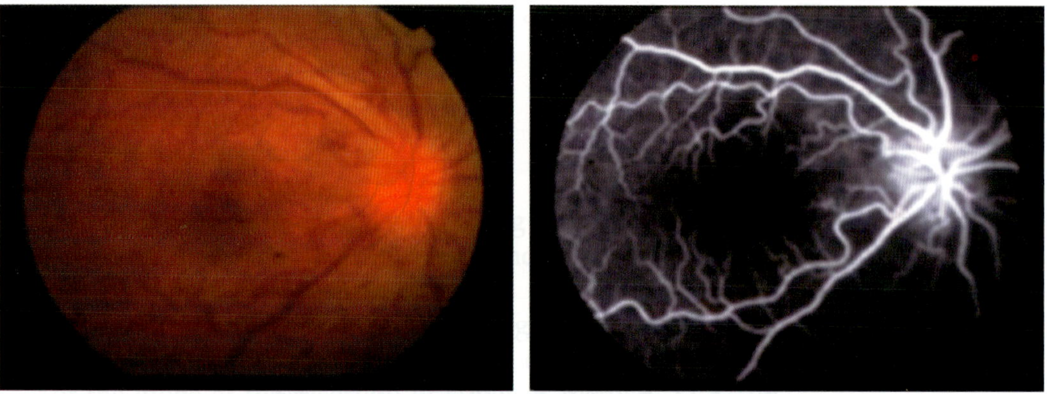

Fig. 3.17: Fundus photograph and FFA of active optic neuritis (*Courtesy:* Dr Anand Saxena)

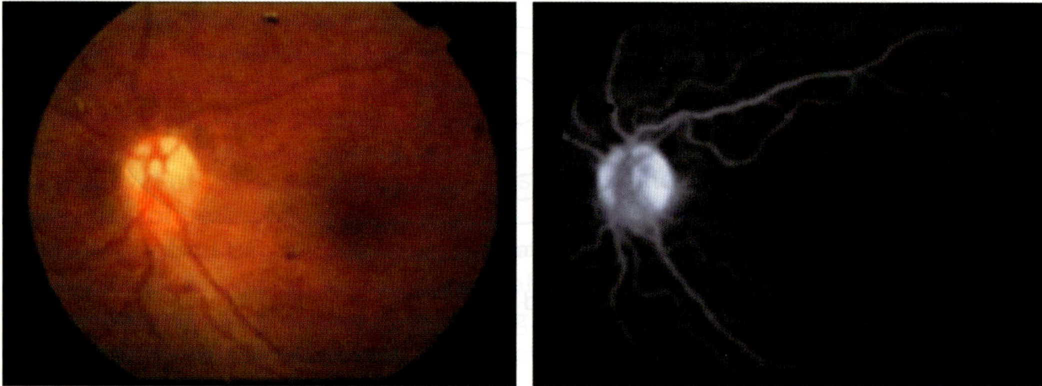

Fig. 3.18: Fundus photograph and FFA of postneuritic pallor (*Courtesy:* Dr Anand Saxena)

(b) **Color:** The disk is hyperemic. There may be small hemorrhagic spots on the disk and peripapillary are (Fig. 3.17).

(c) **Margins** are blurred with edema of the retina round the disk.

(d) The appearance of the disk following recovery is different from active lesion. It can be normal, pale. Pallor may be partial or complete (Fig. 3.18). The cup remains obliterated. Generally pallor of disk is associated with sheathing of the retinal veins.

ii. **Retina**

(a) The surrounding retina is edematous.

(b) There may be peripapillary **splinter, hemorrhages and superficial exudates**.

(c) The **macula may show star formation**.

(d) There may be **cells in the vitreous** in front of the inflamed disk.

(e) In case of neuritis secondary to retinitis or choroiditis, there is evidence of such disorders in the retina.

Optic neuritis in children

1. Incidence of optic neuritis in children is less than in adults. In children it is equal among boys and girls.
2. Presentation of optic neuritis in children differs from those seen in adults.
3. There is no difference in pathogenesis in the two age groups.
4. Optic neuritis in children is more often bilateral causing diminished vision in both eye hence is reported early than unilateral involvement.
5. Papillitis is more common than retrobulbar neuritis in children.
6. Infective process is more frequent cause of neuritis than demyelination.
7. Viruses are major cause of neuritis than bacteria in children. Viral optic neuritis sets in two to three weeks after onset of systemic viral infection.
8. Children with optic neuritis rarely develop multiple sclerosis which is common in adults.
9. Postvaccination neuritis is more frequent than reported. Antiviral vaccines cause optic neuritis more frequently than antibacterial. The postvaccination neuritis is self-limiting, sets in two to there weeks after the vaccination and is generally bilateral. Complete visual recovery is common in postvaccination neuritis.
10. Visual recovery in children is better than in adults.
11. Children respond better to steroid than adults.

Diagnosis

Diagnosis of typical optic neuritis in all ages is not difficult, if following features are found:

1. Unilateral fast fall in vision over days with recovery over weeks
2. Dyschromatopsia
3. Diminished color sense
4. Diminished brightness
5. Afferent papillary defect
6. Pain on movement of the eye
7. Early filling of the cup
8. Cells in the vitreous in front of the disk.

Difficulty arises in **atypical** cases which present as optic neuritis without being so, where vision does not improve over months, i.e. in case of **meningioma of sheath of optic nerve**, **pituitary tumors** which are confirmed by X-ray, CT and MRI.

Differential diagnosis

There is a long list of conditions that masquerade as optic neuritis. They are **early unilateral disk swelling, ischemic optic neuropathy, compressive optic neuropathy, metabolic neuropathy** and **toxic neuropathy**.

Management of optic neuritis is controversial because of spontaneous recovery. Still following guidelines may give better results.

1. All cases associated with infectious process should get specific antibiotic therapy alone or with steroid.
2. All cases of optic neuritis in one eyed person, bilateral neuritis and severe loss of vision in unilateral cases should get mega dose of steroids.
3. All cases of moderate loss of vision should get oral steroids.
4. It should be kept in mind that steroids do not have any effect on final vision; they are given to shorten the period of visual recovery and reduce the ocular discomfort. Role of steroids in prevention of recurrences is not well documented.

Etiology of optic neuritis

The term optic neuritis does not denote a specific disease. It means inflammation of optic disk due to any of the following:

1. **Infection:** Infection can reach the optic nerve from:
   i. Blood stream
   ii. Neighboring structures
      (a) Central nervous system
      (b) Paranasal sinuses
      (c) Orbit
   iii. Intraocular structure.

The infective organism can be any of the microbes from viruses to multicellular parasites.

The common organisms are

Bacteria: Tuberculosis, syphilis, Borrelia (Lyme disease)

Virus: AIDS, herpes zoster, measles, mumps, influenza, infectious mononucleosis, cytomegalovirus.

Fungus: Relatively rare.

Parasites: Cysticercosis, toxoplasmosis, malaria, trypanosomiasis, toxocariasis.

2. **Demyelination:** Multiple sclerosis, Devic's disease, disseminated encephalopathy-myelitis, Schilder's disease.
3. Heredofamilial: Leber's neuropathy
4. Miscellaneous conditions:
   i. Exogenous toxins
   ii. Drugs
   iii. Vaccines
   iv. Venoms
   v. Diabetes
   vi. Thyroid orbitopathy
   vii. Vasculopathy
   viii. Sarcoid

Some specific forms of optic neuritis.

Devic's neuromyelitis optica

Devic's neuromyelitis optica has two components:

1. Optic neuritis.
2. Transverse myelitis.

The condition is common. It is a demyelinating disorder like multiple sclerosis but not related to it. It is known to have multisystem involvement like multiple sclerosis.

The differential points between multiple sclerosis and Devic's disease are

i. Age—neuromyelitis optica is fairly common in first decade while multiple sclerosis is mostly seen in adults.
ii. Multiple sclerosis generally produces unilateral optic neuritis.
iii. Bilateral neuritis along with transverse myelitis is not seen in multiple sclerosis.
iv. Cerebellum is not effected in Devic's disease.
v. Gliosis is not seen in neuromyelitis optica.
vi. Besides optic neuritis and myelitis Devic's disease may have evidence of brain-stem involvement in the form of extraocular muscle palsy and nystagmus.
vii. MRI does not show plaques in white matter in Devic's disease.

Clinical feature of Devic's neuromyelitis

Optic neuritis

Sudden bilateral loss of vision, one eye is affected earlier than the other. When both get involved, one eye has more visual loss than the other. There may be a gap of few hours to weeks. The loss of vision is due to involvement of the optic nerve. **Retro-chiasmal path is not involved**. The loss of vision is not influenced by Uhthoff phenomenon. The loss of vision is sudden and painless. The loss of vision is generally severe. The child may complain of total loss of vision. Recovery of vision starts seven to ten days following maximum loss of vision. It takes weeks to months to improved to its original level. Level of recovery of vision is unpredictable. Some may have good recovery, others may not be so fortunate. Over all prognosis of vision is poor.

Fundus picture

The fundus picture varies between normal fundus, to picture of fully developed optic neuritis. On a long run most of the disks pass into postneuritic optic atrophy.

Myelitis

Transverse myelitis may **precede** or **follow** neuritis. The gap between the two is variable, rarely there may be simultaneous involvement. The myelitis causes various degrees of paraplegia. The **paraplegia** may be in extension or inflexion. Some recovery from paraplegia is the rule, some residual deficit is common.

Cranial nerve involvement in Devic's disease is due to involvement of brainstem. Besides extraocular muscle palsy there may be **conjugate gaze palsy**, **pupillary**

anomaly. Pupillary anomalies can either be afferent or efferent. **Nystagmus** is seen in limited cases.

Diagnosis is straightforward with bilateral loss of vision and variable paraplegia.

Management

There is no specific treatment. Intravenous administration of steroid shorten the period of recovery, may reduce severity that helps in retaining better vision. The child may have to be on low dose of oral steroid for months with usual precautions.

Ischemic optic neuropathy

Ischemic optic neuropathy is a major cause of **sudden painless uniocular** loss of vision that may terminate in blindness in **elderly person** of **both the sexes**. It is a **vascular phenomenon** that results in obliteration of at least one of the **posterior ciliary arteries**. The main pathology is **infarction of the optic nerve** that results in local ischemia in the substance of the nerve.

According to site of involvement the disorder can be:

1. **Anterior ischemic optic neuropathy**
2. **Posterior ischemic neuropathy**

Out of which former is more common and easy to diagnose.

Better classification is on the basis of etiology

1. Arteritic ischemic optic neuropathy
2. Nonarteritic ischemic optic neuropathy.

Arteritic ischemic optic neuropathy (AION)

The disorder occurs in persons between 65-75 years, a decade later than its nonarteritic counterpart. The main cause in **giant cell arteritis** which not only involves the **short posterior ciliary arteries** but also other large and medium sized arteries that have abundant elastic tissue in their arterial wall.

The commonly involved arteries are

- Proximal part of vertebral artery
- Superficial temporal
- Branches of ophthalmic arteries
- **Intracranial arteries other than ophthalmic are spared.**

Besides **giant cells arteritis,** less common causes are **other collagen vascular diseases**, **syphilitic arteritis** and **arteritis in herpes zoster**.

Symptoms of AION can be divided into:

1. Systemic symptoms
2. Ocular symptoms.

1. Systemic symptoms

The systemic symptoms are **nonspecific**. They are due to ischemia in various muscles other than ocular. They are:

(a) **Scalp tenderness:** Tender temporal vessels can be palpated with pulsation. Absence of pulsation is an ominous sign of obliteration that may cause ischemic necrosis of the scalp.
(b) **Headache** may be temporal, frontal or occipital.
(c) **Polymyalgia:** Generally involving muscles of upper extremity and shoulder joint.
(d) **Claudication of jaw:** Pain during talking or chewing.
(e) **Glossodynia:** Pain in the tongue.
(f) Weight loss, night sweats and fever.
(g) Less common but dangerous involvements are **brainstem lesions, myocardial infarction, aortic leak** and **aortic aneurysm**.

2. Ocular symptoms

i. **Diminished vision: Profound, progressive, painless, uniocular loss of vision** is the commonest symptom. This may be preceded by **amaurosis fugax** and **photopsia**. Loss of vision is mostly felt on waking in the morning.
ii. **Diminished color sense:** Loss of color vision is directly proportionate to loss of vision. In contrast to papillitis where color vision defect is disproportionately more when compared to vision.
iii. **Scotoma: Altitudinal lower field** loss is the commonest scotoma. Other field defects like central scotoma or arcuate scotoma may be seen rarely.
iv. **Diplopia** is a rare symptom.

Signs

(i) **Pupillary changes:** A **relative afferent pupillary defect** is always found which cannot be elicited in case of bilateral symmetric cases.
(ii) **Fundus:** The fundus findings are mainly **seen in the disk**. The changes in the disk can be divided into two phase (Fig. 3.19)—fundus and fluorescein of normal disk and AION.
   a. Phase of edema
   b. Phase of atrophy.
   a. **The phase of edema:** The disk in traditionally called **Sick looking (pallid) edematous disk**. The swelling is generally **sectorial,** less frequently be complete. The swollen part is **ischemic**, the remaining part retains usual pink hue or may be hyperemic. The retinal vessels do not show much change this differentiated AION from **central retinal artery** or **central vein occlusion** both of which have sudden, painless vision in patients in fifth decade with vascular changes.
   Less common features are **hemorrhages** in the nerve fiber layer near the disk and **soft exudates**.
   b. **The phase of atrophy** develops **few weeks after** the attack of ischemia. The edema slowly recedes giving place to pallor in about six weeks. The disk

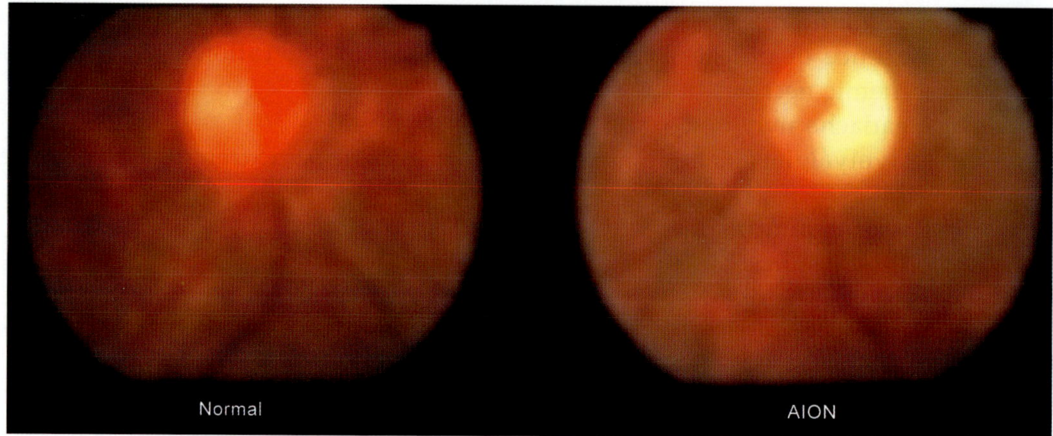

Fig. 3.19: Fundus photograph of anterior ischemic optic neuropathy (*Courtesy:* Dr Anand Saxena)

may develop deepening of cup and the appearance may be **mistaken as glaucomatous**.

Rarely there may be appearance of **pseudofoster Kennedy syndrome**, i.e. edema of the disk on one side and optic atrophy on the other side. The cause of this phenomenon is not well understood.

The changes of involvement is as high as 75% in case of **giant cell arteritis**. Hence the patient should be informed about the possibility of involvement of the other eye. Once AION has been diagnosed in one eye and patient put on heavy dose steroids that may save the other eye.

FUNDUS FLUORESCEIN ANGIOGRAPHY

Due to obstruction in posterior ciliary artery there is delay in choroidal filling the vessels on the disk too show delayed filling the filling delay is more in giant cell arteritis.

Investigation

(i) ESR: A single investigation that is most important in diagnosis of arteritic AION is **raised ESR**. In giant cell arteritis the ESR may be raised as much as **100 mm**. All patients suspected to have AION due to giant cell arteritis should under go ESR evaluation on the **first visit** and if found raised the patient should be advised **temporal artery biopsy** and put on heavy dose of steroid. This may protect the other eye, help improvement in the original eye and reduce chances of systemic complication.

(ii) **C-reactive protein** is generally raised.

(iii) **Temporal artery biopsy** is a simple outdoor procedure. This gives histopathological conformation of giant cell arteritis even when ESR is not raised or C-reactive protein is normal.

Diagnosis

Diagnosis of arteritis AION is straight forward in a patient past sixth decade with sudden, painless uniocular loss of vision with symptoms suggestive of giant cell arteritis and raised ESR.

Differential diagnosis consists of all causes of **uniocular sudden loss of vision**.

They are: Papillitis, central artery occlusion, impending central vein thrombosis, papillophlebitis, compressive optic neuropathy and nonarteritic ischemic optic neuropathy.

Treatment

Once diagnosis of giant cell arteritis has been clinically confirmed by raised ESR the patient should be put on:

i. IV methylprednisolone in dose of 250 mg infused over a period of one hour, every six hours for three days.
ii. This is followed by **oral prednisone** in a dose of 80 mg/day that is tapered gradually. Fall in ESR value is a good indicator of improvement. Steroids should be administered with usual precaution in consultation with general physician.

Nonarteritic ischemic optic neuropathy

Nonarteritic ischemic optic neuropathy is yet another cause of **painless**, **unilateral**, **severe loss of vision** that may sometimes culminate in blindness and involve the other eye as well, in elderly patient in fifth and sixth decade. These patients generally have systemic **vasculopathies** in the form of—**hypertension**, **arteriosclerosis**, and **diabetes**. The condition is **not related to collagen vascular diseases**. It is also seen following **shock** and **massive loss of blood**, may have evidence of **nocturnal hypotension**.

Predisposing factors

The ocular condition that **predispose** the disorder are **small disk**, **chronic glaucoma** and **aphakia**. The small disks in the other eye is at risk of developing the condition.

The exact mechanism of production of the disorder is not well understood. It is thought to be due to **hypoperfusion of the optic disk** secondary to lesion in ciliary circulation. This has been conformed by **fluorescein angiography** and **color Doppler**.

The patients do not have amaurosis fugax, diplopia or other symptoms of giant cell arteritis like fever, malaise and jaw claudication.

The loss of vision stabilizes at a subnormal level in seventy percent of eyes only a few will have further gradual loss of vision. The other eye may get involved over months or years.

Lower altitudinal field defects are common.

Though the disorder is thought to be vasculopathy involving the **posterior ciliary circulation**, the retinal vessels also show changes in the form of thinning once the optic atrophy sets in. The chances of development of myocardial infarction and cerebrovascular accident are less common as compared to its arteritic counterparts.

Diagnosis

Diagnosis is mostly **by exclusion**. Patients with hypertension, atherosclerosis and diabetes with small disk are at higher risk. Hence all patients in fifth decade with small disk should be under observation and asked to keep systemic diseases under control.

Differential diagnosis

Differential diagnosis consists of all case of painless, sudden, unilateral diminished vision in fifth and sixth decade. Most important disorder to be differentiated is **arteritic ischemic optic neuropathy** because it needs large dose of steroids to save the other eye.

Table 3.3: Comparison between AION and NION

	Arteritic	*Nonarteritic*
Age	Sixth and seventh decade	Fifth and sixth decade
Sex	Slightly more in females	Equal in both sexes
Systemic disease	Collagen vasculopathy, i.e. giant cell arteritis	Systemic vasculopathy, i.e. hypertension, diabetes, atherosclerosis
Ocular disease	Noncontributory	Small disk, aphakia, glaucoma
Loss of vision	Unilateral, painless, sudden	Unilateral, painless, sudden
Recovery of vision	Almost nil	May improve
Involvement of other eye	75-80%	Slightly, about 40%
Other symptoms	Weight loss, myalgia, fever, jaw claudication, amaurosis fugax, diplopia	None
Fundus changes	Pallid edema, segmental ischemia, splinter, hemorrhage.	Moderately swollen disk
Systemic complications	Myocardial infarction, cerebrovascular accident, aneurysms of arteries of middle order	Not related
ESR	More than 100 mm	Within normal range or up to 40 m
Temporal artery biopsy	Disruption of internal elastic membrane, granulomatous change with giant cell formation	May show arteriosclerosis
Response to steroids	Nil, saves the other eye	
Treatment	Nil	Steroid with caution

Treatment

No specific and effective treatment has been evolved. The patients with small disk, aphakia and glaucoma with systemic vasculopathies should be instructed to be under supervision of physician and ophthalmologists.

Compressive optic neuropathies

These are a group of condition that are caused by **mass lesion**, may be vascular, i.e. **aneurysms** of the vessels in close proximity of the optic nerve or **growths**, i.e. **tumors** which may be **primary**, **extension from neighboring structures** or **secondary**.

Any part of the optic nerve from chiasma to the globe may be compressed. The signs and symptoms depend on location of the growth, size of the growth and expansion of the growth.

The clinical signs depend on location of the growth that may be:

1. **Intracranial**, may involve the chiasma by vascular or mass lesion.
2. **Intracanalicular:** Meningioma, Paget's disease, osteopetrosis, hyperostoses, metastasis from prostate.
3. **The intraorbital compressive lesion** can be **intraconal**, **extraconal** or both. Lesions near the apex of the orbit are more likely to compress the optic nerve than those situated anteriorly. Commonest cause of compressive optic neuropathy at the orbital apex is **thyroid orbitopathy** followed by **pseudotumor orbit**.

The growth can be intrinsic—arising from substance of the nerve and extrinsic—pressing from outside the nerve.

The compressive lesion present as

1. **Diminished vision:**
   (i) Slow progressive loss of uniocular vision and corresponding field defect.

Chronic loss of vision without improvement over weeks is most likely to be a compressive lesion rather than chronic optic neuritis.

   (ii) Slow progressive binocular loss of vision.
   (iii) Acute loss of vision due to sudden increase in the size of the lesion, commonest being hemorrhage in the tumor.
2. **Proptosis**
3. **Extraocular muscle palsy**.
4. **Pupillary changes: Afferent pupillary reflex** is the commonest pupillary change in compressive optic neuropathy.
5. **The field defects** in compressive optic neuropathy depend on site of the lesion.
   (i) **Central field defects** are seen in lesions in orbital and intracanalicular portion of the optic nerve.
   (ii) **Junctional scotomas** are seen in lesions of anterior horn of chiasma.
   (iii) **Bitemporal hemianopias** are seen in lesion of the chiasma.

Field of the apparently normal other eye should be charted that may have a suspected field change.

6. **Funds**
   (i) Fundus may be **normal** when the lesion is posteriorly placed.
   (ii) Growths in orbit are most likely to present as **unilateral disk edema**.
   (iii) Intercanalicular growth cause **primary optic atrophy** more often.
   (iv) Eyes with disk swelling may end in **postpapilledematous optic atrophy**.
   (v) Other fundus change include presence of **optociliary vessels (opticociliary)**, i.e. small vessels joining the retinal circulation to choroidal venous circulation.

Optociliary vessels are present in:

Meningioma of sheath of optic nerve, optic nerve glioma, wide angle glaucoma, papilledema of long duration, central retinal vein thrombosis

Differential diagnosis

The common condition that are confused with compressive optic neuropathy are:

1. **Under 50 years of age:** Optic neuritis due to infection, inflammation or demyelination. They respond to systemic steroids.
2. **Over 50 years:** Ischemic optic neuropathy.
3. The patient who do not have either ischemic neuropathy or inflammatory process and vision does not improve after 3-4 weeks should be investigated for compressive lesion.

Other conditions that require exclusion are—**metabolic** and **drug induced** optic neuropathy, **vascular neuropathy**, **impeding central vein thrombosis**, **papillophlebitis**, **drusen of optic nerve in children**, **cysticercosis of optic nerve**.

Management is treatment of the primary cause, which includes orbital decompression, neurosurgical intervention, radiation and sometimes steroids.

Traumatic optic neuropathy

It is generally presents as **unilateral loss of vision** following **craniofacial trauma**. The trauma is said to be **direct** if it involves the optic nerve directly, i.e. following penetrating injury of the orbit or brain. It is called **indirect** when the primary site of impact is **frontal bone** and its shearing force travels backwards to the optic nerve or the brain moves backwards exerting pull on the optic nerve. Any part of the visual pathway may be involved in such an injury. The term traumatic optic neuropathy is used to denote neuropathy due to trauma to the nerve anywhere from back of the globe to chiasma.

The direct trauma disturbs the normal tissue planes and cause anatomical disruption of the nerve with resultant loss of function.

The indirect trauma does not infringe the tissue plane, the loss of function is due to **energy absorbed** by the nerve.

Fracture of the frontal bone, walls of the orbit and the apex are the common causes of traumatic optic neuropathy. It is not uncommon to get traumatic optic neuropathy following seemingly **trivial injury** on the frontal bore especially in children. In case of severe head injury, the patient looses consciousness following injury. The overwhelming features of head injury generally overshadow loss of vision in such cases. Loss of vision is noticed when the patient has partially recovered from head injury.

The mechanism of traumatic optic neuropathy differs from site to site.

In the orbit: The nerve may be avulsed at the back of the globe or its blood supply may be disrupted presenting fundus picture similar to central artery occlusion or ischemic optic neuropathy. There may be hemorrhages round the disk.

In the optic canal: Optic canal is the **most common location** where the optic nerve gets damaged. The lesion can be produced by any of the following singly or in combination.

1. Hemorrhage and edema in the substance of the nerve.
2. Hemorrhage and edema disrupting the blood supply of the optic nerve.
3. Fragments of bone following fracture of the optic canal, may impinge upon the substance of the nerve.
4. Retrocanalicular and prechiasmal lesion are either due to mechanical disruption or loss of blood supply to the visual path.

Clinical features

i. Commonest presenting feature is **unilateral loss of vision** following head injury.
ii. As has been pointed out earlier the loss of vision is noticed only when more serious manifestations of the head injuries have subsided.
iii. The loss of vision may be the first sign of head injury when the injury is mild.
iv. The loss of vision may develop three to four weeks after the injury.
v. The loss of vision may be loss of two to three lines on Snellen's chart or may be as low as loss of perception of light.
vi. Lower the initial vision, poorer is the prognosis.

1. **Field changes**
   i. Loss of central field is seen in lesion between the anterior horn of chiasma and the globe.
   ii. Loss of vision in one eye and hemianopia on the other side denotes junctional injury to the chiasma.
   iii. Bitemporal hemianopia denotes involvement of the central part of the chiasma.
   iv. Injury to tract and radiation are not considered to be part of traumatic optic neuropathy. They develop corresponding homonymous field defect.
   v. Injury to occipital cortex may results in cortical blindness.
2. **Pupillary change: Relative afferent pupillary reaction** may be the first demonstrable sign of traumatic optic neuropathy. It can be elicited in an unconscious person also.

3. **Fundus changes: The fundus change depends upon the location and severity of the trauma.**
   (i) A lesion involving the posterior part of the nerve in the orbit or in the canal may not be reflected in the lesion for many days to weeks. After three four weeks the disk may develop pallor that may be partial or total.
   (ii) A lesion just behind the globe may present as:
      (a) Nerve swelling
      (b) Central retinal artery occlusion
      (c) Ischemic optic atrophy.
   (iii) A complete transverse lesion presents as primary optic atrophy after few weeks.
   (iv) An avulsed nerve generally presents with a large blotch of hemorrhage in place of the disk or all round the disk.

Investigation

Routine X-ray skull or paranasal sinuses are not sufficient to show the exact pathology.

CT gives most conclusive evidence and location of the lesion.

MRI is better alternative for soft tissue lesion but has poor results in canalicular lesion.

Management

Management of traumatic optic neuropathy is unsatisfactory and frustrating.

1. The first line of management in management of head injury.
2. Traumatic neuropathy without severe head injury is treated by:
   (i) Mega dose of steroids
   (ii) Decompression of optic canal.

Mega dose of steroids

The ideal drug would be methylprednisolone. The alternative is intravenous dexamethasone. The doses are 20-30 mg/kg/day and 3-5 mg/kg/day respectively for first forty-eight hours, then tapered in usual fashion.

Decompression of optic canal has not proved to be equally effective in all cases.

Drug induced optic neuropathy

The list of drugs and chemicals that have been held responsible for optic neuropathies is long. Some of the commonly used drugs are also known to cause optic neuropathy. Commonly used drugs responsible for neuropathy are **ethambutol**, **isoniazid**, **streptomycin**, **chloramphenicol**, **fluroquinolones**, **barbiturates**, **chloroquine**, **halogenated hydroxyquinolones**, **metronidazole**, **heavy metals**, **oral contraceptives**, **methyl alcohol**. Surprisingly some of the commonly used **vaccines** too have been blamed to cause optic neuropathy, they are—BCG, anti-rabies vaccine, mumps-measles-rubella vaccine and anti-diphtheritic.

Out of all the drugs mentioned above **ethambutol** is the commonest drug that causes optic chronic neuropathy in many people and **methyl alcohol** is the commonest cause of acute neuropathy.

The drug induced optic neuropathy is a **bilateral**, **simultaneous** and **symmetric** condition except for methyl alcohol all have a chronic course. The severity depends on dose of the drug used, duration and idiosyncrasy towards the drug. Associated malnutrition and hypovitaminosis specially B-complex group may be contributory factors. The systemic conditions that predispose the condition are diabetes, arteriosclerosis, **low serum zinc**.

The exact mechanism of production of the disorder is not well understood. The most commonly accepted theory is that the seat of involvement is the **retina**. The axons of maculopapillary fibers and ganglion cells are involved.

The clinical features are

1. **Visual**
   (i) **Vision:** Progressive loss of bilateral central vision.
   (ii) **Color vision** is diminished.
   (iii) Seeing bright or colored spots of light.
2. **Field changes:** Common field changes are central scotomas.
3. **The fundus picture** is variable, may be normal or may show advanced secondary optic atrophy.

Diagnosis

Careful history of drug treatment in a case of bilateral neuropathy often leads to diagnosis.

Management

1. The first step in management is to **discontinue** the offending drug and replace it with best alternative in consultation with physician. Sometimes **reduction in dose** is sufficient. The best examples is ethambutol neuropathy which is dose related. It is less frequent when administered in dose of 15 mg/kg/day and the risk rises with dose above 20 mg/kg. Most of the conditions improve when the dose is reduced to 7.5 mg-10 mg/kg/day.
2. The next step is to improve the nutritional status of the patient.
3. Restriction of alcohol and tobacco enhances improvement.
4. Supplementing B-complex and zinc too have beneficial effect.
5. Injection of hydroxycobalamin and methyl cobalamin too have been suggested.

Leber's hereditary optic neuropathy

Leber's optic neuropathy is a **hereditary** form of bilateral optic neuropathy, seen mostly in **males**, i.e. 80%. The disease is **transmitted by females** because it involves **mitochondrial DNA** that is found in ovum and not sperm. Hence men do not transmit the disease. The heterozygotous female can transmit the trait to the sons and carrier state to daughters. About half of the carriers develop the disease. The disease is most commonly seen **second decade**. Women are affected in third to fifth decade.

The disease is **bilateral**, starting in one eye within few weeks, the other eye gets involved in the similar manner.

The disease has an **acute neuritic phase** that is followed by gradual loss of vision only to terminate in **atrophic phase**.

1. **Vision:** The loss of vision is variable unless loss of vision in simultaneous in both eyes. Diminished vision in one eye may go unnoticed because it is painless without redness or other neurological defects. The fall of vision is rapid and within weeks it comes to about 6/60 or less and may get stabilized at this level or may deteriorate. A small percentage of eyes may have recovery of vision. The mechanism of improvement of vision is not known.
2. **The pupillary reaction** is variable. In unilateral cases, there is afferent papillary defect which is also seen in bilateral asymmetric diminished vision.
3. **The fundus:**
   (i) **May be normal** in the acute neuritic phase.
   (ii) May have combination of **microangiopathy round the disk** that may result in **telangiectasia** and prominent nerve fiber layer round the disk. The telangiectatic vessels do not leak on fluorescein angiography.
   (iii) In late stages, the disk develops **pallor** that may be localized to temporal side or may involve the whole of the disk.
   (iv) Rest of the fundus does not show any change.
4. **The field changes** are generally central or centrocecal.
5. **Management:** There are no neurological defects but there may be **conduction defect in heart**.

There is no known specific treatment. As the disease starts in the prime of life, proper vocational training and low vision aids are helpful.

Other causes of disk swelling

There is a long list of conditions that present as disk swelling and may be mistaken as either optic neuritis or papilledema. The causes of disk swelling other than papillitis and papilledema may be **unilateral** or **bilateral** with or without loss of vision. The loss of vision is painless. The commonest field change is central field loss. Most of them have systemic manifestation that could be **metabolic**, **autoimmune** or **infective**.

1. Diabetic optic neuropathy (papillopathy)

It is a far less than the diabetic maculopathy. It is seen in **insulin dependent diabetics**, hence is more common in juvenile diabetes.

Vision

The patient have **unilateral loss of vision** which soon becomes bilateral. The loss of vision is mild to moderate, gradual in onset and painless.

Fundus

Fundus changes include **swollen disk** with **telangiectatic vessels** on the surface that may be mistaken as Leber's optic neuropathy.

Field changes

The field changes are central, centrocecal or may be arcuate. The field changes are generally permanent, may sometimes be reversed.

No specific treatment is required except control of diabetes.

2. Optic neuropathy in thyroid ocular diseases

This is a form of **compressive neuropathy** where the swollen recti trap the optic nerve at the apex of the orbit. It may be associated with proptosis. Absence of proptosis does not exclude neuropathy.

The symptoms are gradual loss of central vision with corresponding field changes. The appearance of the disk is variable, ranging between normal to swollen and atrophic disk.

Treatment is basically directed towards proptosis by steroid, decompression of orbital apex or radiation. Extraocular muscle palsy is treated by steroid and exposure of cornea is treated by antibiotic and lubricants.

3. Papillophlebitis

This is a disorder of **ill understood etiology** of **young adults** that presents with **unilateral disk swelling** that is confused with optic neuritis or early papilledema. The disk swelling is associated with variable loss of central vision and field changes. The condition is considered to be a **vasculitis**. The two theories prevailing currently are:

(i) It is inflammation of central retinal vein.

(ii) It is a localized form of **Eale's disease**. The fundus changes comprise of **swollen hyperemic disk** with **peripapillary superficial hemorrhage**. As the picture resembles true papilledema, **CT skull** should be done to exclude intracranial space occupying lesion and compressive lesions of optic nerve. Fluorescein angiography helps to differentiate from Eale's disease. The condition does not respond to steroid.

4. Impending central vein thrombosis

The picture is similar to papillophlebitis except for the fact that it develops in **older persons**. The fundus picture consists of swollen disk with scattered superficial hemorrhages. Sometimes optociliary vessels may develop. There is moderate loss of vision.

No treatment is required except those used to manage vasculopathy, i.e. diabetes, hypertension, arteriosclerosis, autoimmune diseases. Role of oral aspirin is doubtful.

Retrobulbar neuritis

Retrobulbar neuritis is a term that denotes inflammation of the optic nerve from anterior horn of chiasma to the globe, **sparing the disk**. The disease has been traditionally divided into two groups:

1. Acute retrobulbar neuritis
2. Chronic retrobulbar neuritis.

The two conditions have hardly any common etiology, pathology or clinical features except loss of function of the optic nerve, i.e. central vision, defective color sense and central field changes.

1. Acute retrobulbar neuritis

Acute retrobulbar neuritis is the retrobulbar **counterpart of papillitis**. The etiopathogenesis and clinical features have striking similarity except a few, i.e. a lesion situated away from disk may not be reflected on fundus examination.

In acute retrobulbar, the **papillomacular fibers** are more commonly involved. However other forms, i.e. **perineuritic** or **transverse neuritic** form are not very infrequent.

Symptoms

The disease begins with:

1. Acute unilateral loss of central vision. Generally the loss of vision is marked.
2. Pain on movement of the eyeball especially in up gaze.
3. The patient may notice tenderness at the upper part of the globe.
4. Loss of color sense.
5. Loss of stereopsis.

The disease begins in one eye and may remain confined to it or the other eye also gets involved. The involvement of the other eye may be simultaneous, or may begin few days after one eye has been involved. Generally there is asymmetry in clinical features. The eye involved later may have more profound loss of vision than the first, the condition may fluctuate between apparent cure to severe loss of vision.

The clinical features

The signs comprise:

1. Uncorrectable diminished vision.
2. Externally normal eyes except:
   i. Tenderness at insertion of superior rectus.
   ii. Relative afferent pupil in:
      a. Unilateral involvement
      b. In bilateral involvement when the vision in one eye is far less than in the other eye.
3. Field changes: **Central** or **centrocecal** absolute or relative scotoma, both for white or colored targets. **Red sensation is more depressed than others.**

4. **Fundus changes:** Fundus changes depend upon location of the lesion in relation to entry of central retinal artery and duration of the disorder. The lesion anterior **to entry of central retinal vessels** generally present with picture similar to that seen in papillitis. Lesions behind this level are not reflected in the fundus picture and the fundus looks normal. In late stages the picture may change to pallor of the disk irrespective of its location. The pallor may be confined to temporal area or may involve the whole of the disk.

Etiology

Multiple sclerosis is the **most common** cause of retrobulbar neuritis world over. Other causes are **tuberculosis**, **syphilis**, other acute systemic diseases or infections spreading from **paranasal sinuses. Sphenoidal sinusitis** is commonest sinus infection responsible for acute retrobulbar neuritis. The other cause **periosteitis** of the orbital apex.

Investigation

Most important investigation is MRI of the brain. Other investigations ordered are X-ray, PNS, X-ray chest, ESR, VDRL. The commonest MRI finding is periventricular white matter lesion.

Treatment is same as that of papillitis.

Multiple Sclerosis

Multiple sclerosis is one of the main causes of lesions of **visual path**. Besides visual path it can involve many other locations of the nervous system, i.e. **corticospinal tract**, **posterior columns**, **brainstem**, **cerebellum**.

The other ocular involvements besides visual path are—**internuclear ophthalmoplegia**, **nystagmus**, **cranial nerve palsy and neuromyelitis**. Surprisingly it also involves non-neural elements of the eye reselling in **uveitis**, **periphlebitis** and **retinitis**.

The exact cause of multiple sclerosis is not well understood. The main pathogenesis consist of **demyelination** and **perivascular inflammation** in patchy distribution. The condition has remission and recurrence that may be as long as three decades.

The common decade when the disease manifests is **third decade**. The disease is **more common in women**. Due to some unexplained factors the disease is frequent during **pregnancy**. The disease is more common in **colder countries**.

The disease has variable manifestations. The commonest presentation is **optic neuritis** that may either be **papillitis** or **retrobulbar neuritis**. Besides these two, any part of the visual path may be involved in multiple sclerosis with corresponding field changes and pupillary changes. Bilateral involvement is not uncommon which may be simultaneous in both eyes or the other eye may follow within few days to weeks.

About **one-third of the eyes** with multiple sclerosis induced optic neuritis show **complete recovery**. About thirty percent of eyes will have **partial recovery** while in remaining the disease progresses relentlessly. The improvement when possible become evident within a fortnight of the onset. The improvement of neurological deficits takes longer time. The end result is **postneuritic optic atrophy**.

Besides involvement of visual pathway there may be other ocular lesions simultaneous with optic neuritis, which may follow or rarely they may precede optic neuritis. There is a definite relation between optic neuritis and multiple sclerosis. 35% of patients with so called idiopathic optic neuritis develop multiple sclerosis. Conversely same percent of patients with multiple sclerosis develop optic neuritis.

The nonocular lesions are:
Facial anesthesia, ataxia, vertigo, tremors, paraplegia, quadriplegia, bladder dysfunction.

Diagnosis

Multiple sclerosis is rarely diagnosed during first episode. Variable neurological signs with recovery and recurrence over weeks to months without any positive clue, should arise possibility of multiple sclerosis.

The commonly ordered investigations are MRI of the brain that should include brainstem and cerebellum that shows nonspecific demyelination. Analysis of CSF may show raised IgG level.

Management

Management depends on course of disease.

In acute exacerbation or relapse, the drugs of choice is **IV methylprednisolone** 1 gm/day for seven days to be followed by either tablet methylprednisolone in tapered dose or oral prednisolone 60-80 mg/day with usual precaution and gradual taper.

Milder attacks are treated by oral steroids.

In case of progressive disease where steroids are ineffective or are not tolerated. The patients are put on **cyclophosphamide** or **methotrexate** in consultation with physician.

Nystagmus may require **baclofen** and **clonazepam**.

2. Chronic retrobulbar optic neuritis (toxic amblyopia)

Logically any retrobulbar neuritis of long duration should be called chronic retrobulbar neuritis but the term is mostly used for a condition that is attributed to **deficiency of vitamin B_{12}, thiamine** and **poisoning by cyanide present in tobacco. The main pathology lies in the ganglion cells of the retina that lead to degeneration of nerve fibers.**

Some of the characteristic features are:

1. They are seen mostly in **males** in **third to fifth decades**. The condition develops after smoking regularly for about **five to six years**. Surprisingly it is **less common in cigarette smokers**. It is more common in persons who smoke **shag in pipe** or **cigars**. Generally these persons indulge in **heavy alcoholic**

drinks as well. The relation between **tobacco and alcohol** is not well established. The disease can occur in persons who are mostly alcoholic and smoke relative less and vice versa.

2. The condition has a protracted course of **diminished central vision** which is painless. Level of vision depends on duration of the disease. In initial stages there may only be loss of one or two lines on Snellen's chart that may deteriorate to 20/200 or less. Loss of perception of light is not known. The vision is known to recover when the person gives up both tobacco and alcohol but never up to normal level.
3. The condition is **bilateral**, rarely simultaneous or symmetric.
4. The condition is always associated with **central scotoma** involving the macula as well as blind spot. The **centrocecal scotoma** is club shaped or eggs shaped with wider are towards the blind spot. The cause of scotoma is involvement of papillomacular fibers. The scotoma generally has constant density which is **more for red** than for white target. Occasionally there may be scattered denser scotomas among the centrocecal scotoma on the papillomacular bundle. The arc known **as nuclei. They represent areas of less vision**.
5. Pupillary reactions are generally **retained**. If there is vast difference in vision in two eyes, the eye with poor vision may show afferent pupillary response.
6. **Fundus:** In initial stages have fundus picture does not show any abnormality, later the disk may develop temporal pallor.

Diagnosis

Gradual, bilateral diminished vision with centrocecal scotoma with history of heavy smoking and alcohol consumption in person between third and fifth decade confirms the diagnosis.

Differential diagnosis consists of all cases of gradual bilateral loss of vision with central scotoma, i.e. Leber's optic neuropathy, drug induced neuropathy and macular degeneration.

Management

Once diagnosis has been confirmed, the patient is advised to abstain from tobacco and alcohol which is not always possible for the patient to comply.

The treatment consists of intramuscular injection of hydroxycobalamin 1000 mgm every fifth day for four shots. Supplementation of thiamine and folic acid is said to hasten recovery. It takes about one to two months to recover the vision after the treatment has been started. Vision does not return to normal if optic atrophy has already sets in.

Methyl alcohol poisoning

Like most of the toxic neuropathies the pathology lies in the **ganglion cells of the retina** resulting in secondary optic neuritis.

2. The axons can be blocked either at the ganglion cells of the retina or anywhere between the nerve fiber to lateral geniculate body.
3. Rarely there may be degeneration across the synapse at lateral geniculate body, i.e. in the retrogeniculate path.
4. The optic nerve does not have Schwann cells, hence regeneration of axons is not possible following insult to the tissue.
5. There is loss of myelin sheaths (demyelinization)
6. Obliteration of capillaries.
7. Variable proliferation of glial tissue. Absence of glial proliferation leads to deepening of the cup while increased proliferation leads to heaping of the disk (secondary optic atrophy).

The degeneration of the optic nerve can be:

1. **Wallerian degeneration** also known as **ascending degeneration**.
2. **Non-Wallerian degeneration** also knows as **descending** or **retrograde degeneration**.

The Wallerian degeneration

The lesion starts in the retinal ganglion cells and proceeds towards the lateral geniculate body as degeneration of the axons within the optic nerve and the tract. The myelin sheaths of the fibers are lost. The degeneration can be **generalized** or **focal**. The loss of myelin sheath is followed by proliferation of astrocytes. Ascending optic atrophy is generally secondary optic atrophy.

The descending degeneration starts in any of the following structures—optic tract, chiasma or nerve itself and proceed towards the ganglion cells of the retina.

Ophthalmoscopic classification of optic atrophy

On the basis of color of the disk, extent of glial proliferation, the optic atrophy has been divided into two classes, i.e. **primary optic atrophy** and **secondary optic atrophy**. Incidences of primary optic atrophy is far less than secondary optic atrophy.

The characteristics of the primary optic atrophy are:

1. The disk margins are sharply outlined.
2. The margin does not merge with the surrounding retina.
3. The color of the disk is chalk white.
4. Hardly any visible vessel is present on the disk.
5. The lamina is better visualized than even in normal eye.
6. The cup is deep but the C:D ratio is normal.
7. The caliber of the retinal vessels may vary according to the status of the central retinal artery. In case of central artery obstruction or trauma, they are attenuated.
8. The retinal vessels are free from sheathing.
9. The surrounding retina does not show any change that can be correlated to optic atrophy.

10. The field changes depend upon the location of the lesion and vision present.
11. The vision is generally greatly reduced.
12. The optic atrophy represents a chronic process in the retrobulbar or intracranial part of the optic nerve that has not been preceded by edema.

Some of the common causes of primary optic atrophy are:
Tabes, hydrocephalus, intracranial meningioma, retrobulbar neuritis, trauma, sellar and parasellar tumors, Leber's optic atrophy.

Secondary optic atrophy

The term secondary optic atrophy too denotes ophthalmoscopic picture and not the cause. It is the effect of acute inflammation or vascular lesion in the or near the disk. It is also due to disease of retina and choroid. In such instances it is called **consecutive optic atrophy**.

The secondary optic atrophy can be **generalized** as following: Papillitis or papilledema or **localized** which are generally referred by the shape of the pallor that ensues, i.e. **temporal pallor**, **bow tie atrophy**, **altitudinal pallor**, **wedge shaped pallor**.

The pathogeneses involved in secondary optic atrophy is excess of proliferation of astrocytes, connective tissue and blood vessels in the optic nerve.

The characteristics of secondary optic atrophy are:
1. The disk margins are ill defined.
2. The disk margin merges with the surrounding retina.
3. The physiological cup is obliterated.
4. In the early stages especially in papilledema the optic disk may be slightly raised above the surface of the surrounding retina.
5. The color of the disk is neither as pink as normal nor as white as in primary optic atrophy. It is called **dirty white pallor**.
6. The retinal vessels show sheathing.
7. The retina may have evidence of pathology, i.e. patch of choroiditis, retinitis, etc.

Consecutive optic atrophy

It is a **secondary optic atrophy** that is secondary to lesions in the retina or in the macula. The common causes are: **Retinitis pigmentosa**, **cerebromacular degeneration**, **diffuse chorioretinitis**, **localized chorioretinitis**, **central retinal vein obstruction**, **trauma**, and **extensive photocoagulation**.

The characteristics of consecutive optic atrophy are:
1. The disk margin is ill defined.
2. The color of the disk is waxy pale.
3. The physiological cup is retained.
4. The lamina may be obscured.
5. The retina shows evidence of chorioretinal inflammation.

Bow tie atrophy

Thus is seen in **mid chiasmal lesions** with bitemporal hemianopic field defect. The atrophic area is wider on the periphery. The superior and inferior part of the disk retains normal appearance. The condition is bilateral. **Optic tract lesions** also produce similar lesion. The bow tie atrophy develops in the eye contralateral to the involved radiation with hemianopia.

Temporal pallor is an **ill defined term** that may be confused with normal paleness of the disk on the temporal side. The term temporal atrophy should be used when there is localized paleness of the disk with localized features of consecutive lesion or a lesion in between the macula and the disk is present.

Altitudinal pallor: This type of localized optic atrophy follows **acute ischemic optic neuritis** of any type. In initial stage there is altitudinal swelling of the disk that is replaced by pallor. Later the condition is associated with altitudinal field loss.

Wedge pallor is seen in strictly localized lesion, i.e. **occlusion of branch of central retinal artery, choroidal rupture, juxtapapillary choroiditis, and localized photocoagulation**.

Foster Kennedy syndrome

This consists of **primary optic atrophy** on one side and **papilledema** of various stages on the contralateral side. The syndrome is rare but when present is highly suggestive of **sphenoidal ridge meningioma**, **frontal lobe tumor** and **olfactory meningioma**. Beside these other conditions that have been reported to cause the disorder are **frontal lobe abscess**, **craniopharyngioma with forward extension**, **glioma of intracranial part of optic nerve**, **aneurysm of internal carotid** and **arachnoiditis**.

The **optic atrophy** on the side of the tumor is **primary in nature**. It is due to direct compression of the optic nerve that produces field change on the same side. According to position of compression, the field changes can be central if away from the chiasma and hemianopic when at the junction of the chiasma.

The papilledema on the contralateral side is due to **raised intracranial tension** and may be seen in various stages of evolution of papilledema, i.e. impending, full blown, chronic or atrophic. The ipsilateral nerve is not capable of developing papilledema.

The end result may be ipsilateral primary optic atrophy and contralateral post-papilledematous optic atrophy.

Heredofamilial optic atrophy

All the conditions included in this group have an element of optic neuritis too in initial stages, hence they are also known as **optic neuropathies**.

They are seen in **young persons**. They may be present at **birth** or manifest **later** but not later than third decode. Some of them terminate in **bilateral blindness**, few have early fall in vision with improvement in vision, not reaching normal level. The conditions are thought to be **abiotrophies**. They may involve the optic nerve only or may be associated with other neurological and various non-neurological symptoms. The pattern of heritance is variable, i.e. **recessive**, **dominant** or **intermediate**.

The commonly encountered neuropathies are:

1. Leber's optic neuropathy (Leber's disease)
2. Kjer's juvenile neuropathy
3. Congenital optic neuropathy
4. Behr's optic neuropathy
5. Neuropathy with diabetes mellitus.

1. Leber's optic neuropathy

This disorder has been studied extensively by and number of cases reported is largest among other heredofamilial optic neuropathies. The exact cause of the disease is not well understood. It has been thought to be either a **abiotrophies** or a **degenerative process** secondary to abnormal **cyanide metabolism**.

The condition is seen mostly in **males** between **ten years to thirty years**. Carrier women are affected rarely and when affected follow a milder course of events.

The features of the inheritance are as follows:

1. It is transmitted through female line.
2. There is no evidence of transmission from father to his children.
3. Females are cent-percent carries.
4. Half of their sons develop the disease.
5. The mutation is in the mitochondria DNA which is exclusively found in females.
6. The carrier may occasionally have the disease in subtle form.
7. Once a male is confirmed to have disease it is not difficult to predict which male member of the family will inherit the disease. **The son of the sister of affected male is at highest risk.**
8. While eliciting family history of the disease, possibility of maternal uncle having the disease should be elicited.

The disease has two phases:

1. The neuritic phase
2. The atrophic phase.

The neuritis phase begins **abruptly** in **one eye** with features of **optic neuritis**, i.e. fast deteriorating vision with central large and dense scotoma. The other eye gets involved within few days to few weeks. There may be an **afferent pupillary defect** if there is marked difference in vision in two eyes, other wise the pupil reacts normally even in presence of gross loss of vision. The loss of vision may be as low as counting fingers from close quarters, but more common vision is 6/60 or little more. Unlike optic neuritis the vision rarely improves after reaching the lowest level. Only in a small percent of cases the vision may improve after years if total optic atrophy has not set in.

The loss of **color sense** and **stereopsis** may set in earlier than loss of vision.

Fundus changes are typical in neuritic phase. There is hyperemia of the disk with filling of the cup and elevation of the disk. The elevation is never more than +3D. The typical features consist of **telangiectasia near the disk** and **microangiopathy** that may be mild enough to be missed on routine ophthalmoscope examination but become visible on fluorescein angiography. There is no leak on FFA. Occasionally unaffected family members too may show telangiectasia round the disk without onset of diminished vision.

The atrophic phase is variable and prolonged. There is gradual loss of vision that may terminate in total loss of vision. The fundus in atrophic phase is similar to that is seen in retrobulbar neuritis. The Leber's optic neuropathy has been found to be associated with various nonophthalmic features. They are **dystonia, cardiac conduction defect** and **multiple sclerosis** like diseases in females.

Management

There is no known treatment as the disease effects person in prime of life. They may require occupational training and low vision aids.

2. Kjer's juvenile optic neuropathy

This is an **autosomal dominant** heredodegenerative disorder of optic nerve of **unknown origin**. It is a **bilateral** disease. The loss of vision is gradual and generally detected on routine examination. The eyes are externally normal without pupillary changes. The loss of vision is mild to moderate when first examined and range between 6/18 and 6/60. The loss of vision continues for years and then stabilizes. There is **impaired color sensation**. Common defective color are in the range of **yellow-blue**.

There is **central** or **centrocecal scotoma**. The condition may be associated with **progressive deafness, diminished night vision, nystagmus** and **ataxia**. There is no known treatment except low vision aids and occupational training.

3. Simple recessive optic neuropathy

It is also known as **congenital neuropathy** though not diagnosed at birth as the diagnosis is made only after 2 years of age, so the term **infantile neuropathy** is more logical. The commonest age when the child is brought for examination is between three to four years. The loss of vision is severe that may be as low as HM, more common visual acuity is 6/60. As the loss of vision starts at very early age, **nystagmus** is common feature. The child fails to recognize color due to associated **severe dyschromatopsia** or even **achromatopsia**.

4. Behr's recessive optic neuropathy

This generally manifests in the **first decade**. The symptom that brings the child to ophthalmologist is gradual, painless, bilateral, noncorrectable poor vision. The child may have **diminished color vision**. Some children may have **nystagmus**. The disk generally shows **mild to moderate pallor** with corresponding scotoma. The condition generally does not go to blindness. The child remains visually challenged which requires proper rehabilitation.

5. Recessive neuropathy with juvenile diabetes

These children with diabetes are referred to ophthalmologist for diminished vision, which is invariably thought to be part of diabetic retinopathy. These children have **severe loss of vision** and marked **color defect**. The disease is relentless. The fundus shows bilateral **diffuse pallor of disk**. These children do not have nystagmus that is frequent in other heredofamilial optic neuropathies.

Optic atrophy in children

Optic atrophy may occur in any age. Its presence in a child leave the child with many problems associated with blindness and require rehabilitation more than aged.

The optic atrophy can be either **primary** or **secondary type**. Unilateral optic atrophy in children are generally due to **traumatic neuropathy** or **optic nerve glioma**. The optic atrophy is rarely present at birth except secondary to birth trauma and delayed myelination where the vision improves with development of myelination.

Optic atrophy in children can be broadly classified under following heads:

1. **Congenital**
   i. **Cranial anomalies:** Crouzon's disease, oxycephaly, scaphocephaly, osteopetrosis, fibrous dysplasia, congenital hydrocephalus, microcephaly, cerebellar ataxia, Schilder's disease.
   ii. **Heredofamilial and heredodegenerative optic atrophy**, i.e. Leber's neuropathy, Kjer's neuropathy, Behr's neuropathy, neuropathy with diabetes mellitus, lipidosis.
2. **Infectious:** The basic pathology is **basal meningitis** or **encephalomeningitis** due to any of the following—measles, mumps, and chickenpox, congenital neurosyphilis.
3. Neoplasm, tuberculoma, optic nerve glioma.
4. Raised intracranial pressure due to infection or intracranial space occupying lesions.

Tumors of optic nerve

The tumors of optic nerve may be **benign** or **malignant**. The malignant growth may be **primary** malignancy or may be **extension** from other structures or may be **secondary** to other malignancies. The primary growth belong to three distinct groups according to their cell or origin:

1. Ectodermal: Arising from the substance of the optic nerve. These are mostly **gliomas**.
2. Mesodermal: They arise from the sheaths of the optic nerve and are mostly **meningiomas**.
3. Neuroectodermal: **Melanomas**.
4. Phakoma.

Age of the patient has important correlation with the growths of optic nerve.

Tumors of **childhood** are generally **benign**. The tumors of **adults** may be **malignant.**

Size and **site** of the growth too have important bearing on final outcome of the tumor.

Locationwise the tumor may be **intraocular**, **intraorbital** and **intracranial**.

The tumors of the intraocular part of the nerve, i.e. the disk is rare than those involving other parts.

The common growths of the disk are:

1. Benign:
   i. Drusen
   ii. Melanocytoma
2. Malignant: These are generally extension form retina or choroids, i.e. **retinoblastoma or malignant melanoma.**

Rarely gliomas and meningiomas form the retrobulbar part may extend in the disk. The drusens and melanocytomas generally do not produce symptoms, they are discovered on routine examination. The infiltrative tumors are vision threatening, may cause blindness due to retinal detachment or glaucoma. They are risk to life as well.

The tumors of the intraorbital part

1. Glioma of the nerve
2. Meningiomas of the nerve.

The main features are:

1. Axial proptosis
2. Diminished vision
3. Pupillary changes
4. Changes in the disk
5. Motility disorder.

Tumors of intracanalicular part are generally extension either from orbital growth or chiasmal growth.

The tumors of intracranial parts may involve the **retrocanalicular** part of the nerve, **the chiasma** and the **retrochiasmal part**. The symptom depend on the location of the tumor, its size, and its infiltration in the neighboring structures while the intraorbital tumors are predominantly benign in nature, many of the intracranial tumors are malignant/invasive. They do not produce proptosis, loss of vision in frequent, so are the field changes depending on the location of the tumor. A prechiasmal tumor causes loss of vision on the ipsilateral eye. Depending on part of the chiasma involved it can be ipsilateral loss of vision with contralateral hemianopia, i.e. junctional scotoma, bitemporal hemianopia when the lesion is mid chiasmal. Papilledema is rare but **optic atrophy** is common. **Nystagmus** is frequent.

Gliomas of anterior visual path (optic nerve and chiasma)

Gliomas of anterior visual path can be:

1. Benign glioma of optic nerve in childhood
2. Malignant glioblastoma of adults.

The first is commonly referred to as **glioma of optic nerve**. These are **benign hamartomas**, may be considered as **congenital** because they are detected within first few years of life. Histopathologically they are **pilocytic astrocytomas**. They are the **intrinsic tumors** of the optic nerve. Association of **neurofibroma type I** is very frequent, about 30-50% of children with optic nerve glioma have neurofibroma or stigma of neurofibroma.

The optic nerve gliomas are divided into two types:

1. Intraorbital
2. Chiasmal

The intraorbital optic nerve glioma is a **unilateral**, **slow progressive**, **benign tumors** of the optic nerve. The typical age of presentation is between **four to eight years** with **diminished vision** and **axial proptosis**.

The loss of vision generally precede onset of proptosis but this is not an infallible rule. The diminished vision is mostly due to involvement of **maculopapillary fibers** in the nerve. The loss of vision may range between losses of few lines on Snellen's chart to no perception of light, the latter is met only when optic atrophy has set in.

Proptosis is axial and variable. In early stages there may just be widening of inter-palpebral aperture, in late stages it may be so marked as to dislocate the globe anteriorly. The proptosis is **noncompressible without bruit** and does not progress in lowering the head.

Ocular movements are not affected but squint is common due to associated amblyopia. **Afferent pupillary defect is the rule**.

There may be **nystagmus**.

The commonest site for the tumor to start is **near the optic canal**. The tumor may **extend back** into the optic canal and **enlarge the optic foramen**. Circular, smooth enlargement of optic foramen is strongly suggestive of canalicular extension of the growth. The growth can be roundish or fusiform.

The fundus picture is variable. Commonest change is **primary optic atrophy**, less common is **postpapilledematous optic atrophy**.

Diagnosis

Diagnosis is not difficult with history of unilateral, gradually increasing painless proptosis, gradual diminished vision in a child in first decade. Presence of stigmata of neurofibroma goes in favor of diagnosis. Even the siblings and near relatives may show neurofibromatous stigmata without glioma. However, other causes of unilateral proptosis in a child should be excluded because they can be fatal. They are **leukemia**, **neuroblastoma**, **rhabdomyosarcoma**. Generally these are more acute and fast growing than glioma.

Investigation

1. **X-ray**
   i. **Optic foramen for asymmetry:** Generally the size of the optic foramen are equal. In case of optic nerve glioma. The involved foramen is enlarged equally in all direction. X-ray of both the sides is mandatory for comparison.
   ii. Orbit may show a dense shadow behind the globe. The orbit behind the orbital rim shows uniform enlargement.
   iii. **Optic canal:** If the growth reaches the optic canal, the canal too is uniformly enlarged in a funnel shape, the wider end is anteriorly.
2. Ultrasonography shows uniform, oval or fusiform retrobulbar growth.
3. CT and MRI show fusiform, intrinsic retrobulbar growth that may extend in the optic canal.
4. Role of fine needle biopsy has not been established.
5. Visual evoked potential is lost early in optic gliomas.

Management

The management is controversial except the facts that there is no medical treatment available. The argument resolves round the question—should the tumor be surgically removed or left as such? The only argument in favor of surgical intervention is cosmetic to a growing child. Proptosis with squint is embarrassing hence he wants it to be cosmetically corrected.

The surgical modalities available are:

1. Tarsorrhaphy to protect the cornea when there is a mechanical lagophthalmos that leaves the cornea exposed.
2. Removal of the eye along with the growth if the cornea has sloughed.
3. Endoscopic debulking of the growth leaving the optic nerve and blood vessels.

Chiasmal glioma

Statistically chiasmal gliomas are more frequent than optic nerve gliomas but less frequently diagnosed in early stages because there is no proptosis and loss of vision is unilateral to begin with that may not be noticed by the child.

As the chiasma is involved, various types of scotomas are reported:

1. Large central scotoma on one side.
2. Loss of vision on one side.
3. Loss of vision in one side with hemianopia on the other side (junctional scotoma).
4. Bitemporal hemianopia.

The chiasmal gliomas are more invasive than optic nerve gliomas.

They may infiltrate:

1. In the optic canal
2. In the pituitary
3. Hypothalamus

4. Third ventricle, causing internal hydrocephalus, raised intracranial tension, hypothalamic signs of obesity, somnolence, diabetes insipidus, dwarfism, precocious puberty.

They may cause bilateral blindness. The chiasmal gliomas do not respond to surgery only, they may require radiation and/or chemotherapy.

Glioma of anterior visual path in adults

These tumors are less frequent than benign gliomata of the anterior visual path. They are almost always fatal. The life span after onset is less than two years. They cause bilateral blindness. Histopathologically, they are glioblastomas (malignant astrocytoma), and are invasive. In the anterior visual path they develop commonly in the chiasma and infiltrate all round including the optic nerve. Bilateral involvement of the optic nerve is common. The growth is seen in the fifth to sixth decade. Males are more effected. The loss of vision is fast and bilateral that soon ends in blindness. The symptoms may be mistaken as optic neuritis. The disease is not associated with neurofibromatosis. Due to its rapid spread it is frequently associated with other signs of central nervous system involvement.

The life span is very short. There is no known treatment. Though steroids given orally initially for mistaken diagnosis of optic neuritis, may cause improvement of vision, only to lapse into blindness.

Optic sheath meningioma

The meningiomas may arise anywhere in the brain from the arachnoidal villi. The common sites are **parasagittal**, **sphenoidal ridge**, **anterior wall of sella turcica**, and **anterior optic pathway**. The meningiomas of anterior visual path may be chiasmal, intracanalicular or optic nerve. Meningiomas of optic canal constitute 10% of all meningiomas. They are mostly invasive tumor of adults past fifth decade. In adults they are slow progressive, in children they grow fast. Adult females are more affected than adult males in a ratio of 3:1. The signs and symptoms are variable and depend on the location of the tumor. **The meningiomas of intraorbital part** produce gradual, painless loss of vision with central scotoma, proptosis, restricted movements, acquired hypermetropia, afferent pupillary defect and fundus change. The fundus shows variable changes in the disk depending on the site, size and duration of the growth. The disk may be normal, pale or may show postpapilledematous changes. One of the important features is presence of **optociliary shunt** vessel of the disk. Gradual uniocular loss of vision in a woman in fifth to sixth decade with mild proptosis and presence of optociliary vessel is almost diagnostic. Sphenoidal ridge meningioma may cause **Foster Kennedy syndrome**.

Proptosis depends upon the position of the growth, if the growth is subdural the proptosis is axial. Proptosis is invariably associated with restricted upward movement.

The growth near the **orbital apex** causes early compressive signs including loss of vision and optic atrophy.

The intracanalicular growth can either grow inside the canal or may be part of extension from intracranial growth or intraorbital part.

The chiasmal lesion can cause bitemporal hemianopia or junctional scotoma with loss of vision without proptosis.

The differential diagnosis consists of—optic neuritis, compressive neuropathy due to causes other than meningioma, cavernous hemangioma, infiltrative neuropathy.

Diagnosis is confirmed by X-ray, CT and MRI.

Management: Surgical treatment is fraught with loss of vision and recurrences. Radiation gives better result.

Disorder of chiasma (see Figs 3.2 to 3.5)

The chiasma has an unique position in the visual path. Some of the feature are:

1. It is the junction of both the optic nerves.
2. The fibers of optic nerve decussate in the chiasma.
3. There is a 90° rotation of fiber form the optic nerve as they pass through the chiasma on way to optic tract.
4. The decussating fibers from nasal retina do not pass into the opposite tract in a straight line.
   i. The medial nasal retina fibers, cross ventrally from a looping the contralateral optic nerve
   ii. The posteriorly decussating fibers of the nasal retina form a loop in the optic tract.
5. The macular fibers of the same side also decussate in the retina.
   i. The medial fiber cross over the contralateral optic tract.
   ii. The lateral fiber pass straight into ipsilateral optic tract.

The peculiar arrangement of the retinal fibers in the chiasma, i.e. decussating and rotation are the anatomical basis of the field changes. The pressure on the chiasma is less important than ischemia in producing the field changes.

6. The chiasma lies above the diaphragma sella obliquely with posterior border at higher level than the anterior border.
7. The position of chiasma in relation to diagphragma sella is constant in 80% of the cases, i.e. it lies above the diaphragma sella in 10% of cases.
   It is:
   i. Prefixed, i.e. it is anterior to the pituitary gland with a short optic nerve and long optic tract.
   ii. Postfixed when the chiasma lies posterior to the pituitary gland, i.e. a long optic nerve and a short tract.
8. Anteriorly, the chiasma is related to anterior cerebral and anterior communicating arteries.

9. Posteriorly, the chiasma is related to pituitary body, it is infundibulum and tubercinerium.
10. Superiorly, lie the third vertical and hypothalamus.
11. Inferiorly, lie the roots of olfactory tract, hypophysis, cavernous sinus and oculomotor nerve.
12. Laterally, it is related to internal carotid outside the cavernous sinus.

The lesions of structures in its relation may compress the chiasma to produce field defect and visual loss (pituitary tumors). Compressive effect of chiasmal lesion on neighboring structure are less frequent and less pronounced.

Relation of chiasma to arteries around it: In the main arteries that come in relation with the chiasma are **circle of Willis** and **internal carotid.** The chiasma is placed oblique in the circle of Willis. The anterior part of the circle is superior to the anterior part of the chiasma while the posterior part of the circle of Willis is inferior to the posterior part of the chiasma. The posterior communicating artery joins the two parts inferiorly (Fig. 3.20).

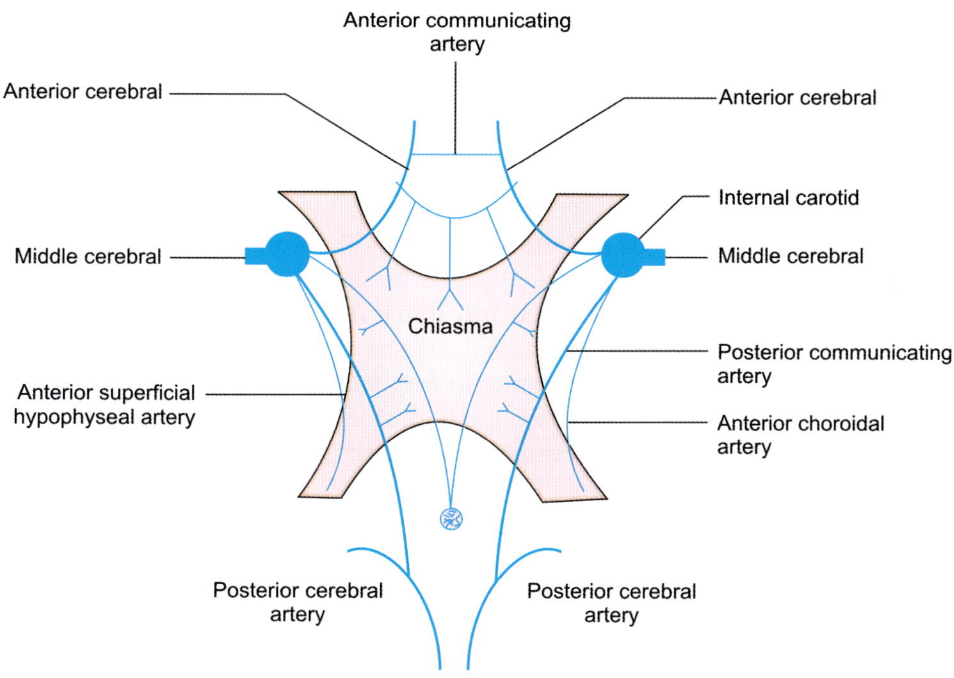

Fig. 3.20: Relation of chiasma to arteries around it

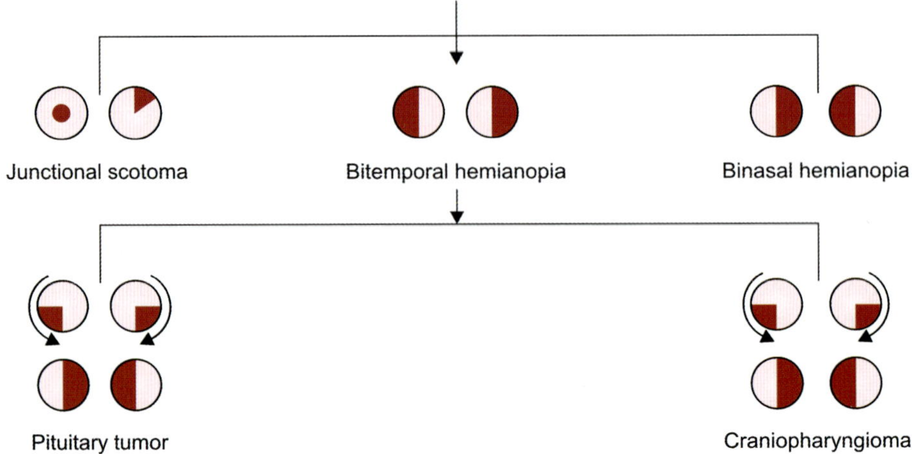

Fig. 3.21: Field changes in lesions of chiasma

The clinical features chiasmal lesion

1. **Field change:** The most important clinical features are variable field changes which the patient may not be aware of unless pointed out. Most of the patient with bitemporal hemianopia may complain of bumping into furnitures in the room and difficulty in driving (Fig. 3.21).
2. **Diminished vision:** Level of vision in chiasmal disorders is variable. It depends on associated dysfunction of visual path. The patient may not complain of diminished central vision even in presence of **bitemporal hemianopia**. **There may be associated color defect**. In late stage there may be gross loss of vision due to optic atrophy.
3. **Pupillary abnormality: Afferent pupillary defect** is a common feature.
4. **Extraocular muscle palsy:** Chiasmal defects themselves do not cause muscle palsy unless the growth responsible for chiasmal pathology infiltrates and cause compression on the nerve. Oculomotor nerve is commonly involved.
5. Pituitary dysfunctions are common feature of pituitary tumors, which are the commonest cause of chiasmal field changes.

Etiologies of chiasmal lesions

The following chart give age-wise common causes of chiasmal lesion

	Age	*Lesion*
1.	Children	Craniopharyngioma Glioma of chiasma
2.	Young adult (20-40 years)	Pituitary tumors
3.	After fourth decade	Meningioma, arachnoiditis, aneurysm.

Flow chart 3.1: Causes of chiasmal and extrachiasmal lesion

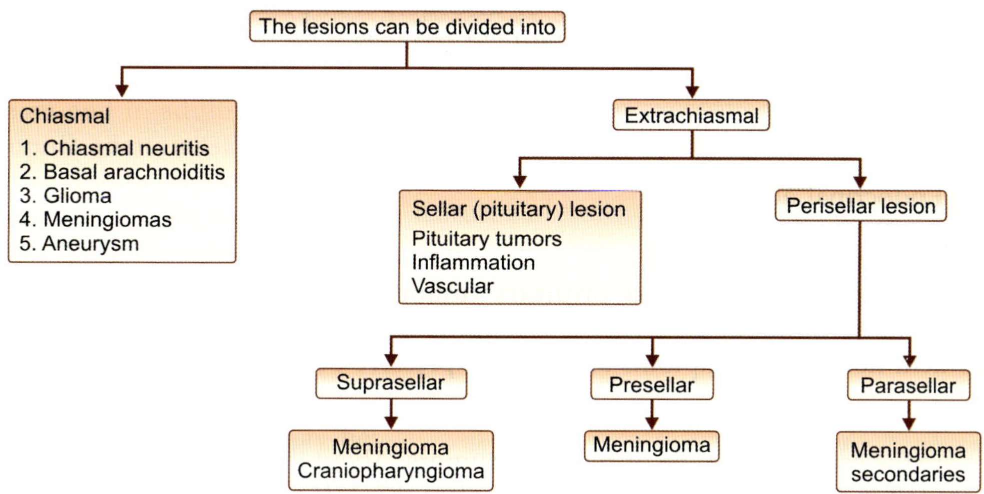

The chiasma may be involved due to lesions of the chiasma it self or due to lesion of the neighboring structure.

The conditions that masquerade as chiasmal field changes:

1. Bilateral sector retinitis pigmentosa
2. Bilateral centrocecal scotoma
3. Bilateral enlarged blind spot
4. Tilled disk.

Disorders of parachiasmal structures

Lesions of the anatomical structure that involve chiasma are:

	Structure	*Lesion*
1.	Pituitary	Benign/malignant tumor
2.	Structures round the sella	Craniopharyngioma
3.	Suprasellar	Meningioma
4.	Circle of Willis	Aneurysms

The common growths that involve the chiasma are:

1. Glioma
2. Meningiomas:
   (i) Chiasmal
   (ii) Suprasellar
   (iii) Presellar
   (iv) Parasellar
3. Craniopharyngioma
4. Pituitary tumors.

The patient may go through **episodes of amaurosis** that may last for few minutes to few hours before passing into **permanent loss of vision**. It takes few months to years before total blindness sets in.

Sudden bilateral loss of vision, bilateral ophthalmoplegia with severe headache is due to hemorrhage in the adenoma.

Field defects

The field changes in pituitary tumors can be divided into two broad groups,

- Early field changes (Fig. 3.22)
- Late field changes (Fig. 3.23).

The **classical** pathogenic field defect is thought to be **bitemporal hemianopia** which is infect a late feature and seen only when the growth presses the middle of the chiasm from below. The field changes depend upon the anatomical position of the chiasm in relation to the pituitary gland and the expansion of the growth, i.e. is it prefixed with short optic nerve or is a postfixed with long optic nerve?

If the growth extends more into the optic nerve on one side, a monocular field defect will develop which may cause central scotoma, temporal scotoma, superior/inferior temporal scotoma. Rarely there may be arcuate defect or attitudinal defect.

The tumor involving the **anterior chiasma** produces **junctional scotomas**, i.e. uniocular central scotoma on one side with contralateral superior temporal scotoma or hemianopia.

The **bitemporal hemianopic** fields may be symmetric or asymmetric. They always **respect the vertical meridian**. They field defect generally starts as superior

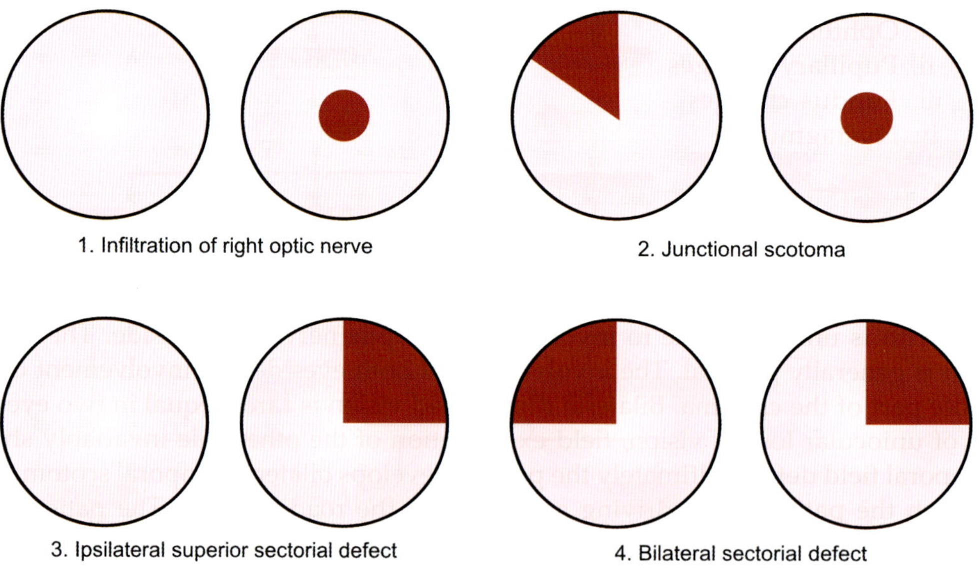

Fig. 3.22: Early field changes in pituitary tumor

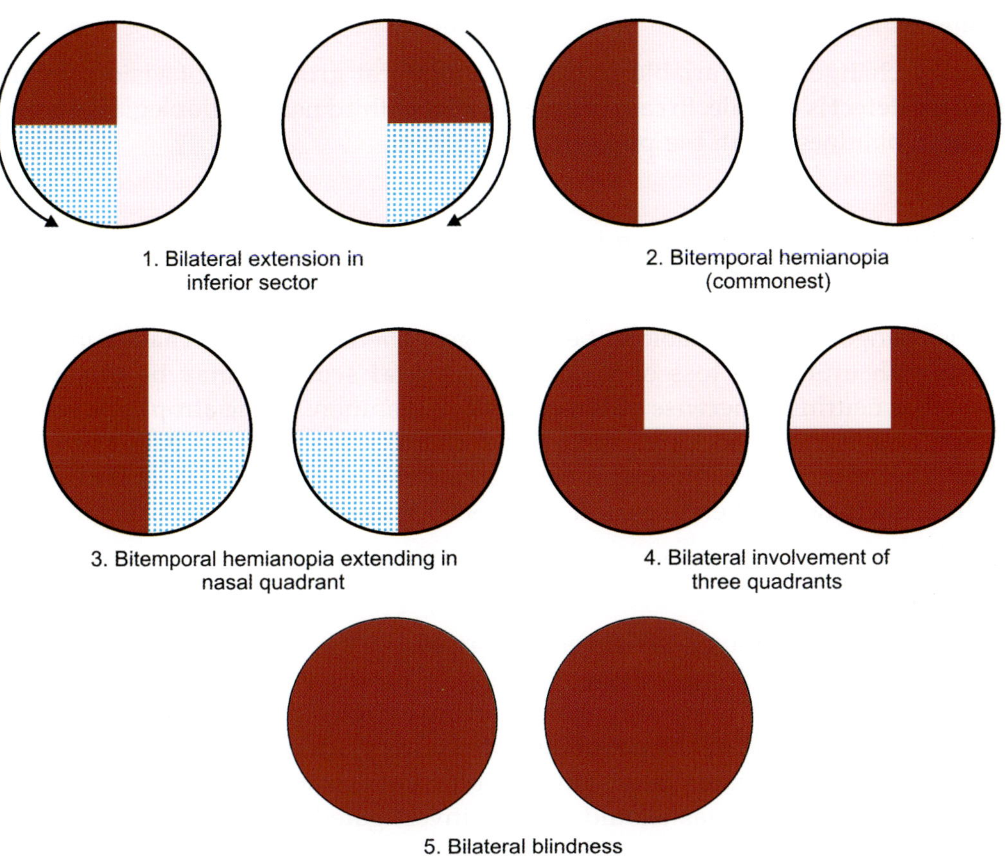

Fig. 3.23: Late field changes in pituitary tumor

quadrantanopic defect on the temporal side. The scotoma follow a predictable course, i.e. from superior temporal quadrant it extends down to involve the inferior temporal respecting the vertical meridian, then it breaks through the vertical meridian to involve the inferior nasal quadrant and extend up to involve the superior nasal quadrant in both eye causing blindness. **The scotoma moves clockwise in right eye and anti-clockwise in left eye.**

Extension of the pituitary tumor in the optic tract causes homonymous hemianopia which is incongruous.

Ophthalmoplegia

Paralysis of extraocular muscles is a **late feature** and is indication of large tumor. The most common nerve to be effected is **third nerve** because of its close proximity to pituitary gland. It may cause **iridoplegia** as well. The other cranial nerves involved are fourth, sixth and fifth. Sudden bilateral ophthalmoplegia with bilateral loss of vision is an ominous sign of pituitary apoplexy.

Pupillary changes

Pupillary changes are variable in case of unilateral gross loss of vision, **afferent pupillary defect** is the rule. In case of involvement of third nerve iridoplegia is common. In case of blindness, both the pupil may be dilated.

Nystagmus

Sea saw nystagmus may be seen in chromophobe tumors.

Fundus changes

Fundus changes are as variable as field changes. There may be **no change** in fundus. A case with uniocular loss of vision and **central scotoma** may be mistaken as retrobulbar neuritis, otherwise **pallor of disk** is common. **Optic atrophy** is generally bilateral and asymmetric. Other optic nerve changes are temporal pallor or **bow tie pallor**, the latter when present means involvement of optic tract. Surprisingly **papilledema is rare**. When present it denotes hydrocephalus and obstruction in third vertical.

Diagnosis

1. An asymptomatic case is generally missed.
2. The hormonal changes draw attention to presence of pituitary tumor.
3. Presence of bitemporal quadrantopic field defect should alert the ophthalmologist about possibility of pituitary adenoma.
4. Bitemporal hemianopia is pathgnomonic but a late feature.
5. Junctional scotomas should also be investigated for possibility of pituitary tumor.

Investigation

The better alternatives are X-ray skull, lateral view, CT is good to detect boney changes and MRI.

The common X-ray findings are:

1. Enlargement of sella
2. Ballooning of sella
3. Thinning of floor of the sella
4. Double floor of sella
5. Destruction of anterior clinoid process
6. Destruction of honey structure of sella
7. Rarely there may be hyperostosis of the sphenoidal bone.

Management

Treatments of pituitary tumors are outside the domain of ophthalmologist. It is a multidisciplinary involvement consisting of neurosurgeon, radiologist and endocrinologist.

Pituitary apoplexy is rare but serious condition that happens due to hemorrhage in a pituitary tumor or an infarct in the substance of the pituitary tumor. The hemorrhage compresses the intracranial part of anterior visual path resulting in:

1. Sever headache
2. Stupor that may end in coma
3. Neck rigidity
4. Bilateral blindness
5. Bilateral ophthalmoplegia
6. Blood in CSF
7. Enlarged sella on X-ray.

The condition is an emergency. The management consists of early diagnosis, high does of systemic steroid, endoscopic decompression and radiotherapy.

Empty sella syndrome

This disorder of pituitary fossa consist of **nontumor enlargement of sella**. In some cases the pituitary gland may be deficient. Clinically these are **two types** of empty sella syndrome:

1. **Primary**, that is due to developmental deficiency of diaphragma sella. The syndrome develops spontaneously in persons with larger than normal sella. It is more common in **young females** who are **obese**. The arachnoid which lies over the sella is pushed into the sella due to normal pulsation of CSF. The sub-arachnoid space is dragged along pressing and flatting the pituitary gland.
   The condition is marked by **intractable headache, visual loss** and **field defects** are common. They may mimic pituitary adenoma in few cases may have normal vision and field.
   Predisposing factors are pseudotumor cerebri and cyst in sella.
2. **The secondary empty sella syndrome** develops following surgery or radiotherapy for pituitary tumors.

Craniopharyngioma

Craniopharyngiomas are **benign congenital tumors** that generally manifests in **childhood**. They are the most common nonglial intracranial tumors in children. They are ectodermal in origin. The common age of presentation is **second decade**, the next peak is seen the sixth to seventh decade. Its presence under one year is very rare. It is an **adamantinoma**. The growth arises from epithelial remnants of **Rathke's pouch**. The craniopharyngiomas are mostly **supraseller.** They may be **prechiasmatic** or **retrochiasmatic** in **position. The tumors can be solid** or **cystic**.

Calcification is very common and almost diagnostic of supra seller cranio-pharyngioma.

The tumors themselves do not produce hormone. The hormonal changes, which are common, develop due to encroachment of the tumor in the pituitary.

The clinical presentation of the tumor is different in two age groups, i.e. **childhood craniopharyngioma and adult craniopharyngioma**.

The childhood craniopharyngioma is more common than its adult counterpart. Average age of diagnosis of the first is under fifteen years. It has been reported in children of one years as well that goes in favor of the growth being congenital.

Symptoms

1. Visual:
   i. Diminished vision
   ii. Field changes
2. Nonvisual:

The clinical features are variable, depend upon size, location, duration and hormonal changes brought about by it. The tumor is slow progressive and remain asymptomatic for long time.

1. The visual loss may go unnoticed for long time and is detected on routine vision testing.
2. Bilateral and loss of vission is detected early.
3. The child has symptoms of raised intracranial tension or symptoms of pituitary dysfunction which brings child for ocular examination and reveal diminished vision, field and fundus changes.
4. The **field changes** look like chiasmal changes, i.e. **bitemporal hemianopia**. The field changes are asymmetric and irregular. The progress of bitemporal hemianopia differs from that of pituitary tumor which starts form superior temporal quadrant and spread to inferior quadrant. The field change of craniopharyngioma starts in inferior temporal and spreads to superior temporal, **anticlockwise in right eye** and **clockwise in left eye**.

The other field changes are variable depending upon the visual fibers involved in the chiasma.

The **common patterns** are:

1. Central or paracentral scotoma in one eye without any change in the other eye. This is commonly seen in prechiasmal lesion.
2. Central, centrocecal or paracentral scotomas in both eyes, with loss of vision in one eye, the other field shows temporal depression.
3. Concentric contraction in both eye.
4. If the tumor invades the optic tract, a contralateral hemianopia supervenes.

Fundus: Optic atrophy is more common than papilledema.

Squint

I. **Concomitant squint** is common due to early loss of vision.

II. **Paralytic squint** results when:
   a. The large tumor compresses the oculomotor nerves.
   b. Secondary to raised intracranial lesion.

III. The nonvisual features are:
   1. **Headache** is common feature in children with craniopharyngioma. That may be independent or raised intracranial tension or with it.
   2. **Vomiting** is mostly due to raised intracranial tension.
   3. Hormonal changes are varied:
      i. **In children**, they are pituitary dwarfism, obesity, gonadal atrophy, Frolic syndrome, arrested sexual growth.
      ii. **In young males:** The person has infantile body structures, lack of secondary sex characters, in females amenorrhea is common.
      iii. **In adults** the nonendocrinal features are similar to those seen in children. The hormonal changes are less marked than in children and young adult but not absent.

The radiological features

The radiological feature of **suprasellar calcification** is diagnostic which is less common in adults. CT and MRI helps to show subtle calcification and show the precise location of the growth, i.e. sellar, pre- or postchiasmal.

Treatment

Surgical removal of the growth is the treatment of choice followed by **hormonal replacement**. The tumors are partially radiosensitive.

Suprasellar meningioma

These are generally **benign, slow growths** that arise form the arachnoid matter of the **tuberculum sella** and **anterior clinoid**. They are tumors of **middle age**, i.e. between 35-50 years. **Women** are effected more than men.

The most common presenting feature is **uniocular fall of vision**. The other eye may develop diminished vision months or years later. **Binocular loss of vision** is less frequent and when present is not equal in two eyes. **Fluctuation of vision** is common. The loss of vision may range between loss of one or two lines on Snellen's chart to perception of light.

Diminished vision is always associated with field changes about which the patient may not be aware of.

The field changes are:

1. Junctional scotoma, i.e. central scotoma in one eye with temporal depression in the other eye.
2. Bitemporal quadrantanopia.
3. Bitemporal hemianopia.
4. Homonymous hemianopia.

Fundus

Disk changes comprise bilateral asymmetric pallor of disk, papilledema is rare and late.

Nonocular symptoms are: Headache, anosmia, mental changes, convulsion. Late cases may develop features of pituitary tumor or hypothalamic changes. The symptoms may changes to worse in pregnancy.

Diagnosis

X-ray skull often does not delineate the tumor unless there is bony hyperostosis.

Presence of hyperostosis is almost diagnostic.

The pituitary fossa is not enlarged.

CT and MRI: High resolution CT and MRI can reveal smallest meningioma.

Treatment

Surgery is the definitive treatment. If surgical excision is done, early chances of visual improvement are more.

Other less effective methods are:

1. Use of estrogen or progesterone antagonist in women.
2. Radiation: The meningiomas are considered to be radioresistant. However, radiation is used to prevent recurrence after incomplete excision of the growth.
3. Stereotactic radiosurgery is coming as a promising method.

Other meningioma of neuro-ophthalmic interest

Besides suprasellar meningioma there are other location where meningioma develop and produce neuro-ophthalmic features. The various sites where meningiomas develop are: **Cerebral hemisphere, wing of the sphenoid, olfactory groove, sheath of optic nerve and apex of the orbit.** Out of which **sphenoidal ridge meningiomas** have maximum ophthalmic features while cerebral have more neurological features and few ophthalmic features.

The characteristics of them are as follows:

1. **Sphenoidal meningioma**
   Features depend upon the location of the tumor which can be:
   - Lateral sphenoidal
   - Medial sphenoidal
   - Mid sphenoidal
     i. **Lateral sphenoidal**
        a. Fullness of temporal fossa due to hyperostosis
        b. Painless, slow, growing proptosis
        c. Fairly good vision
        d. Minimal field change

e. Normal fundus
f. No ophthalmoplegia
g. The meningioma is diffused enplaque.

ii. **Medial sphenoidal**
a. Compress the optic nerve and chiasma
b. Visual loss
c. Field changes
d. Optic atrophy ipsilateral
e. Contralateral papilledema
f. **Foster Kennedy syndrome**
g. Proptosis
h. Superior orbital fissure syndrome consisting of involvement of cranial nerves from second to sixth.

iii. **Middle third sphenoidal:** Features of raised intracranial tension with ophthalmoplegia and papilledema.

Neuro-ophthalmic involvement in intracranial aneurysms (for details see Chapter 14)

About **two percent** of persons have **asymptomatic** intracranial aneurysms. The aneurysms become symptomatic when either they press on various cranial nerves, or neural tracts. Some of the aneurysms are congenital in nature but manifest late in life. The overall incidence of intracranial aneurysm is **more in women**. They develop in both the intracranial arterial systems, i.e. the **carotid system** and the **vertebro-basilar system**.

Shapewise there are two types of aneurysm, i.e. the **saccular** (berry) aneurysm and **fusiform** aneurysms.

The presenting features depend upon:

i. The arterial system involved, i.e. carotid/vertebrobasilar.
ii. The location of the aneurysm
iii. The number—single aneurysm is more common than multiple aneurysms.
iv. Size of aneurysm.
v. Is the aneurysm intact or ruptured. Intact aneurysms behave like **compressive lesions**, the ruptured aneurysm present as compressive as well as **hemorrhagic lesions**.
vi. The fusiform aneurysms are more likely to develop thrombosis than rupture. They are mostly seen in arteriosclerotic old patients.
vii. **Aneurysm of internal carotid systems** cause uniocular diminished vision, gradual onset of paralysis of extraocular muscle, facial pain, pupillary changes including Horner's syndrome, proptosis, field defects.
viii. The aneurysm of **vertebrobasilar system** cause cranial nerve palsy, defects in corticospinal, and spinothalmic tracts.

Salient features of important intracranial aneurysms

Location of aneurysm	*Neuro-ophthalmic features*
1. Carotid system	
i. Anterior communicating artery	a. They are the commonest location of intracranial aneurysm b. Uniocular gradual loss of vision c. Abrupt lateral temporal field defect
ii. Anterior cerebral artery	Same as above
iii. At the junction of internal carotid and ophthalmic artery	a. Chronic, progressive, unilateral diminished vision b. Central scotoma c. Contralateral depression of temporal field
iv. Supraclinoidal carotid	a. Progressive, ipsilateral diminished vision due to compression of optic nerve b. Contralateral, temporal field defect due to involvement of chiasma c. Contralateral incongruous, homonymous hemianopia due to compression of optic tract d. X-ray skull shows erosion of sella and anterior clinoid e. There may be **calcification of the aneurysm**
v. Intracavernous carotid	a. Multiple cranial nerve palsy b. Diplopia, neuralgia c. Involvement of oculosympathetic d. Diminished vision due to optic atrophy e. May cause bilateral ophthalmoplegia f. Symptoms mimic pituitary adenoma g. X-ray shows erosion of anterior clinoid, sphenoidal sinus, widening of superior orbital fissure h. Rupture of intracavernous carotid aneurysm causes carotid cavernous fistula
vi. **Carotid cavernous fistula**	a. Unilateral pulsating exophthalmos with bruit, chemosis and congestion of conjunctiva b. Diminished vision c. Secondary glaucoma d. Ophthalmoplegia
vii. **Posterior communication artery**	a. The posterior communicating artery joins the carotid system with vertebro-basilar system via posterior cerebral artery.

Contd...

Contd...

	b. The oculomotor nerve is closely related to the artery. The nerve is lateral and parallel to the artery. c. The aneurysm generally arises at the junction of internal carotid and posterior communicating artery. d. The commonest neuro-ophthalmic feature is painful, isolated, unilateral third nerve palsy, which involves pupil. e. Lumbar puncture may have blood mixed CSF. f. Recovery is rare and late in contrast to diabetic third nerve palsy which is also isolated palsy where pupil is spared. g. Involvement of fourth and sixth nerve are rare. h. Un ruptured aneurysm cause compressive lesion, which are slow to develop. i. Ruptured aneurysm causes acute features.
2. **Vertebrobasilar system**	
i. **Basilar artery**	a. Commonest site of theurysm is bifurcation of the basilar artery. b. Both saccular and fusiform aneurysms are almost equally found. c. Third nerve palsy is the commonest feature. d. Third nerve palsy may be associated with homonymous hemianopia, cerebellar ataxia, nystagmus, hemiparesis and gaze palsy.
ii. **Posterior cerebellar artery**	a. Rare. b. When present may have third nerve palsy. c. Visual loss when the aneurysm rushers.

Retrochiasmal lesions

The retrochiasmal visual path consist of **optic tract, lateral geniculate body** and **optic radiation**. Broadly the retrochiasmal lesion can be divided into two parts, i.e. **pregeniculate** and **retrogeniculate** or **geniculo-calcarine path**.

The lesions of optic track and lateral geniculate body are infrequent. It is difficult to differentiate lesion of posterior part of the tract and lateral geniculate body.

Contd...

b. Homonymous quadrantanopia
c. Macular sparing
d. Macular splitting
e. Preservation of temporal crescent in hemianopia

ii. **Other ocular features**
a. Good vision
b. **Cortical blindness**
c. Optic kinetic nystagmus

iii. **Neurological features**—Nil

Macular sparing

Macular sparing is seen in lesions of bilateral occipital cortex. It is considered to be present when at least 5° of central field is retained in both the eyes, towards the hemianopia. The exact cause of macular sparing in occipital lesion is not well understood (Fig. 3.25). Most probably if is multifactorial. Commonest lesion that causes macular sparing is **vascular**, the other cause is **trauma**. The probable causes of macular sparing are:

1. Dual blood supply from terminal branches of middle cerebral and posterior cerebral arteries.
2. Large area of macular representation in occipital cortex, small lesion may spare enough neurons to retain macular vision.
3. Dual innervations as a cause cannot be ignored.

Cortical blindness

Cortical blindness is not very rare, many a times it is dismissed either as malingering or mental derangement because the condition is **sudden in onset without any external signs** and the **fundus does not reveal any lesion** that may explain such gross loss of vision.

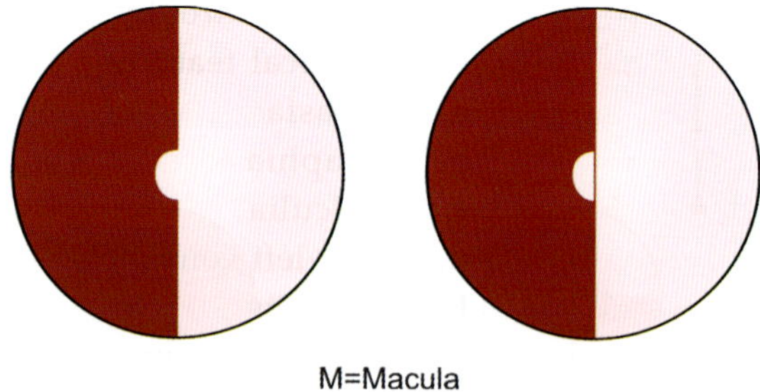

M=Macula

Fig. 3.25: Field changes in macular sparing

The syndrome consists of triad of:

1. Bilateral blindness (amaurosis)
2. Normal pupillary reaction
3. Normal fundus.

The blindness is sudden, equal is both eyes; profound, painless and **the eye is white.** The vision may be reduced to counting finger from close quarter. Most of the time perception of light is retained but **projection of light may be faulty**.

The patient complains as if the lights in the room have been switched off or a curtain has come down between the patient and the surrounding.

In spite of such a gross loss of vision the **patient often denies blindness**. This in called **Anton's syndrome**. The patient attempts to walk unaided only to tumble against the nearest object. The patient resents being assisted by others.

Fortunately **complete or partial recovery** is the rule in large of cases. The time lapse between onset of blindness and recovery is variable. It may be weeks or months before maximum vision has been regained. Unfortunately the patient never regains the preattack vision.

The recovery of vision follows a fixed pattern. The first visual sensation to change toward good is **improvement in brightness of the light**. This is followed successively by **form and movement. Recovery of color is last.**

Those who do not regain vision are most likely to die due to multiple vascular lesion.

The condition can be seen at **any age**. Even children are known to suffer from cortical blindness mostly due **to trauma or infection**. In neonates the commonest cause is **neonatal asphyxia. Venoms** and toxins have been reported to cause cortical blindness, otherwise common age group is **after sixty years**. The patients generally suffer from **atherosclerosis, hypertension**. The patient may have **undergone cardiac surgery, cerebral or coronary angiographies**. So far no case has been reported following fundus fluorescein angiography but a possibility cannot be ruled out. The other cause in **manipulation of neck**.

In spite of gross loss of vision the patient may complain of **photopsia**. **Mental changes are common**.

The lesion has to involve both the visual cortex. The cause in 80% of cases is vascular in the form of an obstruction. The common site of obstruction at the **end of the basilar artery**, which is the common origin of both the posterior cerebral arteries, the main arterial supply to the visual cortex.

The other causes are **hypoxia, hypotension, asphyxia, occipital migraine, occipital tumors** and **degenerations cause gradual onset**.

The condition is mostly **monosymptomatic**, i.e. loss of vision**. There are no neurological signs and symptoms** that may be directly traced to cortical blindness because the visual cortex does not contain any other sensory or motor tracts.

There are no reasons that may explain mental changes except that CT and MRI invariable show lesion in the parietal cortex that have been confirmed many a times on autopsy.

The differential diagnosis consists of:

1. Malingering
2. Amaurosis fugax
3. Ischemic optic neuropathy
4. Acute chiasmitis
5. Severe bilateral optic neuritis
6. Migraine
7. Basilar migraine.

Management

No specific treatment is required. The systemic hypertension, diabetes should be managed by usual drugs.

Amaurosis fugax

Amaurosis fugax is **transient, monocular, painless loss of vision**. The condition **may alternate between two eyes**. The disorder is seen in **elderly patients of any sex**. The basic pathology is **transient ischemic attack** in the **internal carotid** due to thrombus formation in the extracranial course of the internal carotid. The carotid responsible for the episodes have **atheromas** in their lumen. The other predisposing causes are—**arteriosclerosis, hypertension, diabetes, hyperviscosity condition, giant cell arteritis** and **migraine**.

The pathogenesis is an embolic phenomenon in **ophthalmic-retinal circulation**. Sometimes **middle cerebral artery** too may be involved. Complete embolization leads to obstruction of central retinal artery or its branches. Amaurosis fugax may be caused by spasm in the vascular tree, as the spasm passes off vision improves.

The episode is described variously by patients. The patient may feel a curtain to descend or ascend in front of the eye and pass off in the reverse order. Though complete obscuration is the rule, some patients may have partial obscuration. It takes few seconds for obscuration to set in but take 5 to 30 minutes for the curtain to pass off. Due to transient short period of symptoms the fundus pictures are not well documented. The picture looks like central retinal artery spasm. **The pupil is dilated during the episode**.

About 40-50% of eyes with amaurosis fugax go blind due to vascular causes. About same percentage of patient **develops cerebral stroke**. Mortality rate is high among these patients. Some patients with amaurosis fugax also have contralateral weakness of limbs and paresthesia.

Diagnosis is based on **clinical history** of monocular, transient, painless loss of vision in elderly persons. Tender scalp and raised ESR point toward possibility of giant cell arteries. A bruit over carotid is common. The other causes of uniocular causes should be excluded.

Causes of uniocular loss of vision are:

- Amaurosis fugax
- Ischemic optic neuropathy
- Papilledema
- Central retinal vessel obstruction
- Migraine
- Anemia
- Policythemia
- Coagulopathies
- Hypotension.

Management

There is no definitive treatment of amaurosis fugax. Some patients may improve with endartectomy, which should be preceded by ultrasonography, Doppler. The medical treatment consists of management of systemic hypertension, diabetes, raised lipids. **Oral aspirin** for long time under supervision have proved to reduce chances of blindness, stroke and death.

Malingering

Malingering is a functional (nonorganic) ocular condition. It has been defined variously. The most commonly used definition is, **wilfully misleading the existence or seriousness of a disease or disability for purpose of a conciously desired gain or purposeful feigning of a condition for advantage.**

Malingering can be seen in from 5-7 years to fifth, sixth decade; it is more common in young adults.

It is generally sudden in onset. The onset may be traced back to an incidence that is related to some sort of compensation or the person wants change in place of work or type of work.

When the patient exaggerates the condition, the condition is called **positive malingering**. Less common is a situation when the person plays down the disease, i.e. avoid dismissal, or gain a job, etc.

The loss of vision is not associated with pain or redness.

The loss of vision may be **binocular** or **uniocular**. In both the cases it can be **total** or **partial**. The condition generally does not linger long even without treatment or may improve by some religious rites or folk medicines only to relapse. This phenomenon is more common in hysteric persons.

Before labelling a person malinger one should exclude other genuine possibilities of bilateral painless loss of vision, i.e. amblyopia, central serous retinopathy, kerato-conus, cystoids macular dystrophies, glaucoma, opacities in media. It will be realized that none of the above mentioned conditions are of sudden onset.

The ophthalmologist should listen to the history carefully and pretend to agree with the patient and be sympathetic. The malinger while moving in the room does not miss the obstacle but deliberately and gently bumps into the obstacle without hurting.

On examination the eyes are externally normal. The pupillary reaction in both eye have brisk direct and indirect light reaction. Sometimes a malinger may instil cycloplegic purposely and deny doing so. Accommodation and convergence is normal. The extraocular muscle have full range of movement. Either there is no error of retraction when refractive error is present it is correctable but the patient denies improvement, the fundus is normal.

Excluding diminished vision is most arduous task:

1. **Patient with partial loss**
   i. Vision improves by few lines on Snellen's chart when a nonmalinger is moved towards the Snellen's chart. A malinger denies such improvement.
   ii. Bilateral partial loss of vision are the most difficult to mange.
   iii. Monocular partial loss is managed as monocular gross loss.
2. **Monocular gross loss**
   a. Producing high anisometropia
      i. The patient is asked to close both the eyes.
      ii. A strong plus lens is put in front of eye with good vision.
      iii. A plain glass is put in front of the eyes with so called blind eye.
      iv. The patient is asked to open both eyes simultaneously and asked to read the Snellen's chart. He cannot see through the strong plus lens. So if the reads with both eyes open he is reading through the plain glass. This clinches the diagnosis. Now close the eye with plain glass and demonstrate to the patient that whatever he has read has been done by the so called blind eye and his bluff has been called off.
   b. Causing diplopia
      i. The so called blind eye is closed.
      ii. A strong prism is held in front of the other eye, apex bisecting the pupil. The patient confesses that he has diplopia.
      iii. The so called blind eye is uncovered.
      iv. The entire prism is shifted so as to cover the whole of the eye.
      v. If the patient complains of diplopia he has good binocular vision.
   c. Causing refixation movement
      A ten dioptre prism base out is put in front of normal eye causes shift of both eyes with a refixation of other eye.
3. **Binocular gross loss**
   i. Patient with true blindness will have absent or sluggish pupillary reaction.
   ii. Stretch out one hand of the patient and ask the patient to touch the index finger of the outstretched hand. A blind person will be able to do it because this does not depend on vision. A malinger will hesitate to do so.
   iii. Ask the patient to put his signature on a paper. A blind will readily oblige once his pen and paper has made contact. A malinger will deliberately distort the signature.

iv. A strong light thrown in the eye will cause reflex tearing in seeing eyes.
v. Menace reflex: A threatening gesture will force the malinger to move the head and close the eyes.
vi. A mirror is held in front of the eyes about 18-24 inches in front and then tilted. The position of the eyes are observed as the mirror moves. The eyes of a blind will not change position with tilting of the mirror.
vii. Optokinetic nystagmus: Nystagmus produced by optokinetic drum cannot be suppressed in a seeing eye.

Management

Management of malingering is difficult. In fact it does not fall in the domain of ophthalmology. It is best managed by psychiatrist. The aim is to outwit the patient and convince that his/her vision is not lost. Occupational malingering is more difficult to manage.

BIBLIOGRAPHY

1. Aaberg TM. Fluorescein angiography in principle and practice of ophthalmology, Vol-II. 1st edn. Peyman GA, Sanders DR, Gold berg MF (Eds). Jaypee Brothers Medical Publishers, New Delhi 1987;905-34.
2. Aderson D, Khalim M. Meningioma and ophthalmologist. A review of 80 cases. Ophthalmology 1981;88:1004-09.
3. Andrew BT, Wilson CB. Suprasellar meningiomas surgery 1988;69:523-28.
4. Appen RE. Devencei G, Ferweda J. Optic disk vasculitis. Am Jr Oph 1980;90:353-57.
5. Arnold AC. Ophthalmic manifestation of multiple sclerosis. Semin Ophthal 1988;3: 229-43.
6. Beck RW. The optic neuritis treatment three years follows results. Arch Oph 1995;113: 136-37.
7. Chou PI, Sadun AA. Chenye clinical experience in management of traumatic optic neuropathy. Jr Neuro-ophthalmology 1996;16:325-36.
8. Dhaliwal U. Cortical blindness and snakebite unusual sequela of I Jo, 1999;47;191-92.
9. Duke Elder S, Scott, GI. The optic nerve: General consideration in system of ophthalmology, Vol. XII. Duke-Elders and Scott GI (Eds). Henry Kimpton London 1971;11-18.
10. Dutton JJ. Glioma of the anterior visual pathway. Surv Oph 1994;38:427-52.
11. Ellenberger C, Messner KH. Papillophlebitis Benign retinopathy resembling papilledema or papillitis. Ann near of 1978;3:438-40.
12. Glasser JS. Ischemic optic neuropathy in neuro-ophthalmology. 3rd edn. Lippincot-Willians and Wilkims, Philadelphia 1999;163.
13. Hayreh SS, Pathogenesis of oedema optic disc. A preliminary report. BJO 1964;48:522.
14. Hayreh SS, Podhajsky PA, Zimmerman B. Ocular manifestation of giant cell arteritis Am Jr Oph 1998;125:509-20.
15. Hebbar K6. Optic atrophy in Neuro-ophthalmology. 1st edn, Natchair G (Eds). Arvind Eye Hospital, Madurai 1301-12.
16. Hoyt WF, Baghdassarian SA. Optic glioma of childhood natural history and rationale of conservative treatment. Br Jr Oph 1969;53:793-98.

17. Levin LA, Beck RW, Joseph JP. The treatment of traumatic optic neuropathy. The international optic nerve trauma study. Ophthalmology 1999;106:1268-72.
18. Lopez PF, Smith JL. Lebers optic neuropathy new observation. Jr Clin neuro-ophthalmic 1986;6:144-52.
19. Martyn LJ. Optic atrophy in pediatric ophthalmology. Vol 1. 2nd edn. Hartey RD (Eds). WB Saunders company, Philadelphia 1983;817-19.
20. Mukhejee PK. Congenital put of the optic disc in current ocular therapy. 5th edn, Fraunfelder FT and Roy FH. WB Saunders company, Philadelphia 2000.
21. Mukherjee PK. Pseudo Foster Kennedy syndrome in clinical examination in ophthalmology. 1st edn. Elsevier, New Delhi, 2006;361.
22. Optic neuritis study group clinical profile of optic neuritis. Arch oph 1991;109:1673-78.
23. Steinsapir KD, Gold berg RA. Traumatic optic neuropathy. Sur Oph 1994;38:487-578.
24. Tabaddor K. Neonatal craniopharyngioma. Am J. Dis child 1974;128.
25. Tandon Radhika, Verma L. Papilledema in clinical practice in ophthalmology. 1st edn. Saxena S (Eds). Jaypee Brothers Medical Publishers, New Delhi, 2003.
26. Wilson WB. Meningiomas of anterior visual system. Sur Oph 1981;26:109-27.
27. Wray SH. Visual field pathology in manual of ocular diagnosis and therapy. 3rd edn. Deborah Pavan (Eds). Langston Little Brown 1991;336-37.

4 Pupillary Changes in Neuro-ophthalmic Disorders

The pupils are two naturally present apertures in the iris, one in each eye, though they look to be placed centrally in fact they are slightly shifted medially. A gross shifted of pupil from its usual position is called **corectopia**. The normal pupil is circular, a distorted pupil is called **dyscoria**. The size of normal pupil at rest is 2 to 2.5 mm. A small pupil is called **miotic pupil** and the process is known as **miosis**. A large pupil at rest is called **mydriatic pupil** and the process of dilation of the pupil is called **mydriasis**. Miosis due to neurological and pharmacological causes are associated with spasm of accommodation, i.e. **cyclotonia** and mydriasis due to neurological causes and para-sympatholytic drugs is associated with abolished or reduced accommodation and, i.e. **cycloplegia**. A combination of neurological mydriasis and cycloplegia is called **internal ophthalmoplegia**. The **term iridoplegia** denotes absence of movement of the pupil to light and near.

- All parasympathomimetic drugs are miotic as well as cyclotonic.
- All parasympatholytics are mydriasis as well as cycloplegics.
- Sympatheticomimetic (sympathomimetic) drugs are only mydriatic.

Generally, the two pupils are of equal size within a small variation. A difference in size is called **anisocoria**, i.e. one is larger or smaller than the normal.

It is rare to have one neurologically small pupil and the other neurologically large pupil.

The size of the pupil is due a delicate balance between constrictor and dilator of the pupil.

The important point in anisocoria is to decide whether the larger or the smaller pupil is abnormal.

The rule is as follows:

1. It the anisocoria is more in bright light, the larger pupil is abnormal.
2. If the anisocoria is more in dim light, the smaller pupil is abnormal.

The ability to bring the diverging rays to focus on retina is called accommodation. If the pupillary reaction to near (accommodation) is better than light, the condition is referred to as **light near dissociation**.

Features of pupillary abnormalities

Feature	*Probable cause*	*Probable location*
1. Corectopia	Congenital, lesion at mesencephalon	Mesencephalon
2. Dyscoria	Congenital, trauma, iritis	Iris
3. Miosis	Physiological, mitoes	Local
	Iritis	Iris
	Horners	Cervical sympathetic
	Irritation of third nerve	Midbrain
4. Mydriasis	Physiological	
	Mydriatic	Local
	Irritation of cervical sympathetic	Neck
	Paralysis of third nerve	Infranuclear
	Lesion of anterior visual path.	Optic nerve
5. Internal ophthalmo-plegia	Total third nerve palsy	Infranuclear third nerve
	Use of parasympatholytic drugs	Local
6. Iridoplegia	Mydriatics	Iris
	Blind eye	Anterior visual pathway
7. Light near dissociation	Argyll Roberson syndrome	Pretectal
	Adies pupil	Ciliary ganglion
	Parinauds syndrome	Mesencephalon
8. Amaurotic pupil	Optic atrophy	
	Total retinal detachment	Retina and optic nerve
	Absolute glaucoma	

Examination of the pupil is one of the simplest clinical methods that are either not done properly or the findings are misinterpreted.

The basic mechanisms involved in pupillary reaction are:

1. It constricts to light and near object.
2. It dilates in dark and looking at a distant object.

The pupillary reaction is influenced by: Ambient light, brightness of source of light, accommodation exerted, age, refractive state of the eye, drug ingested or instilled in the eye, local disease in the eye, congenital anomalies, balance between sympathetic and parasympathetic paths and intact afferent and efferent visual path.

A bright light in the examination area may constrict the pupil, a pupil may become large in dark room. A too faint source of light may give false impression of sluggish pupillary reflex to light. Holding a source of light too close to the eye causes accommodation and resulting in small pupil. Pupil of newborn and old persons are smaller than young adults, hypermetropic eyes have smaller pupil while myopic eyes have larger pupil. Instillation of mydriatic or miotic change the size of the pupil as per nature of the drug used. Central sedatives cause constriction of the pupil, Central stimulants and parasympatholytic drugs dilate the pupil. Iridocyclitis and trauma cause miosis, glaucoma and optic atrophy cause mydriasis.

Abnormal pupil impart clue to lesions of:

1. Pathway for light reflex
2. Parasympathetic path
3. Sympathetic path
4. Cortical path.

The two major types of pupillary reflexes of neuro ophthalmic importance are:

1. Light reflex
2. Near reflex.

Besides these, there are a few more pupillary reflexes which do not have much neuro-ophthalmic value, they are:

1. Vagotonic
2. Vestibular
3. Orbicularis
4. Trigeminal
5. Cochlear
6. Psychosensory.

The pathway of the light reflex

To understand the pupillary reflexes, it is better to know the visual pathway and its variation in relation to path for light reflex and near reflex.

The visual pathway for each eye starts at the end organs, i.e. the rods and cones. The visual sensations are transmitted to the brain in three stages.

The three neurons (Fig. 4.1) are:

1. **The neurons of the first order** are located in the bipolar cells of the inner nuclear layer of the retina with their axons in the inner plexiform layers.
2. **The neurons of the second order** begin in the ganglion cells of the retina. The axons of these cells form the nerve fiber layer of the retina, which in turn pass into the optic nerve → chiasma → optic tract → lateral geniculate body.
3. **The neurons of the third order** begin at the lateral geniculate body and pass into the optic radiation to end in the visual cortex.

The fibers from the temporal half of each retina reach the lateral geniculate body without crossing over to the other side. The fibers arising from the nasal half cross-over to the other side at the chiasma to reach the optic tract of the other side, hence the fibers of each optic tract contains temporal fibers from one eye and nasal fibers from the opposite eye. This arrangement is continued in the lateral geniculate body and the optic radiation (Fig. 4.2).

3. **The third neuron** extends form Edinger-Westphal nucleus to **ciliary ganglion**.
4. **The fourth neuron** extends from the **ciliary ganglion to the sphincter pupillae in the iris**.

Some points worth remembering

1. A lesion of the optic tract and beyond after the fibers of light reflex (pupillomotor) have left the visual pathway will not produce pupillary change. There will be diminished vision and field change.
2. The pupillomotor fibers lie superficially in the third nerve between its exits from the brainstem and entrance in the cavernous sinus. A compressive lesion of this part of the third nerve will involve the pupil.
3. A diabetic third nerve palsy will spare the pupil.
4. In the cavernous sinus the pupillomotor fiber becomes central, hence a compressive lesion large enough to cause total third nerve palsy at this level cause pupillary changes.

The pathway of near reflex

The near reflex consists of three components. They are:

1. Constriction of pupil—**miosis**
2. Increased tone of ciliary muscles—**accommodation**
3. Contraction of medial rectus—**convergence.**

Near reflex

The near reflex path is not so precisely established as visual path or light path. **It is not a true reflex**, it is better called **synkinetic reaction**. It is a **parasympathetic path**.

The three components of near reflex are—**accommodation, convergence** and **miosis**. The components are inseparable but can be abolished individually, i.e. accommodation by plus lenses and cycloplegic; miosis by mydriatic and convergence by base out prisms.

All the component are controlled by third nerve.

The pupil of both the eyes constrict simultaneously by looking at a near object.

The reflex may be initiated ether by convergence or by accommodation.

The afferent path of convergence is—Medial rectus → Third nerve—Mesencephalic root of fifth nerve → Perlia's nucleus → Edinger-Westphal nucleus (Fig. 4.4).

The afferent path of accommodation is rods and cones (looking at a near object) → Optic nerve → Chiasma → optic tract → Parastriate area → Occipitomesencephalic tract → Perlia's nucleus → Edinger Westphal nucleus (Fig. 4.5).

The efferent path for both accommodation and convergence is common. It begins in the Edinger-Westphal nucleus, passes through the main trunk of the third nerve, pass in the lower division, from their to ciliary ganglion or accessory ganglion and end in constrictor muscle iris.

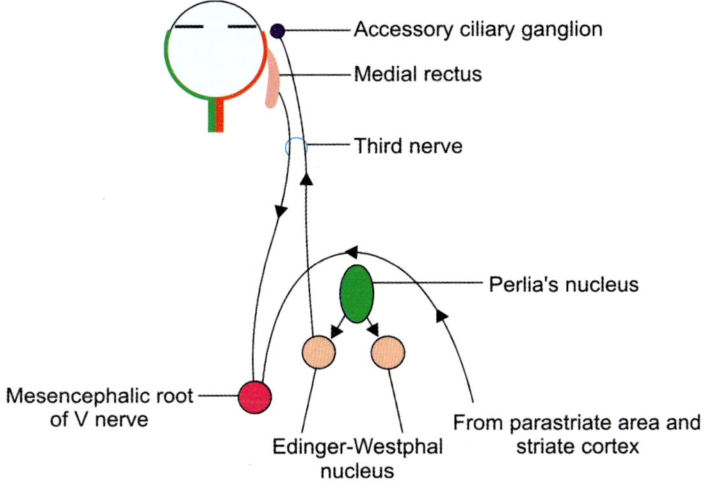

Fig. 4.4: Path of convergence

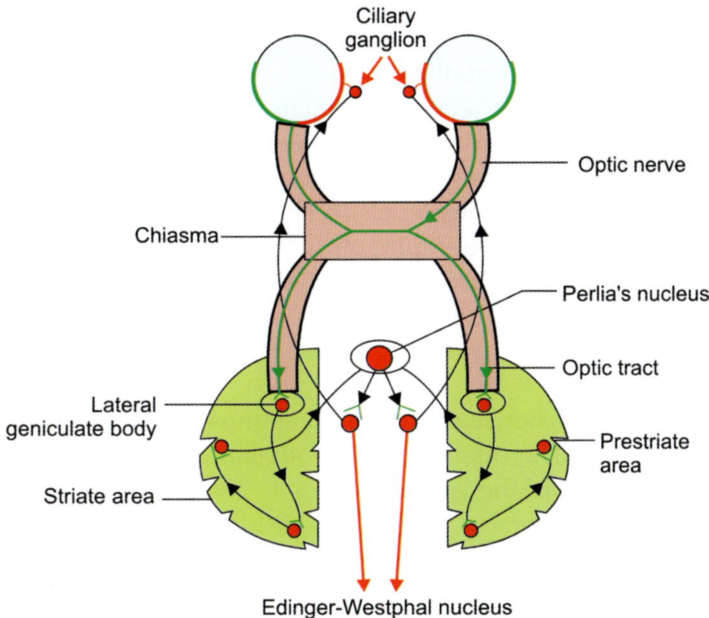

Fig. 4.5: Pathway of accommodation

The sympathetic path of pupillary reaction:

1. This path is better understood than path of near reflex.
2. It is **an adrenergic** path.

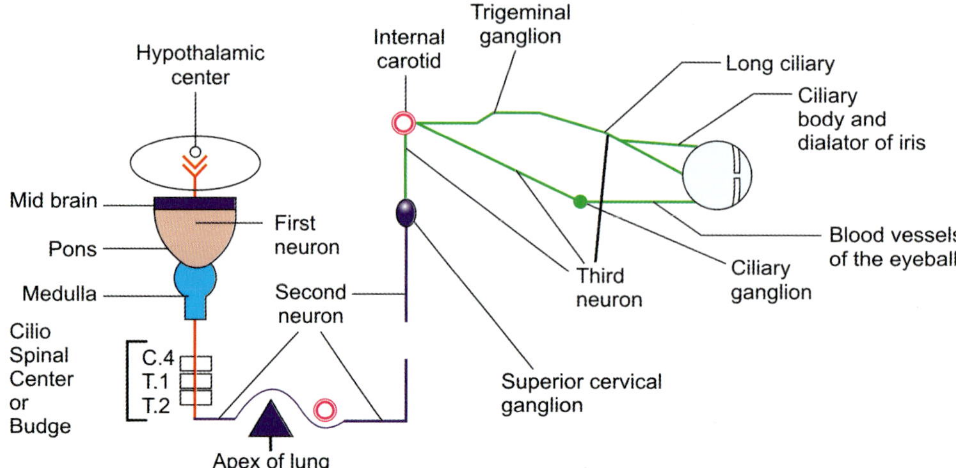

Fig. 4.6: Arrangement of sympathetic supply to the eye

3. It has a long course extending from the **hypothalamus** to the **dilator pupillae**, **Muller's muscle** and the **blood vessels** of the eye. The course of the path is like an elongated hair pin.
4. The path is **three neuron** path.
5. It contains **preganglionic** as well **postganglionic fibers** (Fig 4.6).
6. The preganglionic and postganglionic reactions behave differently to directly acting and indirectly acting adrenergic drugs. This phenomenon is used to differentiate between various levels of Horner's syndrome.
7. The direct acting drugs are—epinephrine, phenylpherine and ephedrine.
8. The indirect acting drugs are—cocaine, hydroxy amphetamine (paredrine) and 6 hydroxy dopamine.

The sympathetic path starts in the posterior hypothalamus in a **presumed to be nucleus**.

The first neuron extends between the hypothalamus and ciliospinal center of Budge at the level of C8 and T2. The fibers from hypothalamus pass through pons, medulla and intermediolateral part of the spinal cord.

The second neuron extends from center of Budge to superior cervical ganglion. During this course, the nerve passes over the apex of the lung in close proximity to subclavian artery and is liable to be injured during surgery in this area. This is the path where it may be invaded by tumor of the apex of lung.

The third neuron extends from the **superior cervical ganglion** to the dilator fibers of iris. This is a long course, which passes along the internal carotid artery to enter the cranium and reach **gasserian ganglion** to pass along the **ophthalmic division** of the fifth nerve, then to the **nasociliary** and **long ciliary nerves** to reach the ciliary body and dilators of iris. Some sympathetic fibers before reaching the eyeball pass through

Flow chart 4.1: Abnormalities of pupil: The lesion can either be in the afferent or efferent path (Fig. 4.7)

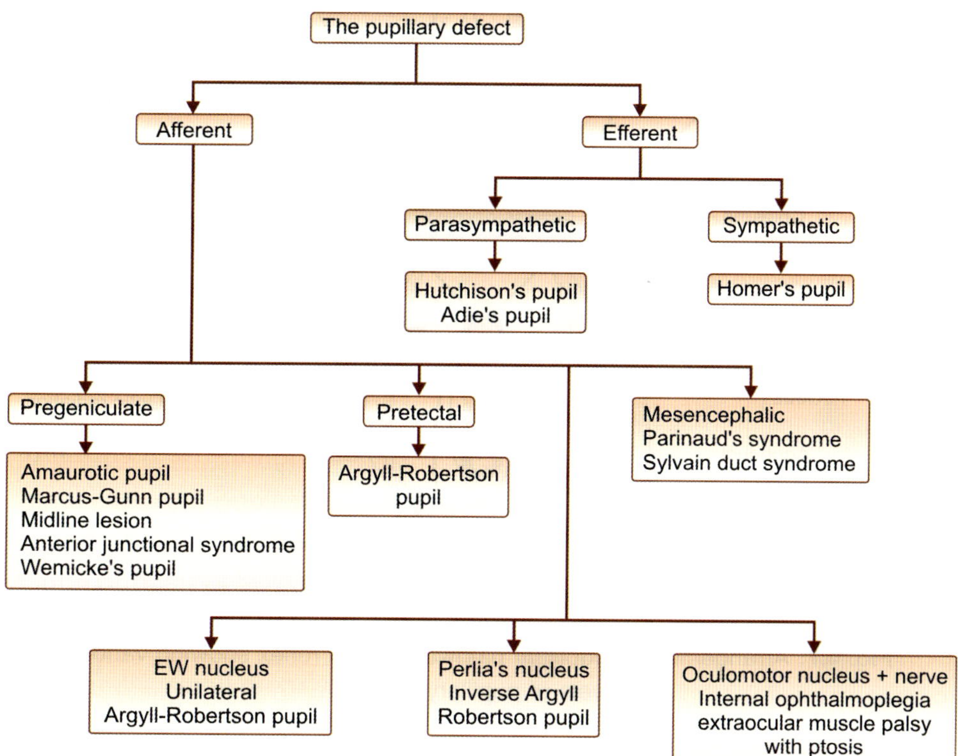

the ciliary ganglion as well they **do not relay in the ganglion**. These fibers are destined to supply **the blood vessels** of the eyeball.

The first and the second neuron constitute the preganglionic fibers. Fibers and neurons beyond are postganglionic.

Characteristic of afferent pupillary defect

1. The afferent pupillary fibers leave the visual path before the lateral geniculate body, hence lesion beyond geniculate body, do not produce changes in light reflex but vision will be defective depending upon severity with corresponding field changes (Flow chart 4.1).
2. Pupillary light reaction can be normal even in absence of vision because the afferent pupillary light fibers leave visual path anterior to lateral geniculate body.
3. Lesion of pregeniculate path or pretectal lesions produce change in light reflex.
4. The afferent conduction defect manifest as:
   i. Decreased amplitude of contraction of pupil to light.
   ii. Latency of contraction is prolonged.

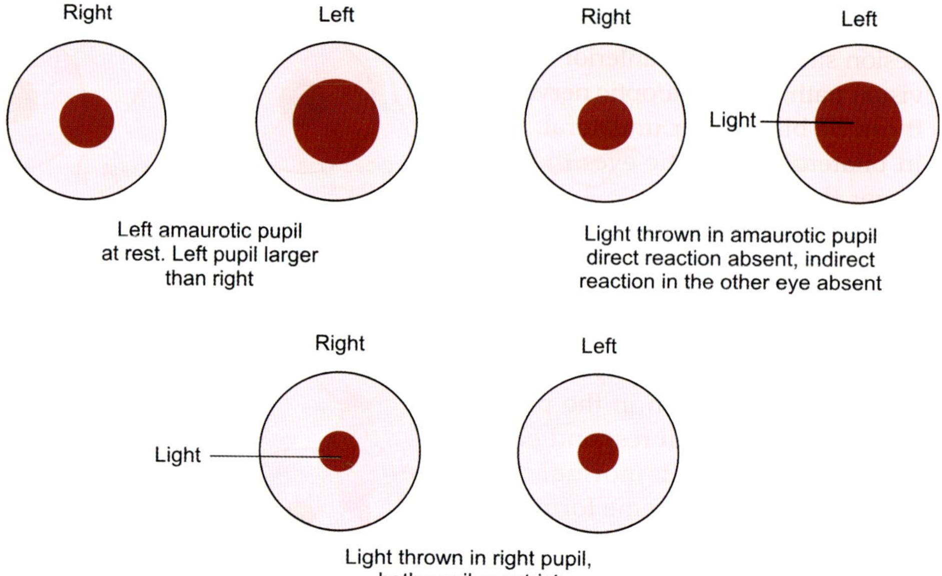

Fig. 4.9: Amaurotic pupil

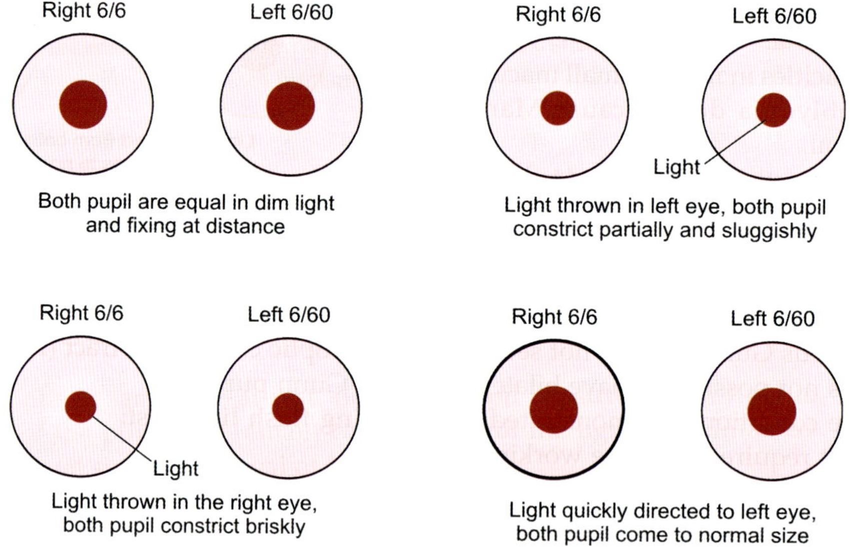

Fig. 4.10: Marcus Gunn pupil

Pupillary change in mid chiasmal lesion (Fig. 4.11)

Such a lesion interrupts the heminasal pupillary fibers leaving the temporal fibers uneffected, hence a small beam of light directed from nasal side that stimulates the

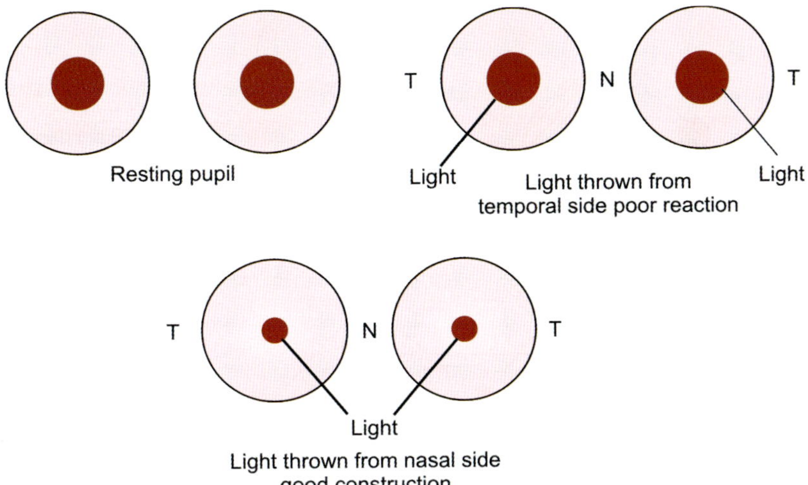

Fig. 4.11: Pupillary change in midchiasmal lesion

temporal retina causes more pupillary constriction than light thrown from temporal side.

Pupillary changes in anterior junctional lesions

In this syndrome, the optic nerve of one eye and anterior part of the chiasma on the same side are affected. Both the pupil are of the same size in this case the side of involvement, has Marcus Gunn pupil while the contralateral side has chiasmatic hemianopic pupil.

Wernicke's hemianopic pupil

This is a **rare** form of pupillary reaction which is **generally missed** unless specifically looked for. It is **difficult to elicit**. The lesion to cause Wernicke's hemianopic pupillary change is **situated in the optic tract** before the pupillary fibers have separated. The eyes are **hemianopic**, the **field defect is incongruous** and the **pupils are equal in size**. It is elicited by stimulating the seeing and nonseeing hemiretina separately by narrow bean of light. When the nonseeing retinal half is stimulated, there is either no reaction or very sluggish reaction. A lesion placed more posteriorly after the pupillary fibers have left the optic tract will cause incongruous hemianopia, diminished vision, equal pupils and no pupillary changes.

Pupillary changes in pretectal lesion (Fig. 4.12)

Pretectal lesions **cause light near dissociation**, i.e. the lesion produces defective light reflex with intact or almost intact pupillary changes for near. The visual path remains intact. This happens due to the fact that light reflex fibers reach the Edinger Westphal nucleus dorsally and the near reflex fibers are relatively ventral. The visual path is away from both. A normal eye should have brisk light reflex with brisk near reflex.

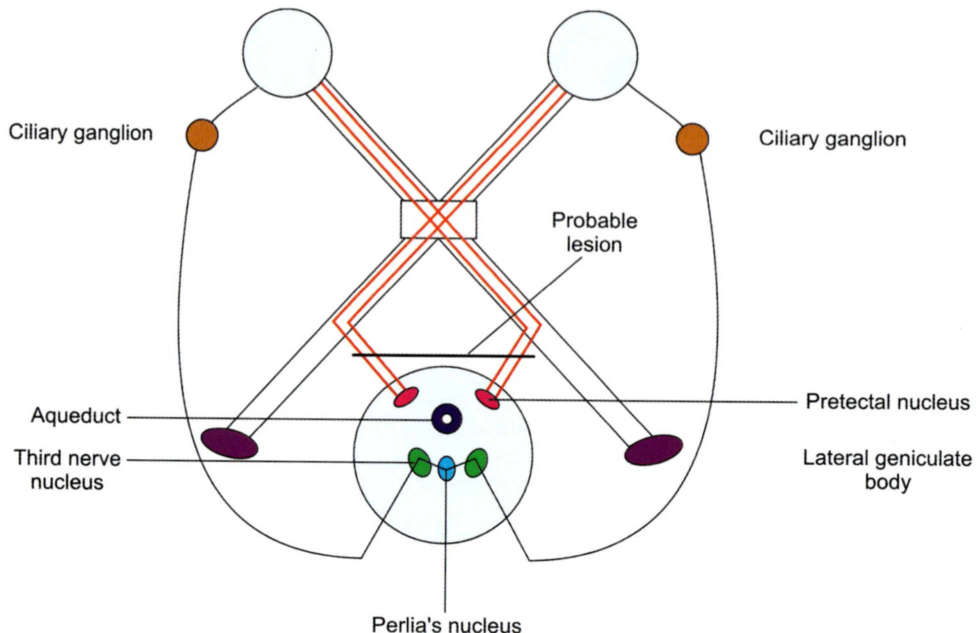

Fig. 4.12: Lesion causing typical Argyll-Robertson pupil

There is no condition where the light reflex is brisk and near reflex in defective. The reverse, i.e. absent or very poor light reflex with intact near reflex (accommodation) is called **light near dissociation**.

The lesions can be present between the pretectal nucleus and the Edinger-Westphal nucleus or more peripherally.

The causes of light near dissociation are:

1. Classical Argyll-Robertson pupil
2. Incomplete Argyll-Robertson pupil
3. Unilateral Argyll-Robertson pupil
4. Adie's pupil
5. Parinauds syndrome
6. Sylvian aqueductal syndrome
7. Long standing juvenile diabetes
8. Trauma
9. Herpes zoster
10. Aberrant regeneration of third nerve.

The systemic conditions that cause light near dissociation are:

1. Neurosyphilis
2. Juvenile diabetes

3. Pinealoma
4. Primary amyloidosis
5. Myotonic dystrophy
6. Herpes zoster

Other causes are—encephalitis, brain tumor, alcoholism, sarcoidosis.

Argyll-Robertson pupil (Fig. 4.12)

Association between Argyll Robertson pupil and neurosyphilis was so common that presence of former was almost diagnostic. With the advent of antibiotic to treat neurosyphilis the incidences has come down drastically and the condition has become rare and other causes of ARP have come to light.

Features of classical Argyll-Robertson pupil are:

1. Bilateral condition
2. Pupil are:
   i. Small
   ii. Irregular
   iii. Anisocoria
   iv. Do not dilate in dark or by mydriatic.
3. Light reflex is either absent or is very poor.
4. Accommodation reflex is brisk.
5. Vision is good.
6. Convergence is present.
7. Not associated with paralysis of extraocular muscles.
8. Patchy atrophy of iris is frequent.
9. Heterochromia of iris is seen in some cases.
10. Orbicularis reflex is intact.
11. The miosis is suspected to be due to enhanced sensitivity to cholinergic impulse.
12. The exact location of the lesion is not well settled. It is said to be due to involvement of inter nuclear fibers between the pretectal nucleus and Edinger Westphal nucleus.
13. Unilateral Argyll-Robertson pupil are less common than bilateral. They may be the incomplete form of bilateral involvement and are known to become bilateral.
14. Inverse Argyll-Robertson pupil is also rare. There is absent near reflex with defective convergence and intact light reflex. The lesion is most probably in the Perlia's nucleus.

Efferent pupillary defects

The efferent defects can be either in **parasympathetic path** or in **sympathetic path**. The lesions of parasympathetic innervations can be anywhere between the midbrain to the ciliary ganglion. The lesions cause diminished pupillary constriction to light and accommodation. The pupil is generally large. It may involve the ciliary body also.

The examples of parasympathetic pupillary changes are:

1. Hutchinson's pupil
2. Adie's pupil.

Horner's syndrome is the only one condition that produce sympathetic efferent pupillary defect.

Hutchinson's pupil

Hutchinson's pupil (pupil of coma) is an important sign of fast increasing intracranial pressure with deteriorating consciousness. This is due to **internal ophthalmoplegia** associated with compressive lesions of the third nerve. As the intracranial pressure rises the uncus of the temporal lobe is pushed down, and the third nerves is compressed against either the pteroclinoid ligament or dorsum sella. The fine pupillomotor fibers in the third nerve, which are placed on the periphery and have thin myelination are more sensitive to increasing pressure. Hence they are the first to be involved in increased intracranial pressure.

The sequence of changes are:

1. The pupil on the side of the intracranial lesion is miotic due to irritations of the third nerve fibers (Fig. 4.13).
2. As the pressure increase this pupil dilates.
3. As the pressure still increases the other pupil follows the same sequence.
4. Ultimately both the pupils dilate.
5. The pupillary changes may revert if a timely decompression is done.

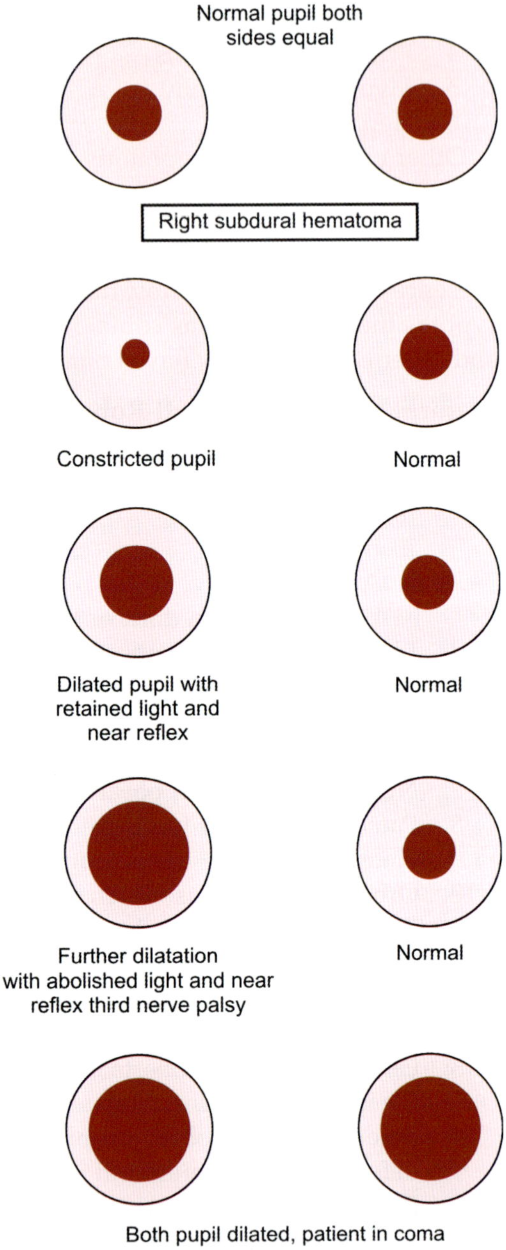

Fig. 4.13: Various stages of Hutchinson's pupil

Holmes Adie's pupil (Tonic pupil)

In contrast to Hutchinson's pupil, the Adie's pupil is a benign condition.

Characteristics of Holmes Adie's pupil

1. The conditions is **generally unilateral**.
2. Some cases do become bilateral over years.
3. It is seen in second to third decade.
4. There is no predilection for side involved.
5. **Women** are affected more than men in a ratio 7:3.
6. The **pupil is large**.
7. The patient may not be aware of it's presence but occasionally may complain of unilateral blurred far as well as near vision due to paralysis of accommodation.
8. The pupil either does not react to light or reacts slowly.
9. The pupils constrict slowly to prolonged near vision and dilates equally slowly when near efforts no more in play.
10. The iris may show segmental paralysis.
11. The iris shows vermiform movement on slit lamp.
12. The pupil is **supersensitive** to cholinergic drugs. Normal pupil does not constrict to instillation of 0.125% pilocarpine or 2.5% methacholine. The Adie's pupil constricts in half an hour following instillation of either of the drugs.
13. The tonic pupil dilates with mydriatic well.
14. The consensual reflex to the contralateral eyes is present.
15. The lesion is either in the **ciliary ganglion** or **short ciliary nerves**.
16. Adie's pupil with diminished deep tendon reflexes is called Adie's syndrome.
17. **Riley-Day syndrome** is seen in children with congenital dysautonomia. The pupil is tonic but super sensitive to weak solution of methacholine.

The exact cause of tonic pupil is not known. Most of the time it is considered idiopathic. **Other causes** too have been attributed to the condition, they are: Viral infection, trauma to ciliary ganglion, radiation, aberrant regeneration of third nerve, ischemic episodes of vessels in the orbit.

Sympathetic efferent pupillary change

Only Horner's syndrome causes sympathetic efferent pupillary defect. Unlike Adie's pupil that has only pupillary changes, Horner's syndrome has more manifestation than pupillary changes.

It can be **congenital** (rare) or **acquired** (common). It can be **partial** or **total**. Partial Horner's syndrome is more common than total.

Characteristic of Horner's syndrome are:

1. It is **unilateral** condition.
2. Changes in **lids** consist of:
   i. Mild ptosis of upper lid not more than 2 mm.
   ii. **Upside down ptosis of lower lid:** The lower lid margin rises by one to two millimeters.

iii. Interpalpebral aperture is narrow. **This gives an appearance of enophthalmos.**

3. **Globe:** There may be true retractions of globe.
4. **Pupil:**
   i. Miosis—mild
   ii. Anisocoria—more for dark, painful stimulus or sudden loud sound
   iii. Light near reflexes is maintained
   iv. Pupil does not dilate with cocaine, dilation by hydroxy amphetamine and epinephrine depends upon the level of the lesion.
5. Vision—normal.
6. Movement of the globe:
   i. Horner's syndrome without other neurological involvement have normal range of movement of extraocular muscle.
   ii. Horner's syndrome with neurological involvement have defective ocular movement in the form of:
      i. Midbrain **Fovile's** lateral medullary syndrome.
         (Posterior inferior cerebellar artery syndrome) that consists of:
         a. Horner's syndrome
         b. Ipsilateral sixth nerve weakness
         c. Ipsilateral facial analgesia
         d. Loss of taste in anterior 2/3rd of tongue
         e. Ipsilateral facial weakness
         f. Ipsilateral hearing loss
         g. The lesions is at the level of dorsal pons.
      ii. **Raeder's para trigeminal** syndrome: Pain in the distribution of first and second division of trigeminal along with Horner's syndrome on the same side, seen in middle-aged males, mostly due to migraineous dilation of internal carotid.
      iii. **Wallenberg's syndrome**
         a. Horner's syndrome
         b. Facial pain and hypoesthesia on the same side
         c. Ipsilateral ninth, tenth and eleventh cranial nerve palsy
         d. Cerebellar ataxia.
         The lesion is at the level of tagmentum of medulla.
      iv. **Cavernous sinus lesion**
         a. Horner's syndrome
         b. Ipsilateral third, fourth and fifth nerve palsy.
         c. Loss of sensation on the distribution of first and second division of trigeminal nerve.
7. The condition is generally painless unless associated with Raeder's para-trigeminal syndrome or Wallenberg's syndrome.

8. Anhidrosis (anhidrosis) on the same side of the face, unless the lesion is below the bifurcations of common carotid.
9. Warm dry skin of the face on the same side.
10. Dilatation of conjunctival vessels.
11. Ocular hypotony.
12. Increased accommodation.
13. Heterochromia of the iris (only in congenital Horner's syndrome)
14. The lesion of the Horner's syndrome can be anywhere between the hypothalamus to the orbit.

Localizing the level of the lesion

Clinical presentation and response to pharmacological tests depend upon the level of the lesion.

The level of the lesions have been clinically divided into:

i. **Central**, when the lesion is either in the brainstem or cervical spinal cord.
ii. **Preganglionic**, the lesion is in the chest or in the neck.
iii. **Postganglionic**, the lesion is above the superior cervical ganglion that is situated at the level of transverse process of C1 and C2.

The central and preganglionic lesions carry poor prognosis of life. The post-ganglionic lesions are benign, mostly vascular and are not threat to life.

Steps of localizing the lesion

1. Clinical evaluation:
   i. Anisocoria more in dark.
   ii. Absence of anhydrosis means that the lesion is above the bifurcations of the common carotid hence it is postganglionic and involves the third neuron.
   iii. Presence of neurological features of midbrain syndrome means that the lesions is central and preganglionic.
2. Pharmacological: The pharmacological test is divided into two parts:
   i. Screening for presence of Horner's syndrome
   ii. Confirming the level of the lesion.

The pharmacological basic of the test are:

a. There is loss of sympathetic neurotransmitter at the synapse.
b. The adrenergic receptors in the dilator muscles of the iris become sensitive to sympathomimetic amines.
c. In central and preganglionic lesions, such sensitivity is absent.

The drugs used are:

1. Cocaine—5%-10%
2. Epinephrine—1:1000 (0.001%)
3. Phenylepherine—10%
4. Hydroxy amphetamine—10%

To conduct the test **the drug should be instilled in both the eyes**. The noneffected eye serves as control.

The first drug to be tested should be cocaine.

There should be a gap of at least 48 hours between instillation of cocaine and other drugs.

Cocaine test

One drop of 5% cocaine is instilled in each eye. Second drop is repeated after one minute. The result is seen after 45 minutes.

Cocaine dilates the normal pupil but not the pupil of Horner's syndrome. Non-dilatation of pupil confirms presence of Horner's syndrome because cocaine acts only in presence of intact sympathetic path.

Hydroxy amphetamine (paredrine)

One percent paredrine is instilled in each eye and repeated after few minutes; both pupils are observed for size. If both the pupil dilates, the smaller pupil has Horner's syndrome of first or second neuron. If the small pupil does not dilate, it has Horner's syndrome of third neuron. In short paredrine will dilate the pupil in preganglionic lesion. The test is not reliable in congenital Horner's syndrome.

Epinephrine will not dilate pupil of central type of Horner's syndrome, poorly dilate pupil in preganglionic lesions and widely dilate pupil in postganglionic lesion.

Phenylephrine 10% will dilate the pupil in all lesions, least in central, moderate in preganglionic and best in postganglionic lesion.

Other investigations

X-ray, CT of chest and neck to exclude apical and mediastinal growth in adults and neuroblastoma in children.

Treatment

Horner's syndrome itself does not require any treatment but life threatening conditions like midbrain stroke, intracranial tumors, malignancy of lung, neuroblastoma require specialized management.

Reverse Horner's syndrome

Irritation of oculosympathetic system anywhere between the hypothalamus and eye will produce a condition of **lid retraction** mostly the upper lid, the lower lid is minimally effected, **mydriasis** and **exophthalmos**, constriction of conjunctival vessel, excessive sweating and cold skin. Same effect in milder form can be caused by instillation of 10% phenylphrine in persons with sympathetic over activity. The condition does not require any treatment. Lid retraction may be corrected by partial removal of Muller's muscle (Fig. 4.14).

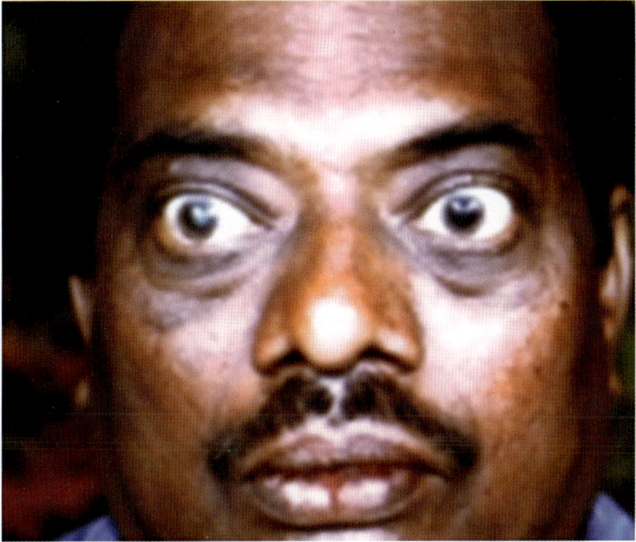

Fig. 4.14: Lid retract due to drugs mydriasis

Spasms of the pupil

The pupil may become **spastic** and **miotic** or **spastic** and **mydriatic** due to increased tone of sphincter pupillary or dilator pupillary. In both the instances light reflex is retained.

Causes of spastic miosis are:

1. Traumatic miosis
2. Prolonged use of miotics
3. Horner's syndrome
4. Meningitis and encephalitis
5. Pontine hemorrhage
6. Hemorrhage in third ventricle.

Causes of spastic mydriasis are:

1. Traumatic mydriasis
2. Use of parasympatholytic agent (both light and near reflexes are lost)
3. Mediastinal and pulmonary tumors
4. Aneurysm of aorta.

Pharmacological differentiation of fixed dilated pupil (Flow Chart 4.2).
Sometimes, it is difficult to find out the cause of pupillary dilatation.
The following scheme is helpful:

Paradoxical pupil

This is a rare phenomenon of unknown origin where the pupil constricts in dark. The probable cause are: Achromatopsia congenital stationary night

Flow chart 4.2: Pharmacological differentiation of fixed dilated pupil

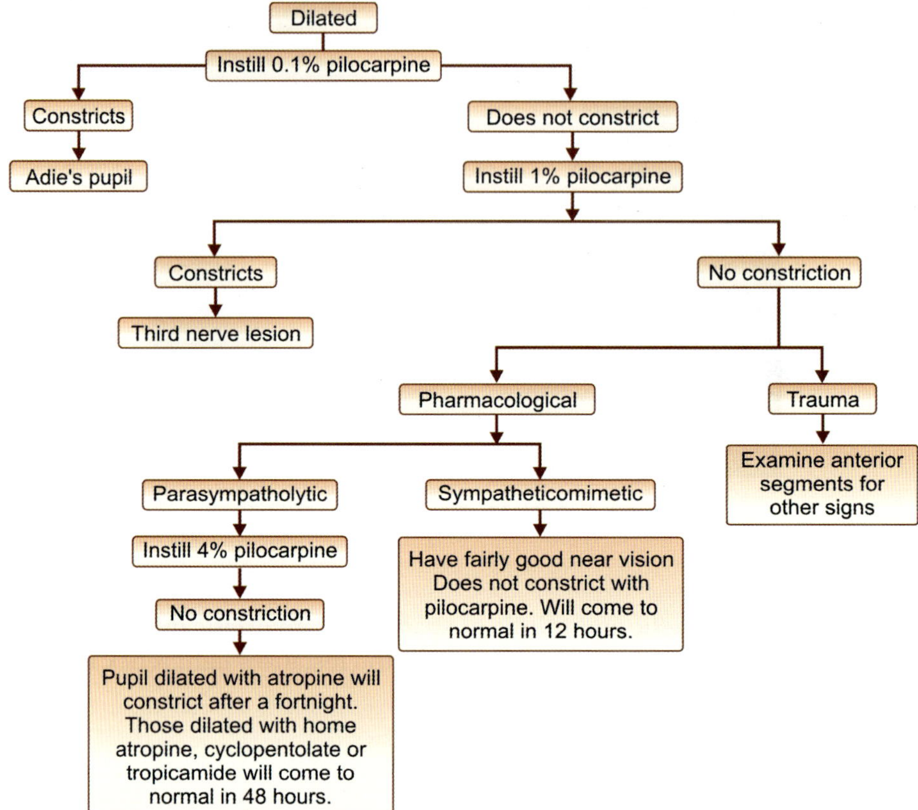

blindness, optic nerve hypoplasia or coloboma, albinism retinitis pigmentosa, macular dystrophy.

BIBLIOGRAPHY

1. Denniston AKO, Murry PI. Oxford Handbook of Ophthalmology, 1st edn, Oxford University Press, New Delhi 2007.
2. Gilman S. New man SW. The autonomic nervous system in Mante and Gatz's. Essentials of Clinical Neuroanatomy and Neurophysiology, 7th edn, Jaypee Brothers Medical Publishers, New Delhi 1980;182-86.
3. Harihara Subramanian N. Pupil and its reaction in Neuro-ophthalmology. 1st edn. Natchiar G (Eds). Arvind Eye Hospital, Maduri 4-13.
4. Karna S. Pupil evaluation in step by step neuro-ophthalmology. 1st edn, Jaypee Brothers Medical Publishers, New Delhi 2006;72.
5. Kumar SM. Neuro-ophthalmology, 4th edn, Arvind Eye Hospital, Maduari, 2007.
6. Martin LJ. Pupillary abnormalities in pediatric ophthalmology, Vol-2, 2nd edn. Harley RD (Eds). WB Saunders company Philadelphia 1982;783-88.

7. Nichols EB. Evaluation of autonomic denervation in textbook of ophthalmology. 9th edn. Scheie HG and Albert DM (Edn). WB Saunders company Philadelphia 1977; 144-46.
8. Singh Inderbir. Autonomic nerve supply of some important organs. In textbook of human neuroanatomy. 6th edn, Jaypee Brothers Medical Publishers, New Delhi 2002;243-45.
9. Thompson HS, et al. Unequal pupils. A flow chart for sorting out anisocoria. Sur oph 1976; 21:45-48.

5 Neuro-ophthalmic Disorders of the Lids

The lids have two functions

1. Opening of the eye, i.e. widen up of the interpalpebral fissure from zero to widest possible width. This function is essential for vision. It keeps the pupillary area exposed. The other purpose is to let evaporation occur from the corneal and conjunctival surface, this keeps the cornea cool and also helps evaporate part of the tear. The widening of the interpalpebral fissure is brought about by **levator palpheral superior** and **Muller's muscle** via *third nerve* and *cervical sympathetic* respectively.
2. Closing of the lids, i.e. narrowing of the interpalpebral fissure from maxim to zero width. The main purpose is protective. This also helps in spreading of the tears. This is brought by **orbicularis** via *seventh nerve*. The two functions of movements of the lids are diagonally opposite to each other.

In normal person, there is an equilibrium between the protractors and the retractors.

1. The **retractors** of the lids are—**the levator** and the **Muller's muscle**.
2. **The protractor** of the lid is *orbicularis*.

When the eyes open, the force closing the lids is lowest while the eyes are closed, the tone of the levator and the Muller's muscles are minimal.

Break down of any of the two kinetic functions due to neurological lesions produces neuro-ophthalmic manifestation of disorders of the lids.

The lesions can be **central** or **peripheral**. They can be due to lesions of:

1. *Cranial nerves*
   - Third nerve—Ptosis and synkinetic movements of the lid.
   - Seventh nerve—Lagophthalmos
2. *Oculosympathetic*
   - Horner's syndrome
   - Lid retraction
3. *Central*
   - Cortical ptosis
   - Supranuclear facial palsy
   - Blepharospasm
   - Decreased blinking

The cranial nerve lesions of the lids can be:

1. Supranuclear
2. Nuclear

3. Fascicular
4. Basilar
5. Trunk

The lesions of the **cervical sympathetic** causing lid anomalies can be anywhere from **hypothalamus** to **terminal ends** of the sympathetic chain. They are generally unilateral (see Fig. 4.6).

Some peculiarities of nerve supply to the lid:

1. Levator is the only muscle that has **independent representation in cerebral cortex** hence it is possible to have isolated ptosis.
2. Supranuclear control of lid opening is through **corticobulbar** and **extra-pyramidal tracts**.
3. Specified areas in temporal, frontal and occipital, cortex are also associated with mechanism of lid opening.
4. The peripheral control of lid opening is through third nerve and assisted by oculosympathetic.
5. Both levators are supplied by a **central caudal nucleus** hence nuclear lesion of third nerve causes **bilateral ptosis**.
6. The levator shares a common twig with **superior rectus** hence it is common for superior rectus palsy to be associated with ptosis.
7. Neurological ptosis need not be associated with paralysis of other extraocular muscles. Causes of such isolated ptosis are selected lesion of caudal nucleus of third nerve and supranuclear lesions.
8. Proximity of the caudal nucleus of the fourth nerve nucleus may cause superior oblique palsy with nuclear ptosis.
9. Once the fibers have left the nucleus of third nerve, the lesions are unilateral and the ptosis is generally associated with paralysis of other muscles supplied by third nerve.
10. The lesions in cavernous sinus are associated with palsy of other muscles.
11. The movements of the upper lids are governed by **Herings law**, hence they are identical and coordinated.
12. There may be contralateral widening of interpalpebral aperture in an attempt to lift the ptotic lid of neurological cause. This is due to Hering's law of equal innervations.
13. The **oculosympathetic** supplies only **Muller's muscle** in the upper lid and its counterpart in the lower lid.
14. The lid closure is controlled by bilateral corticobulbar and extrapyramidal tracts.
15. The **supranuclear lesion of seventh nerve** causes the weakness of lower two third of contralateral face and lower lid.
16. The peripheral control of the lid closure is through VII nerve trunk.
17. The fibers of seventh nerve encircle the sixth nerve nucleus partly. Lesions of the sixth nerve in the pons at this level involves ipsilateral seventh nerve causing widening of palpebral fissure.

18. Lesions of oculosympathetic do not involve closure of the eyelids.
19. The basal lesion of the seventh nerve may involve the eighth nerves also.
20. The central lesions have little effect on the orbicularis.

Neurological lesion resulting in difficulty in opening the lid are:

1. **Paralytic ptosis**
   i. Unilateral/Bilateral
   ii. Isolated/Associated in the paralysis of other muscles.
   iii. Associated with jaw winking.
2. Ptosis of Horner's syndrome
3. Myogenic ptosis
4. Blepharospasm/hemifacial spam

The neurological ptosis

The two mechanisms by which neurological ptosis is produced are:

1. Lesions of **third nerve** that can **be supranuclear, fascicular, basal** or **trunk lesion**.
2. Lesions of **cervical sympathetic**.
3. **Mixed** (rare) lesions of cavernous sinus.

Ptosis of third nerve origin

Supranuclear ptosis: Supranuclear lesions are relatively **infrequent**. They can be caused by many etiological factors, i.e. *infection, trauma, raised intracranial pressure,* vascular **thrombosis** or **hemorrhagic**. The pathology lies in the area of **posterior commissure**.

Characteristics of supranuclear ptosis are:

1. The ptosis is generally **mild**.
2. It is **generally bilateral** and **symmetric**, rarely unilateral.
3. Ptosis develops before the onset of unilateral paralysis of extraocular muscles.
4. It is frequently associated with **difficulty in upward gaze** and **miosis**, less commonly **horizontal gaze** disorder.
5. **Cortical ptosis** is unilateral ptosis. If the pupil is dilated, the lesion is in the temporal lobe.

Nuclear

Ptosis due to nuclear lesion is also **rare**. It is **bilateral**, **symmetric**, **mild** and **associated with superior rectus palsy** because both levators are supplied by single caudal nucleus. Each superior rectus is supplied by opposite third nerve nucleus. As the caudal nucleus of levator is near the nucleus of fourth, it is possible to have fourth nerve palsy, along with nuclear ptosis, fourth nerve may be spared in partial nuclear third nerve lesion.

Basal

Ptosis due to basal lesions are associated with **widespread third nerve palsy** along with lesions of **fifth, sixth, seventh** and **eighth cranial nerves**. Basal lesions are

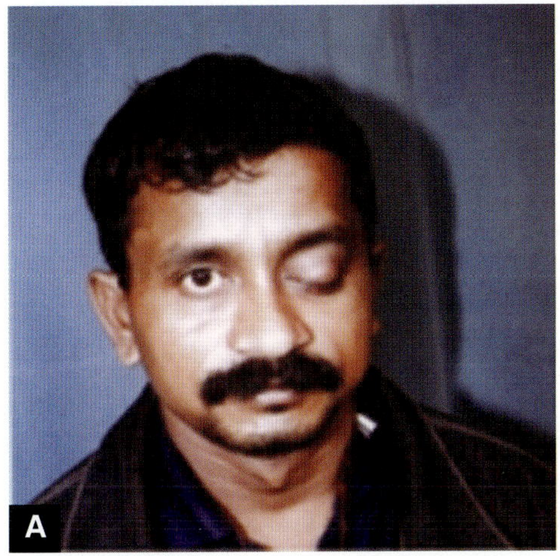

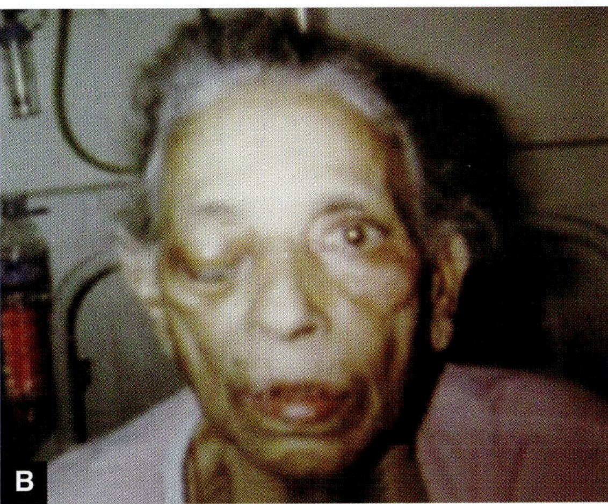

Figs 5.1A and B: Neurological ptosis. A. Total ophthalmoplegia. B. Diabetic third nerve palsy

associated with lesions of **cortiospinal tract**, **red nucleus**, and **superior cerebellar peduncle**.

Trunk

The ptosis due to lesions of the third nerve is seen in the *cavernous sinus, superior orbital* **fissure**, **orbital apex**. It is generally associated with other cranial nerves sub-serving the ocular muscles and the fifth nerve (Figs 5.1A and B).

Ptosis of Horner's syndrome (Sympathetic ptosis)

Horner's syndrome is caused due to lesion of **cervical sympathetic chain** from hypothalamus to twigs to the ciliary ganglion. The incidence is **far less common** than ptosis due to third nerve lesion. The syndrome can be **congenital** or **acquired**, seen at **any age** but is **more common in adults**. It is an **unilateral** disorder.

The characteristics of sympathetic ptosis are:

1. The ptosis is mild, never more than 1 mm to 3 mm.
2. The **lid fold** is retained.
3. There is **no lid lag**.
4. The lower lid is elevated from its normal position. This is called **upside down ptosis**.
5. Drooping of upper lid along with raising of lower lid margin accentuate the narrowing of interpalpebral fissure. This gives an impression of **relative enophthalmos**.
6. The ptosis is not affected by exercise.
7. Ptosis is not modified by Tensilon test.

Other features of Horner's syndrome that are present with sympathetic ptosis are (see Chapter 4)—

1. Real enophthalmos
2. Miosis—Pupil dilates less fast in dark. Reacts equally to light and fix kerning accommodation.
3. Anisocoria is most marked in dim light.
4. Anhydrosis (anhidrosis)
5. Dilatation of conjunctival vessels.
6. Warmth of the skin of face and lid on the affected side.
7. Lowered intraocular pressure
8. Hypochromia of the iris (mostly seen in congenital Horner's syndrome)
9. Brittle and dry hair.
10. Increased amplitude of accommodation.

The lesions can be

1. Central
2. Preganglionic
3. Postganglionic

The central lesions are seen either in the **brain Stem** or in the **spinal cord**.

The preganglionic lesions are found either in the **neck** or **apex of the lung**.

The postganglionic lesions are widely spread over orbit, cavernous sinus, in the middle ear or in the internal carotid artery.

The therapeutic test are generally not useful for management for which exact location and nature of the lesions should be found out by MRI of brain spinal cord, neck and orbit.

Other investigations employed are CT thorax and carotid Doppler.

The commonly used therapeutic tests to find out the level of the lesion in the sympathetic chain are:

1. **Cocaine test**—Pupil does not dilate with cocaine irrespective of the neuron involved.
2. **Paredrine** (Hydroxyamphetamine)—Paredrine test differentiates third neuron lesion from first and second.
3. There is no pharmacological test that can differentiate lesion of first neuron from lesion of second neuron.

Myogenic ptosis

It is better to call them **neuromuscular ptosis**. The ptosis due to neuromuscular disorders can be put in **three broad groups**.

1. Due to myoneural transmission defect at neuromuscular junction.
2. Due to muscular dystrophies where the fault lies in muscle mass itself, i.e. chronic progressive external ophthalmoplegia, myotonic dystrophy, congenital and variants of the above condition.
3. Dysthyroid ocular myopathy.

Myasthenia

Myasthenia is one of the most common causes of **nonneurogenic ptosis** which may initially be diagnosed as neurogenic ptosis in **all ages** in **both sexes** but **women are twice more prone than men**. It may be seen in **neonates** if the mother has myasthenia. In neonates, the respiratory distress and difficulty in swallowing are main features. Myasthenia is a **progressive, chronic disease**. The two initial symptoms are **diplopia** and **narrowing of the interpalpebral fissure** both of which become worse in the evening after days work.

All the cases of diplopia that elude neurological tests with or without ptosis with normal pupil should be considered to be myasthenia unless proved otherwise.

In spite of involvement of many extraocular muscles and muscles of trunk and extremities, there are **no abnormal reflexes. Sensations are normal**. The muscles do not develop atrophic changes. The disease has subacute onset and is an **autoimmune disease**. Antibodies are formed against acetylcholine.

The disease is **self-limiting** in some persons. There is marked variation in muscle involvement even during the same day. It may be associated with **thyroid eye disease**. Association of *thymoma* is frequent. **Familial incidence is seen in 5% cases**. Association of systemic collagen vascular disease are frequent.

Ocular involvements are the main features in 90% of cases. About two third of the patients may be diagnosed on the basis of ocular symptoms of **ptosis** and/or **diplopia.** 80% of persons with ocular involvement are likely to develop paralysis of other skeletal muscles within first two years of onset. Involvement of skeletal muscles after two years is less common so a small group of patients will have only ocular involvement in myasthenia.

Lids

Drooping of lids may be the first sign of myasthenia. It **begins in one eye**, the other may follow, the ptosis in two eyes is **asymmetric**. The severity of ptosis may range from **few millimeters to total ptosis**. In case of unilateral ptosis, the other lid may be lifted as per Herings law. The ptosis may **change sides,** i.e. lid of one eye may droop first, then recover and the other eye may develop the ptosis. The extent of droop may change not only in days but in hours. The drooping is minimal in the morning and gradually increase as the hours pass and may become worse by end of the day. **Variability of the ptosis is demonstrated by the following tests:**

1. *Fatigue tests*

   Note the position of the lid in relation to the upper limbus. Ask the patient to walk briskly for few minutes and observe the position of the lid in relation to upper limbus. In proved case of myasthenia, the effected lid will show enhanced drooping. The contralateral IPA may widen.

2. *Cogan lid twitch*
   Ask the patient to look down for 10 to 15 seconds and then bring the eye to the primary position. This causes **fine tremor** like twitching in the upper lid. The upper lid may become higher than normal only to sag to a ptotic position.
3. *Lid fatigue*
   Sustained up gaze worsens the ptosis.
4. *Cold test*
   Position of the lid is noted in relation to upper limbus. An ice cube is applied to the ptotic lid for two minutes and then removed. This results in elevation of the lid. As the temperature of the lid returns to normal, the lid gradually comes down. Application of heat lowers the lid marginally.
5. *Pharmacological tests*
   - Tensilon test
   - Prostigmine test
   - Therapeutic trial by oral prostigmine and pyridostigmine.

Tensilon test is a sensitive test to clinch the diagnosis of myasthenia but is not infallible. There may be **false negative** or **false positive** results.

Tensilon (edrophonium) is available in multidose vial containing 10 mg edrophonium hydrochloride per ml.

The steps of the test consist of:

1. Evaluate and photographically document the ptosis.
2. Measure diplopia by appropriate test.
3. Get the patients cardiovascular system evaluated before the test.
4. It is better if the test is carried out by a trained anesthetist.
5. Explain the procedure to the patient, take a written consent.
6. 0.6 ml of injectable atropine is given intravenous.
7. After 5 minutes, 0.2 ml of tensilon is injected intravenously through an intravenous drip and flushed with 1ml of saline. Observes the position of the lid and assess lessening or abolision of diplopia, improvement in ptosis is taken as positive result confirming myasthenia (Figs 5.2A and B).
8. If no improvement is noticed, another 0.8 ml of tensilon is injected in the same way and look for improvement. If no improvement occurs, the test is said to be negative.

There may be following variations:

1. Worsening of ptosis and tropia.
2. The contralateral eye develops ptosis.
3. If there is ptosis in the contralateral eye, it becomes worse.
4. The hypertropia changes side, i.e. right hypertropia becomes left and vice versa.

The variations noted above are seen in nonmyasthenia patients.

In absence of tensilon, the test may be done by injecting prostigmine with usual precautions.

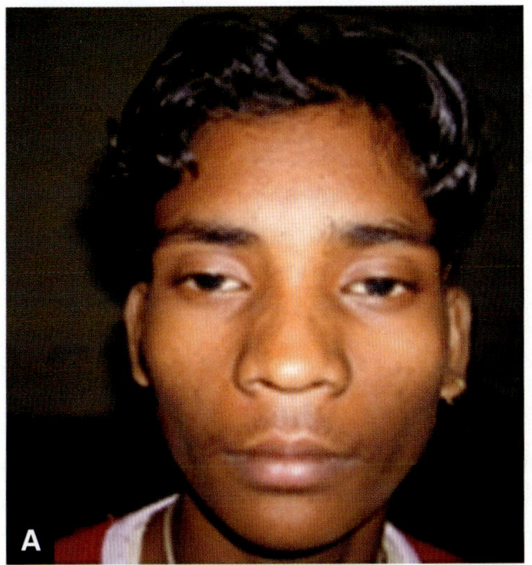
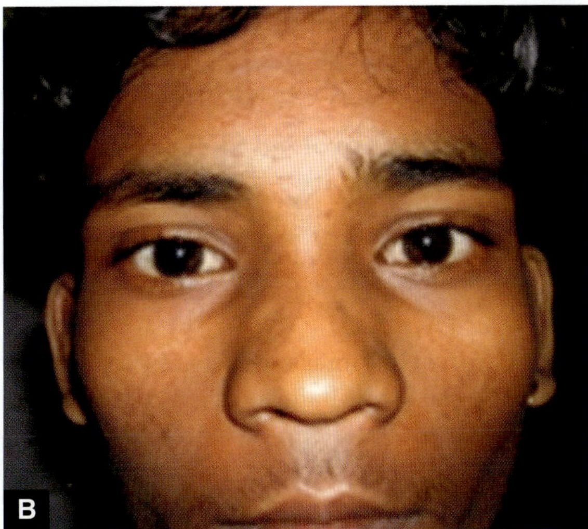

Figs 5.2A and B: Myasthenic ptosis. A. Before injection of prostigmine. B. Abolition of ptosis after injection of prostigmine

Extraocular muscles

1. **Orbicularis** is invariably involved but missed because either it is not tested or under action of orbicularis is neutralized by associated ptosis. Exposure of the cornea is rare, only sign of orbicularis involvement may be moderate ectropion of lower lid.
2. **Other extraocular muscle**—Involvement of other extraocular muscles do not follow any fixed pattern. Limitation of **upward gaze** may be the first clue. Under action of extraocular muscles may be limited to only one muscle or all muscles. Like ptosis the tropia may change direction as well as side. The ensuing paralytic squint may be mistaken as **central gaze palsy, internuclear ophthalmoplegia** and **thyroid eye disease**.

   On a long run, the eyes pass into a chronic state called **fixed form**. It may show **bilateral**, **symmetric ophthalmoplegia with ptosis** which gives negative tensilon test and **confusing forced duction test**. At this stage, the condition is confused with **chronic progressive external ophthalmoplegia**.
3. *Intraocular muscles are always spared* in myasthenia. **The pupillary reaction is brisk** both to light and accommodation. Convergence may be defective due to medial rectus involvement. **The accommodation may be accentuated**.
4. **Nystagmus**—Myasthenoid nystagmus too has been reported.

Skeletal muscles

Many of the skeletal muscles are involved in myasthenia. The relatively smaller muscles of face, neck, and throat are involved more severely and more frequently than larger muscles of limb though they are not always spared. The condition is worsened by infection, excitement, prolonged exercise, menstruation and many drugs. **Quinine** is one of the commonly used drug that worsens myasthenia.

The commonly involved skeletal muscles are:

- **Muscles of face**—This smoothens the forehead creases, gives a mask like appearance and attempt to smile evokes a snarling appearance.
- **Muscles of palate, larynx and pharynx**—Paralysis of these muscles result in regurgitation of food, difficulty in swallowing, distressed breathing and nasal voice.
- **Paralysis of masseters** leads to drooping of the lower jaw.
- Tongue has bilateral furrow.

Differential diagnosis consists of many conditions that are associated with drooping of the lids with extraocular muscle palsy. They are **thyroid eye disease, chronic progressive external ophthalmoplegia, central gaze palsy, internuclear ophthalmoplegia and botulinum toxin**.

Diagnosis

A well-established case of myasthenia is not difficult to diagnose. The diagnosis is made on the basis of history of variable ptosis and diplopia, involvement of orbicularis, sparing of pupil and accommodation.

The diagnosis is confirmed by tensilon test, therapeutic trail by anticholinesterase drugs.

Treatment

1. All cases do not require treatment. Some cases resolve without treatment but there may be recurrence.
2. Most of the cases progress and require management.
3. Ocular components respond poorly to anticholinesterase drugs.
4. The treatment can be divided into:
   i. Systemic drug therapy.
   ii. Ocular therapy.
   iii. Thymectomy.

Drug therapy in myasthenia

1. **Anticholinesterase drugs** form the first line of treatment. Most commonly used drug is *pyridostigmine*. Its effect starts within **30 minutes** but the effect passes off within **3 hours**. This requires it to be administered frequently. The usual dose for adults is 60 mg every four hours during waking hours. The night dose should be a sustained release tablet. Less effective drug is *neostigmine* (prostigmine) available as 15 mg tablet also given every four hourly. The frequency and strength of both the drugs is titrated clinically. It is better to administer an **parasympatholytic** drug alongwith to reduce side effects of anticholinesterase drugs.

2. **Corticosteroids**—Oral steroids are indicated in those patients who do not respond to anticholinesterase drugs. The regime commonly followed is to start a low dose daily initially and increase the dose till the best results are reached. Then the dose is shifted to alternate day schedule and tapered over weeks.
   - **Immunosuppressive drugs**—Azathioprine is used in cases that are resistant to anticholinesterase and steroid. It takes few months to be effective. Other immunosuppressive drugs used are cyclophosphamide and cyclosporine.

Ocular management

Prisms may be given to overcome diplopia however changing pattern and severity of diplopia make their use difficult. In troublesome diplopia, the best alternative is occlusion. The patient on long run learns to close one eye to avoid diplopia.

Surgery

Squint surgery is tried only in case where there is fixed pattern of diplopia that is stable for at least one year.

Thymectomy

Thymectomy may help adults, role of thymectomy in children is not well-established. It does not have much benefit in ocular myasthenia. It must be carried out in specialized centers.

Ptosis associated with jaw winking (Marcus-Gunn syndrome)

This is generally seen in **unilateral congenital ptosis** but may be acquired in **post encephalitis status** and in **cyclic oculomotor palsy**.

The phenomenon consists of (Figs 5.3A and B):

1. At rest (i.e. when the jaw is stationary) the lid covers the upper part of the cornea more than 2 mm.
2. When the jaw is opened, the ptotic upper lid is lifted upwards higher than the other eye.
3. If the month is kept open, the up shoot lessens.
4. There may be a greater up shoot if the jaw is moved towards the affected side.
5. The jaw winking generally diminishes as the child grows and even may vanish.
6. Often there is a positive family history.
7. Inverse jaw winking is a phenomenon, where opening the mouth causes drooping of the lid.

Blepharospasm

Generally, the term blepharospasm is used to denote reflex force full closure of the lids due to irritation of the cornea, the pathway is through the trigeminal. This is generally associated with photophobia and is bilateral, commonly seen in children and not listed in neurological causes of blepharospasm.

i. **Lesion before the geniculate ganglion** produces **unilateral, lower motor neuron facial palsy, diminished tear production** and **loss of taste** in anterior 2/3 of tongue.

ii. **Lesion of the geniculate ganglion** results in facial palsy, hyperacusia, and loss of taste in anterior 2/3 of tongue.

iii. **Lesion below lateral geniculate ganglion** The tear production is normal, there is loss of taste in anterior 2/3 of the tongue and hyperacusia.

The common causes are fracture base of skull, surgery on mastoid, otitis media, herpes zoster and Guillain-Barre syndrome.

7. **In the sylomestoid foramen**—The commonest lesion is Bell's palsy.
8. **In the face**—The commonest cause is *leprosy* (Figs 5.4 and 5.5) followed by trauma, parotitis, tumor of parotid. In forceps delivery, the blade of the forceps may press the nerve on the face.

Bell's palsy

Bell's palsy is **one of the commonest cranial nerve palsies**. It is seen in **all ages**, equally in **both sexes**, has an **acute onset** with **complete** or **partial** recovery even without treatment, recurrence on the same side are not known. In rare instances, the other side may be involved but not simultaneously. It is not associated with any other neurological deficit.

Presence of neurological deficit rules out possibility of Bell's palsy and lesions at a level higher than facial canal should be looked for.

The exact cause of the disease is not known. Various possibilities are:

- Viral infection
- Autoimmune disease
- Vascular ischemia

The basic pathology lies in the trunk of the seventh nerve, which suffers from **interstitial neuritis** that in turn produces **swelling of the nerve trunk**, in the facial

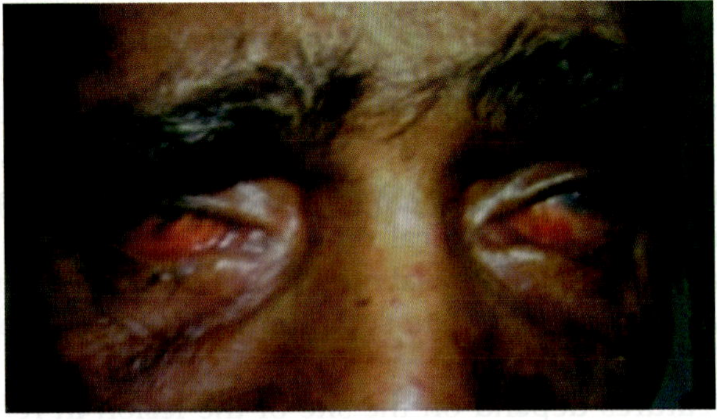

Fig. 5.4: Bilateral lagophthalmos in leprosy without loss of eyebrow

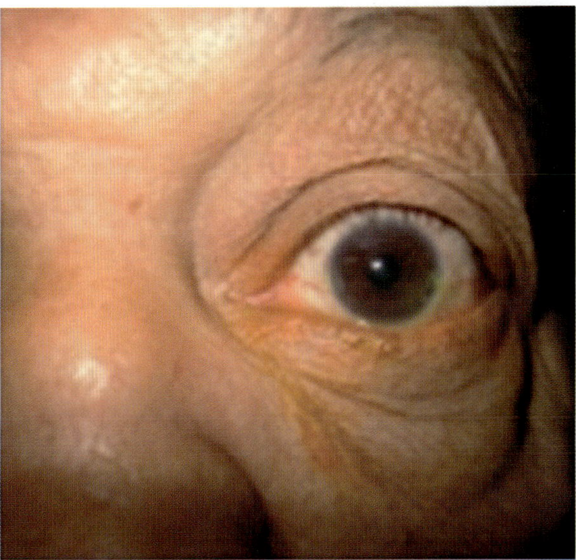

Fig. 5.5: Lagophthalmos in leprosy with loss of eyebrow and lashes (*Courtesy:* Dr Santosh Patel)

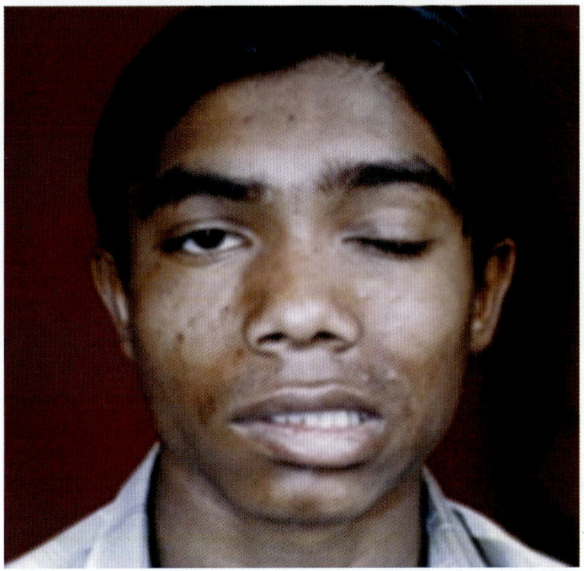

Fig. 5.6: Right-sided Bell's palsy of recent origin. The patient recovered completely with treatment

canal or stylomestoid foramen. The rigid body canal impinges the swollen nerve trunk to produce conduction defect (Figs 5.6 and 5.7).

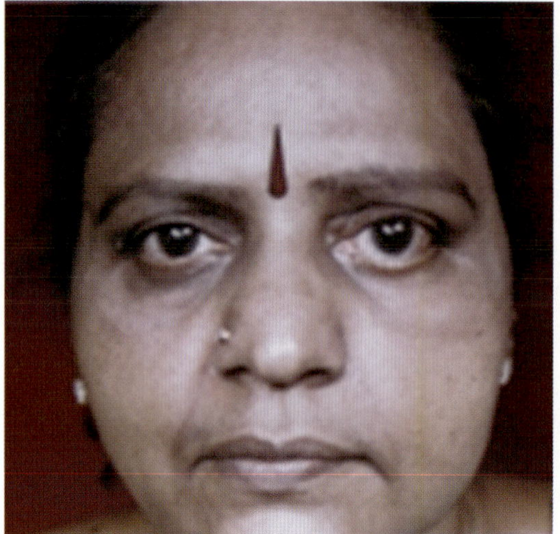
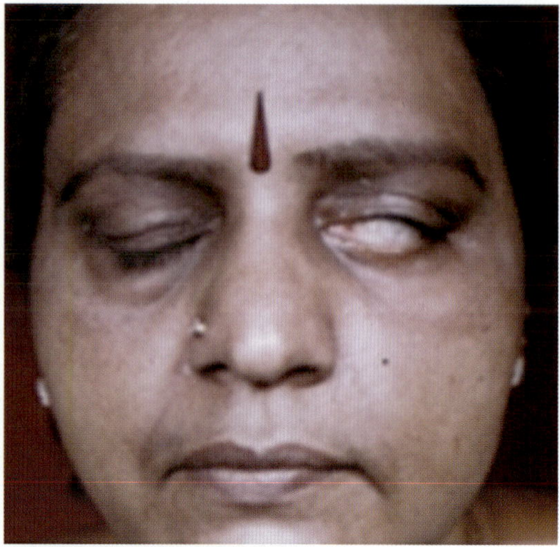

Fig. 5.7: Left-sided Bell's palsy of long standing without recovery

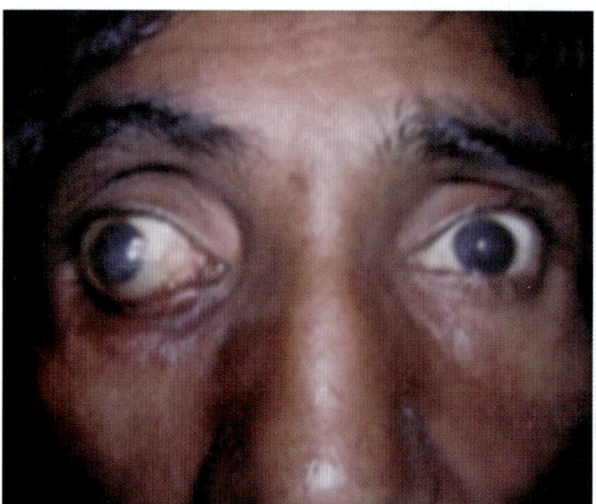
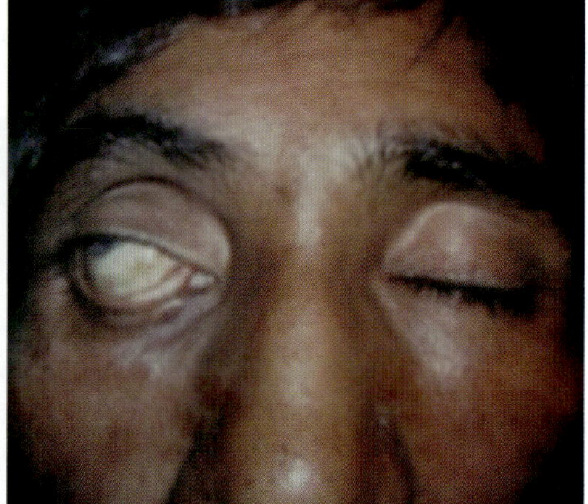

Fig. 5.8: Unilateral lagophthalmos right eye. Note: The right eye is exotrophic from childhood (*Courtesy:* Dr Santosh Patel)

The condition is **unilateral** without any premonitation. The patient generally wakes up in the morning with the **symptoms of watering** and **foreign body sensation** in the effected eye only to discover that he **cannot close the eye well**. The mouth is deviated and the nasolabial fold is smoothened.

The findings depend on severity of the condition. In a fully developed case, the **forehead creases** are **obliterated**. **The arch of the eyebrow is lowered**. **The inter-palpebral fissure is widened.** The lower lid shows various degrees of paralytic **ectropion**. **Epiphora** is copious. The action of orbicularis is absent or minimal. In an attempt to close the lids, the lids fail to move. The eyeballs roll up due to **intact Bell's phenomenon** (Fig. 5.8).

All other extraocular muscles are normal.
The corneal sensation is normal.

The lower conjunctiva is congested. The **cornea** shows desquamation of epithelium in the lower part, may develop frank corneal clear.

If the palsy lasts for few weeks, the lower lid develops **complete ectropion**. The tarsal conjunctiva is everted over the ectropioned lower lid, is hypertrophied, may show dry spots and keratinization. The bulbar conjunctiva in the lower half shows chronic conjunctivitis and dryness. The cornea shows various stages of keratitis, ulceration and opacification. The upper lid may develop blepharochalasis.

Management

Mild to moderate cases do not require much of management except reassurance regarding its benignness and possibility of its complete recovery.

At this stage, all that is required is **frequent instillation of antibiotic** and **lubricating drops**, antibiotic eye ointment at bedtime and dark glasses. Patching of the affected eye is better avoided. Patching does not prevent opening of lids under the pad. This scratches the cornea that keeps moving under the patch resulting in more discomfort.

Soft contact lenses may be prescribed under supervision with usual precaution.

In severe cases, the upper lid may be anchored down by sutures to the cheek.

If lagophthalmos does not improve within seven to ten days and the corneal epithelium is jeopardized, *tarsorrhaphy* is the best choice. It can be *lateral* or *median* tarsorrhaphy. *Complete tarsorrhaphy* is rarely required (Fig. 5.9).

Other indications of tarsorrhaphy in lagophthalmos are:

- Loss of corneal sensation
- Loss of Bell's phenomenon.

Children are not immune to lagophthalmos. Most of them are due to **classical Bell's palsy**. However, more serious condition like **posterior fossa tumors, pontine glioma, myasthenia, otitis media** should be excluded at the earliest.

Ramsay hunt syndrome

It is a **unilateral infranuclear facial palsy** seen in **herpes zoster** infection of the **geniculate ganglion**. It is of acute onset with features of Bell's palsy. Herpes zoster

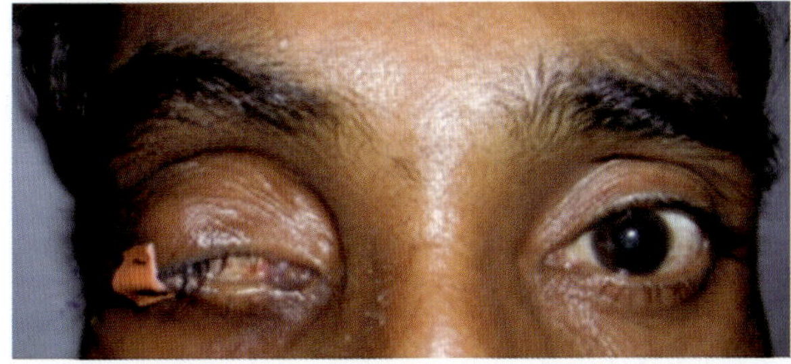

Fig. 5.9: Tarsorrhaphy for lagophthalmos (*Courtesy:* Dr Santosh Patel)

vescicles are seen on the area with sensory supply from seventh nerve, i.e. pinna, external auditory canal, tympanic membrane, buccal mucosa.

Besides lagophthalmos and its manifestation, the syndrome consists of **earache, deafness, tinnitus**. The condition is self-limiting but recovery period is longer than in classical Bell's palsy. Beneficial role of **acyclovir** and **steroids** have not been proved beyond doubt. The ocular management is similar to that of Bell's palsy.

Crocodile tears

This **unusual** and **rare** condition is seen during *recovery from infranuclear seventh nerve palsy* due to **aberrant regeneration of seventh nerve** which transmits the neural stimulation for salivation, this stimulates lacrimal gland to produce tear during eating.

Facial diplegia

Bilateral involvement of facial nerve can be brought about by

1. Congenital anomaly—Mobius syndrome
2. Infection
   - Leprosy
   - Lyme disease
   - Polio
   - AIDS
3. Autoimmune disease—Guillain-Barre syndrome
4. Myogenic—Myasthenia gravis
5. Dystrophic—Mystonic dystrophy
6. Vascular—Basilar artery stroke
7. Trauma—Contusion of brainstem, crush injury face
8. Neoplasm—Glioma of brainstem, leukemia
9. Others—Melkersson-Rosenthal syndrome, sarcoidosis, porphyria

The list of conditions that cause bilateral facial palsy is long. Fortunately, the incidence is relatively low. The two causes that are seen more frequently are—Infection and myasthenia.

Leprotic facial palsy

Out of all the infections, **leprosy** remains the commonest cause of facial palsy world over. Its incidence in underdeveloped nations is higher than in developed countries. About **one-third of patients** with lagophthalmos in leprosy **have bilateral involvement** (Fig. 5.10). The generally accepted view about level of the lesion's is that it is a **peripheral lesion,** i.e. that of the zygomatic branch of the facial nerve. Now it is known that the lesion is more proximal, may even be intracranial.

The condition has all **the features of Bell's palsy** with loss of corneal sensation putting the cornea at higher risk of ulceration. Corneal anesthesia is due to **lesion of fifth nerve** which is independent of seventh nerve involvement.

Melkersson-Rosenthal syndrome

It is a **rare** condition of **bilateral recurrent facial palsy**. The facial palsy may be simultaneous on both sides or may alternative. It is associated with facial swelling.

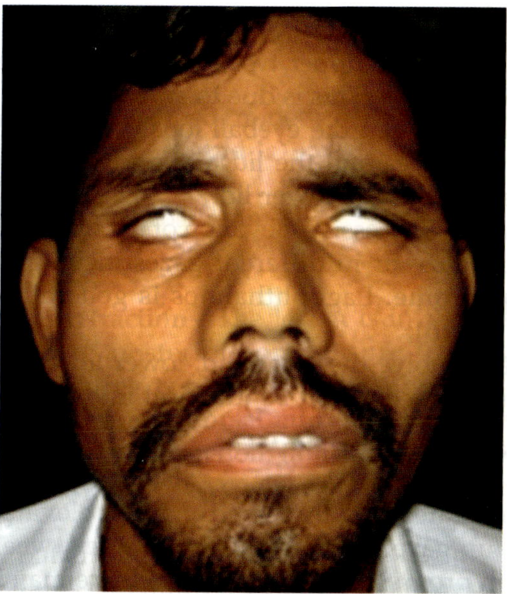

Fig. 5.10: Bilateral facial palsy in leprosy (*Courtesy:* Dr Santosh Patel)

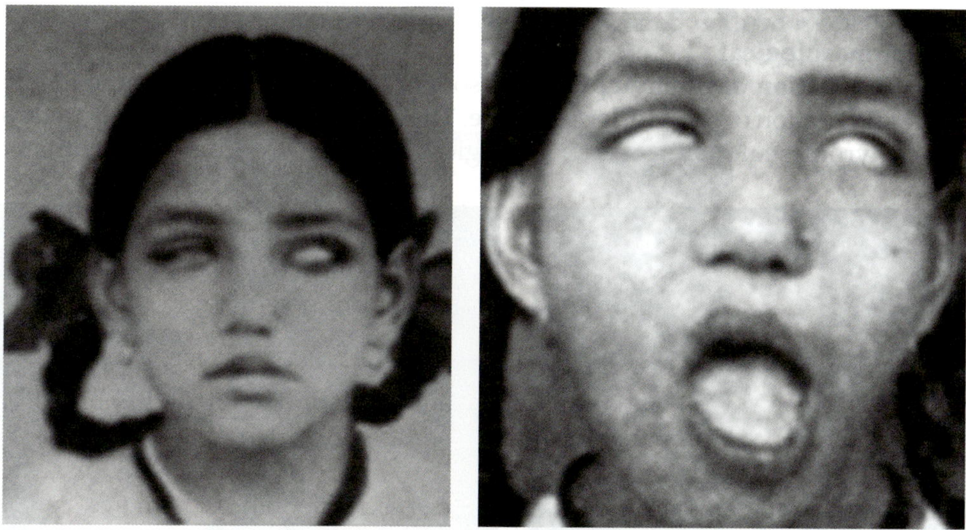

Fig. 5.11: Bilateral lagophthalmos with furrowed tongue in Melkersson-Rosenthal syndrome (*Courtesy:* Editor IJO)

The tongue is transversely fissured. The face has a mask-like appearance. The exact cause is not known. It is most probably a congenital condition but can be acquired as well (Fig. 5.11).

ii. Related to oculosympathetic chain
Claude Bernard Syndrome is due to irritative lesion of cervical sympathetic chain. It is reverse of Horner's syndrome and consists of lid retraction, dilated pupil, excessive sweating, vasoconstriction and lowering of temperature.
All the features are unilateral.

4. **Myogenic**
   a. Commonest cause is thyroid eye disease (Fig. 5.13).
   b. A child born to a mother with hyperthyroid may have lid retraction.

The causes of lid retraction in hyperthyroidism is less due to neurological causes and more due to changes in the muscle of the lid.

BIBLIOGRAPHY

1. Bartley GB. The differential diagnosis of eye lid retraction. Ophthalmology 1996;103:176.
2. Gittinger JW. Blepharospasm in manual of clinical problems in ophthalmology. 1st edn, Gittinger J, Asdourian GK (Eds). little Brown Boston 1988;7-10.
3. Glaser JS. Oculomotor palsies in neuro-ophthalmology. Harper and Row, London 1978;255-80.
4. Harvey JT, Anderson RL. Lid lag and lagophthalmos. A clarification of terminology. Oph Surg 1941;12:338-40.
5. Huppl SL. Eyelid disorder in neuro-ophthalmology, 5th edn, Kline-LB and Bajandas FJ (Eds). Jaypee Brothers Medical Publishers, New Delhi 2004;187-94.
6. Joshna J. Surgical management of lagophthalmos in leprosy. Proceedings of first international symposium on ocular leprosy, Kolkata, 2005.
7. Miller NR. Myasthenia gravis in current ocular therapy, 5th edn. Fraunfelder FT. Roy FH (Eds). WB Saunders company, Philadelphia, 2000;221-22.
8. Mukherjee PK, Dongre RC. A case of acquired facial diplegia, macular edema and lingua plicata. Ind Jr Oph 1975;21:36-39.
9. Wary SH. Diagnosis of Horner's syndrome in manual of ocular diagnosis and therapy. Dehorah (Eds), Pavan Langston, Little Brown 1991;359-60.

6 Neuro-ophthalmic Manifestation of Third Nerve

The third nerve supplies maximum number of extraocular muscles in two groups:

1. Those supplied by upper division, i.e. levator palpebral superior and superior rectus
2. Those supplied by its inferior division
   a. Striated muscle, i.e. medial rectus, inferior rectus and inferior oblique
   b. Intraocular nonstriated muscles, i.e. iris and ciliary body (parasympathetic)

The fascicles of third nerve are closely related to other neural tracts in the mid brain. Hence it has not only ophthalmic features but other neuro-ophthalmic features in its fascicular lesions. Basilar lesions are mostly confined to vascular structures. Cavernous and orbital lesions are associated with other cranial nerves from second to fifth and sympathetic change.

The lesions of third nerve can be:

1. Supranuclear
2. Nuclear
3. Infranuclear:
   i. Fascicular
   ii. Basilar
   iii. In cavernous sinus
   iv. In superior orbital fissure
   v. Orbit

Each level has distinct clinical features that help in localizing the level of the lesion.

1. **Supranuclear lesion**
2. **The nuclear lesions**

The third nerve **does not have a single nucleus** like fourth or sixth nerve. The third nerve nucleus comprises of a **group of sub nuclei** scattered over a large area. Some of them are paired, some of the fibers decussate to supply muscles of opposite side, i.e. levator, palpebral superior and superior rectus. The non decussated fibers go to the ipsilateral muscles. **Nuclear lesions are rare.**

A. **The common** presentation of nuclear lesion of third nerve comprises of:
   i. Bilateral partial paralysis of levator
   ii. Unilateral third nerve palsy with contralateral superior rectus palsy.
   iii. Bilateral third nerve palsy with or without pupillary involvement, sparing the levator.

The above features are so constant that they are called as **obligatory features.**

Isolated total third nerve palsy that includes **iridoplegia**. Iridoplegia is so constant feature of posterior communicating artery aneurysmal leak that presence of reacting pupil with isolated third nerve palsy excludes aneurysm and goes in favor of diabetes.

Diabetic third nerve palsy

Involvement of third nerve in diabetes is **common**. It is **isolated trunk lesion** which is **unilateral,** may be associated with pain. One of the important signs is **intact pupillary response** in spite of involvement of all extraocular muscles supplied by third nerve. (see Fig. 2.10). The lesion is secondary to **microvascular ischemia**. The phenomenon is explained on the basis of peculiar blood supply of the pupillomotor fibers in the **third nerve**. The pupillary fibers are located superficially in the trunk of the third nerve, deriving blood supply from the pial vessels. The main trunk is supplied by the vasa nervorum. In diabetes the vasa nervorum is involved resulting in pupillary sparing third nerve palsy. A compressive lesion will involve more extensive blood supply causing total paralysis of third nerve that includes pupillomotor fibers. Besides diabetes other micro vasculopathies may also cause pupillary sparing third nerve palsy (Figs 6.2 and 6.3).

A patient with long standing diabetes if develops isolated total third nerve palsy with pupillary involvement should be investigated for possibility of a compressive lesion as well, by MRI and MR angiography.

The diabetic ocular palsy is self-limiting fleeting palsy, that recovers within six weeks. It may recur or change side.

Common causes of isolated third nerve palsy include:

1. Infection:
   i. Meningococcal meningitis.
   ii. Tubercular meningitis.
   iii. Syphilitic basal meningitis.

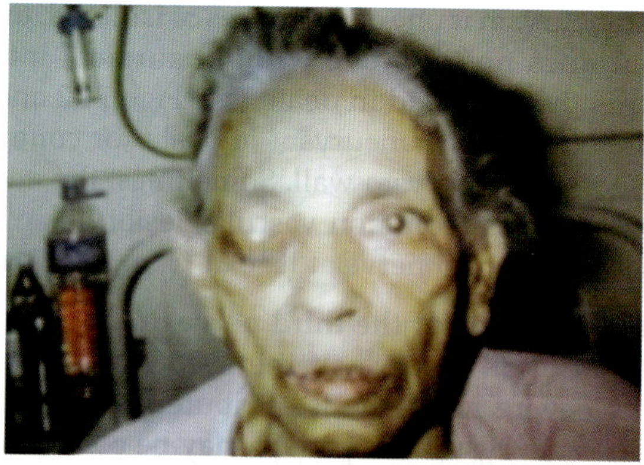

Fig. 6.2: Diabetic third nerve palsy (*Courtesy:* Prof Nupur Chakravarty)

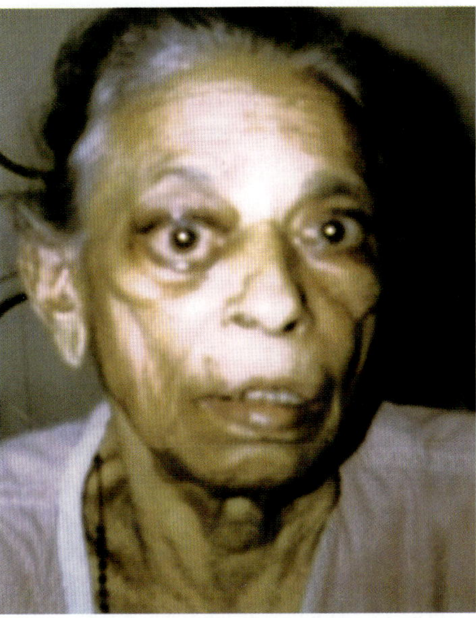

Fig. 6.3: Partial recovery in diabetic third nerve palsy
(*Courtesy:* Prof Nupur Chakravarty)

2. Vascular:
   i. Diabetes
   ii. Hypertension
   iii. Arteriosclerosis
3. Third nerve palsy in down ward displacement of cerebral hemisphere:
   i. The third nerve before entering the cavernous sinus lies on the edge of tentorium cerebelli.
   ii. The inferior surfaces of the temporal lobe overlies this edge of the tentorium.
   iii. An expanding lesion above this level pushes the uncus downwards.
   iv. The downward directed pressure impinges the third nerve against the tentorial edge causing **total third nerves palsy** and **Hutchinson's pupil**. The commonest expanding lesion is **ipsilateral subdural hematoma**. Other causes are intracranial or subtentorial mass. Besides third nerve palsy there may be other neurological signs.

The Hutchinson's pupil is a sign that carries great importance in neurosurgery. It is generally seen in a **comatose patient** following **head injury** due to extra or **subdural hematoma**. It also occurs in ease of expanding tumor, cerebral abscess, apoplexy and cerebral edema (see Chapter 4).

In most of the cases the pupillary changes are ipsilateral to the subdural hematoma, rarely it can occur on the other side also.

The third nerve palsy generally follows onset of pupillary changes.

The pupillary changes consist of:

1. Initial constriction of pupil on one side, generally on the side of the expanding lesion due to irritation of ipsilateral third nerve.
2. Dilatation of ipsilateral pupil which still reacts to light and convergence.
3. Dilatation of pupil further with abolished light and near reflex, due to paralysis of pupillomotor fibers.
4. Development of oculomotor palsy.
5. Dilatation of the contralateral pupil as well.
6. Besides oculomotor nerve palsy the condition may be associated with paralysis of other cranial nerves, i.e. fourth, fifth, sixth and seventh. Homonymous hemianopia is rare, still infrequent are ipsilateral hemiparesis or hemiplegia.

Onset of Hutchinson's pupil is an ominous sign. It requires urgent cerebral decompression.

The phenomenon of Hutchinson's pupil is explained by (see Fig. 4.13)

1. The pupillomotor fibers are situated in the peripheral part of the third nerve.
2. The pupillomotor fibers are thin and poorly myelinated.
3. They are supplied by thin pial blood vessels. All these factors make pupillomotor fibers more vulnerable than the main trunk.
4. **Traumatic third nerve palsy**
   Third nerve palsy in uncal herniation is an indirect effect of cranial trauma. Direct trauma to the third nerve in head injury is not uncommon. It can happen in following condition
   i. The fine roots of the third nerve are torn as they leave the brainstem.
   ii. There is contusion of the distal part of the nerve due to trauma.
   iii. There is intraneural or perineural hematoma formation.
   iv. There may be ischemia or pressure necrosis of the trunk.

(iii) Cavernous lesion

In the cavernous sinus the oculomotor nerve comes in close proximity of *fourth,* **fifth and sixth nerves**. The lesion in the cavernous sinus also involves the *sympathetic* **chain**.

Thus, isolated third nerve palsy is not possible in lesion of cavernous sinus (Fig. 2.8).

The characteristic of the palsy are:

a. **Partial third nerve palsy**—All the muscles supplied by the third nerve are not involved simultaneously or equally.
b. The paralysis of third nerve is never isolated. It is generally associated with paralysis of fourth and sixth nerves.
c. The involvement of fifth nerve is common. This results in either pain or numbness in the distribution of the fifth nerve.
d. The pupil is invariably normal in size and reaction. In case of third nerve palsy it is expected that the pupil will be dilated (Unless it is a diabetic palsy).

Cavernous sinus lesion also leads to paralysis of sympathetic, which should result in a miotic pupil. These two factors neutralize each other hence the pupil assumes an intermediate size which is almost as large as a normal pupil.

The common cavernous sinus lesions responsible for third nerve palsy are:

1. **Vascular**
   i. Thrombosis
   ii. Aneurysm of internal carotid
   iii. Carotid cavernous fistula
2. **Neoplasm**
   i. Pituitary tumors
   ii. Meningioma
   iii. Nasopharyngeal growths
   iv. Metastasis
3. **Infection**
4. **The orbital lesions**

Nerve palsy in the superior orbital fissure and orbit: The third nerve divides into two divisions; the upper and lower just before entering the orbit through the superior orbital fissure (Fig. 2.9), Hence orbital lesions may involve the muscles separately supplied by two different divisions. Larger lesion may involve both the divisions simultaneous. Other nerves, i.e. fourth, fifth and sixth may also be involved. The common causes are—infection, inflammation and neoplasm.

Aberrant regeneration of third nerve

Aberrant regeneration of third nerve results in **paradoxical action** of muscles due to **sprouting of new axons** that instead of terminating in the muscles meant for them, end up in a wrong muscle, may be extraocular striated muscles or intraocular non-striated muscle. The misdirection is confined to the muscles supplied by the third nerve only.

Signs of aberrant regeneration and their eponym

Feature	*Eponym*
1. Upshoot of lid in downgaze	Pseudo Von Graffe's sign
2. Upshoot of lid in adduction	Inverse Duanne's syndrome
3. Absence of light reaction and miosis in adduction	Pseudo Argyll-Robertson pupil

There are **two types** of aberrant regeneration of the third nerve:

1. **Primary:** Seen in intracavernous lesion of the third nerve. The condition has slow development. The common causes are **aneurysm**, and **meningioma**. It is not preceded by acute third nerve palsy. It is less common than secondary aberrant regeneration.

2. **Secondary:** Develops weeks after acute third nerve palsy secondary to trauma or compressive pathology. The other clinical classification is based on whether it involves the lid or the pupil. The first is known as **lid dyskinesis** and the second as **pupil dyskinesis**.

The following combination of movement are possible:

1. **Lid dyskinesis**
   i. Elevation of lid on
      a. Adduction
      b. Down gaze.
   ii. Elevation of globe on adduction.
   iii. Depression of globe on adduction.
   iv. Retraction of globe on action of any of the muscles supplied by third nerve.
   v. Limitated elevation or depression of globe.
   vi. Lid retraction when the patient looks down pseudo-von-Graffes' sign.
2. **Pupil dyskinesis**

Pseudo Argyll-Robertson pupil—No light or near response in primary position but near response is present on adduction or adduction depression.

Aberrant regeneration of third nerve is associated with monocular vertical opto-kinetic response.

Aberrant regeneration of third nerve is not seen in third nerve palsy due to diabetes or demyelination.

Cyclic oculomotor palsy

This is **rare, unilateral** disease seen in **congenital oculomotor paresis**, first noticed in **children** that **lasts for rest of the life**. It is **periodic** in nature and consists of **two cyclic phases,** i.e. the paretic phase and spastic phase.

The paretic phase consists of ptosis, mydriasis, moderate cycloplegia, paralysis of adduction and elevation resulting in exotropia. The cycle lasts for 10 to 30 seconds.

The spastic phase is shorter, comprises of lid retraction on attempt to adduct, there may be twitching of lid in an attempt to adduct, miosis and spasm of accommodation.

Ophthalmoplegia migraine

This is a **rare** condition **seen in children**. The child either suffers from migraine or has a **history of migraine in the family**. The commonest nerve to be involved is third, less common is involvement of sixth. The fourth nerve is involved least. It may be associated with **hemianopia**. The ocular palsy is **unilateral**. The third nerve palsy includes **pupillary palsy**. The palsy is **periodic**. The typical history is onset of migrainous

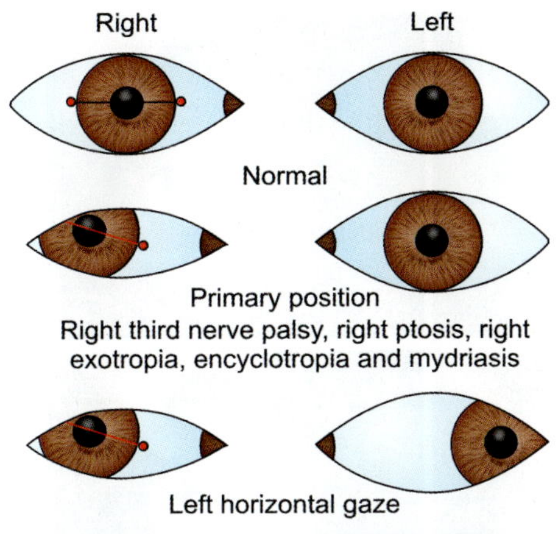

Fig. 6.4: Position of the eyeball in total third nerve palsy

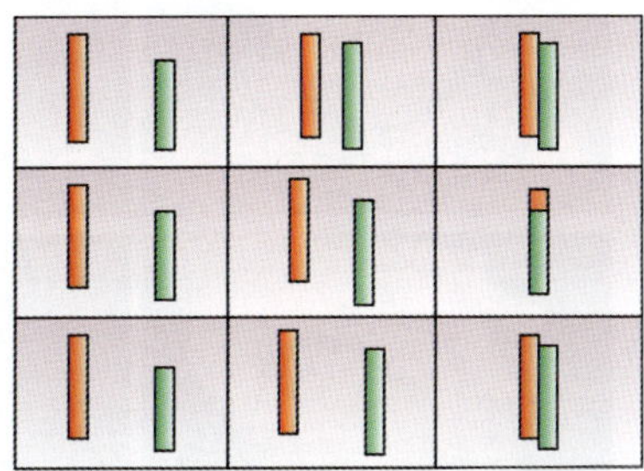

Fig. 6.5: Diplopia chart third nerve palsy right side

headache. At the peak of headache ophthalmoplegia sets-in and the headache abates. The ophthalmoplegia lasts for **few weeks with complete recovery**. Recurrences is common. The exact causes of the conditions is not known. **Edema of intracavernous carotid** has been thought to be the main cause.

Points to be noted in localizing the level of lesion in third nerve palsy:

Clinical features of total third nerve palsy (Figs 6.4 to 6.7)

Signs	*Cause*
• Ptosis	Paralysis of levator
• Difficulty in elevation	Paralysis of superior rectus
• Exotropia	Unopposed action of lateral rectus
• Poor adduction	Weakness of medial rectus
• Intortion in down gaze	Unopposed action of superior oblique
• Limitation of depression	Weakness of inferior rectus
• Spared pupil	Diabetes, hypertension, involvement of sympathetic chain in cavernous sinus
• Mydriatic pupil not responding to light or accommodation	Parasympathetic paralysis

Find out the following:

- Unilateral/bilateral
- Supranuclear (rare) or infranuclear.
- Nuclear (rare) bilateral ptosis.

Bilateral superior rectus palsy is more common than other types.

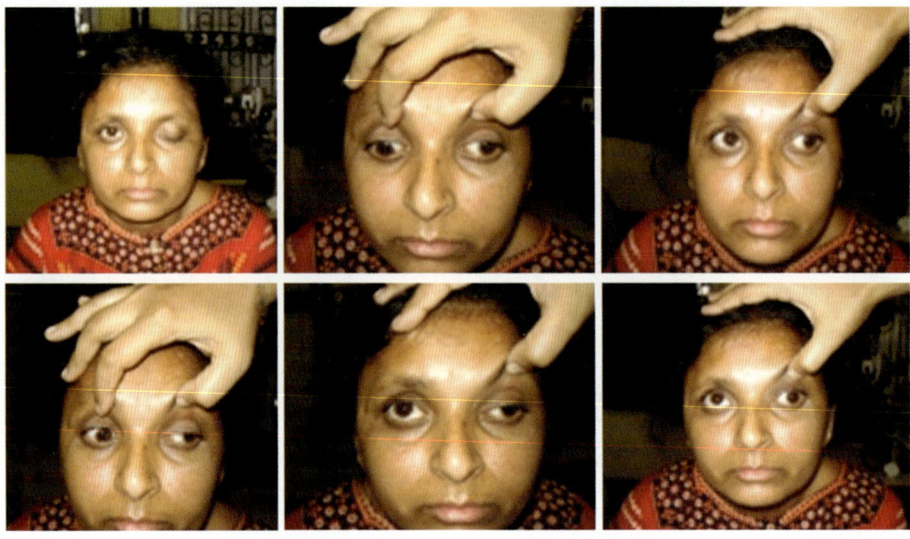

Fig. 6.6: Nondiabetic total third nerve palsy (*Courtesy:* Dr Hetal Yagnik)

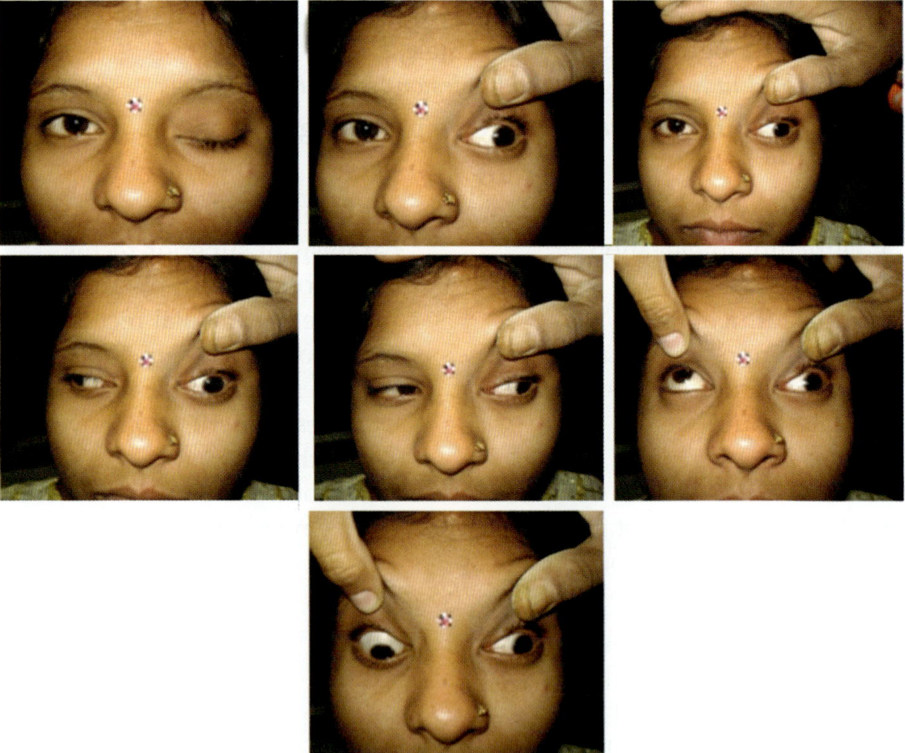

Fig. 6.7: Nondiabetic total third nerve palsy (*Courtesy:* Dr Santosh Patel)

3. If subnuclear

Find out if it is

i. Fascicular generally associated with other neurological defects.

ii. Basal – Isolated:

  a. Diabetic

  b. Compressive.

iii. Cavernous—Generally associated with multiple cranial nerve palsies. Sympathetic involvement with pupillary sparing.

iv. Orbital—May be partial or complete, other nerves may be involved, may have proptosis.

4. Is the palsy, pupillary sparing or pupillary involving.

5. Find out if aberrant regeneration is present. It is never present in diabetic neuropathy.

6. Exclude **myasthenia gravis, dysthyroid status and pseudo tumor orbit**.

Investigations required in third nerve palsy

The **two main groups** of causes of third nerve palsy are:

1. Ischemia
2. Compression
   - Tumor
   - Aneurysm
   - Hemorrhage.

The first produces pupillary sparing neuropathy, the second produces pupillary involving neuropathy.

There are some investigations common for both the groups. However they can broadly divided in following sets of investigation.

1. For pupillary sparing third nerve palsy the commonly ordered investigations are:
   i. Postprandial blood sugar
   ii. Glucose tolerance test
   iii. Fundus examination for:
      a. Diabetic retinopathy
      b. Arteriosclerotic and hypertensive retinopathy.

Diabetes of recent origin does not cause ophthalmoplegia, but ophthalmoplegia may be the first presentation to bring a diabetic to physician first time.

2. Pupillary involved third nerve palsy (Flow chart 6.1).
   i. MRI
   ii. MR angiography
   iii. CT
   iv. X-ray skull for fracture
   v. Four vessel angiography.

Flow chart 6.1: Diagnosis of third nerve palsy

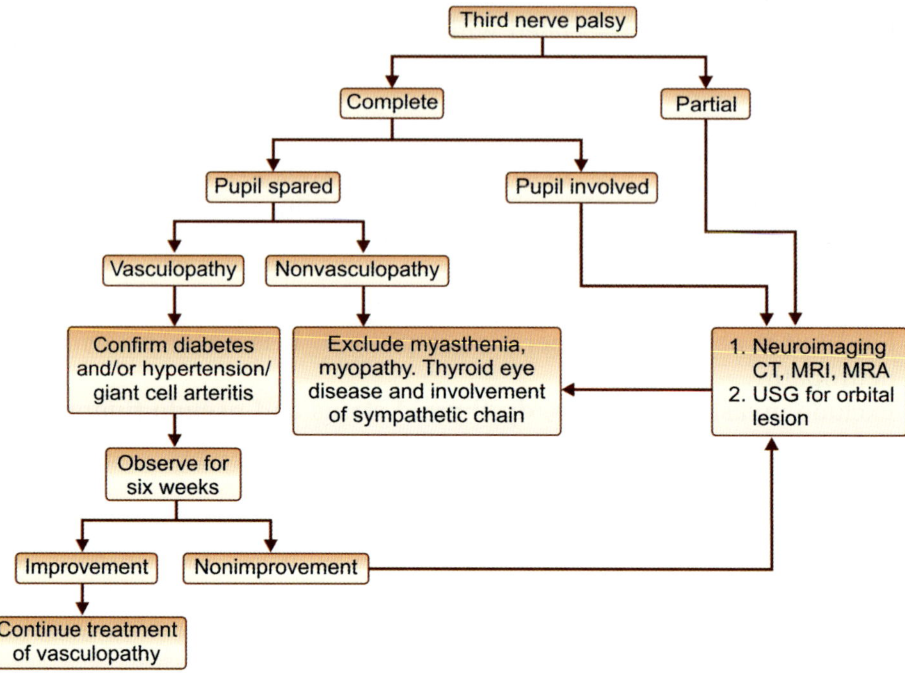

3. Diabetic palsy not improving within six weeks or developing pupillary involvement should have a neuroimaging along with:
   i. ESR for giant cell arteritis.
   ii. Total blood count.
   iii. VDRL, FTA-ABS.
   iv. Antinuclear antibody
   v. HIV test.

Indications of MRI and MRA in third nerve palsy

The MRI and MRA are done to rule out:

1. Neoplasm
2. Aneurysm
3. Demyelination
4. Trauma.

The clinical indications are:

1. Pupil involving third nerve palsy
2. Pupil sparing third nerve palsy
   a. Patient without ischemic vasculopathy, i.e. diabetes, hypertension.
   b. Diabetic third nerve palsy not improving in six weeks.
   c. Incomplete third nerve palsy.

d. Associated with other cranial nerve palsy.
e. Associated with other neurological signs.
f. Trauma.
g. Nontraumatic aberrant regeneration.
h. Third nerve palsy in all child under 10 years irrespective of pupillary changes.

BIBLIOGRAPHY

1. Brazis PW. Localisation of lesions of the oculomotor nerve – recent concepts. Mayo Clinic Proc 1991;66:1029-35.
2. Green WR, Hackett ER, et al. Neuro-ophthalmic evaluation of oculomotor nerve palsy. Arch Oph 1964;72:154-67.
3. Jacobson DM, Trobe JD. The emerging role of MRI in management of patient with third nerve palsy. Am Jr Oph 1982;113:489-96.
4. Jacobson DM. Pupil involvement in patients with diabetes associated oculomotor nerve palsy. Arch Oph 1998;116:723-27.
5. Lee AG, Hayman LA, Brazis PW. The evaluation of isolated third nerve palsy revisited. Sur Oph 2002;47:137-57.
6. Mwanza JC, Georgette B, Ngweme, Kayembe DL. Ocular motor nerve palsy: A clinical and etiological study. IJO 2006;54:173-75.
7. Richards BW. Jones FR, Younge BR. Causes and prognosis in 4278 cases of paralysis of oculomotor, trochlear and abducence. Carnial nerves, Am JO 1992;113:489-94.
8. Rush JA, Young BR, Paralysis of Cranial nerves III, IV and VI causes and prognosis in 1000 cases. Arch Oph 1981;99:76-79.
9. Trobe JD, Isolated pupil sparing third nerve palsy. Ophthalmology 1985;92:58-61.

7 Neuro-ophthalmic Manifestation of Fourth Nerve

Lesion of fourth nerve causes under-action of superior oblique. The nuclear and fascicular lesion differs from trunk lesion (see Figs 2.8, 2.9, 2.12, 2.13 and 2.15). The nucleus and fascicles on the right side of the mid line become left trocheal nerve trunk hence lesion of right nucleus and fascicle cause left sided paralysis. This is not applicable to trunk lesion. Trunk lesions produce ipsilateral superior oblique palsy.

The fascicles are so small and so near the nucleus that it is not possible to differentiate lesions between the two.

The fascicular portion of the fourth nerve does not come in the vicinity of fascicles of any other cranial nerves or nerve tract except:

1. Sympathetic pathway that passes through the dorsolateral tegmentum of the mid brain next to fascicles of fourth nerve. A lesion in this region causes contralateral Horner's syndrome.
2. The caudal end of the third nerve reaches almost up to the upper level of fourth nerve nucleus, hence a large nuclear lesion of third nerve may involve fourth nerve nucleus as well.
3. A large nucleo fascicular lesion causes bilateral palsy.

Less common nucleofascicular lesion can be:

I. Medial longitudinal fascicle causing **ipsilateral internuclear ophthalmoplegia** and contralateral superior oblique palsy.
II. In superior cerebellar peduncle, the lesion causes ipsilateral ataxia, tremors and contralateral superior oblique under action.

Fourth nerve palsy can be **congenital** or **acquired**. Congenital superior oblique palsy is one of the ocular palsies that may go unattended becauses of mild to moderate compensatory head posture that alleviates the symptoms. The fourth nerve palsy can be **unilateral** or **bilateral**, peripheral, i.e. in the cavernous sinus or beyond and is associated with other cranial nerves palsies concerned with ocular movement.

Clinical features of recent unilateral fourth nerve lesion (Figs 7.1 and 7.2)

1. The eye is deviated up, adducted towards the normal side.
2. The face is turned towards the sound side.
3. The hypertropia increase on adduction.
4. The chin is depressed.
5. The head is tilled to the sound side.

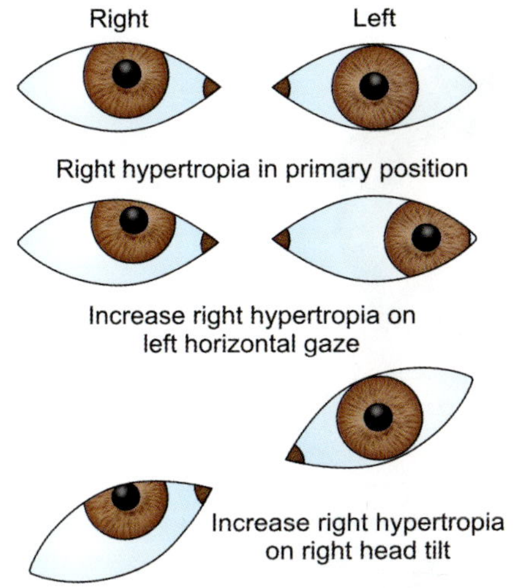

Fig. 7.1: Position of the eyeball in recent unilateral fourth nerve palsy

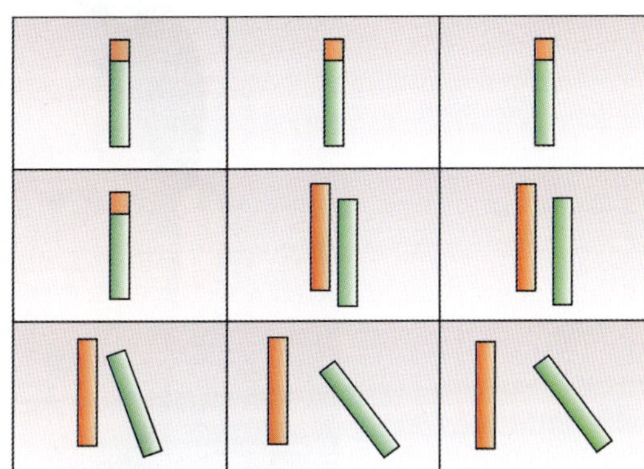

Fig. 7.2: Diplopia charting in recent superior oblique palsy

6. The hypertropia increases away from the side of palsy, i.e. towards sound side.
7. There is excyclotropia diagnosed by ocular torticollis. Compensatory scoliosis is seen in children.
8. The diplopia is homonymous. Vertical separation increases on looking down to sound side and intortion increases.
9. Diplopia is more for near.
10. For right superior oblique palsy there is right hypertropia that increases on left gaze and when the head is tilted to the right. Tested by Bielchowsky test (Fig. 7.1).
11. Some persons with unilateral fourth nerve may not have abnormal head lift.
12. There is overaction of contralateral inferior rectus and ipsilateral inferior oblique. The superior rectus on the sound side shows under action (Fig. 7.3).

Clinical features of bilateral fourth nerve palsy

1. Bilateral fourth nerve palsy is more difficult to elicit and diagnose.
2. In bilateral symmetrical cases the hypertropia is minimal or absent in primary gaze.
3. The eye may present either as esotropia or exotropia, may be even orthophoric.
4. The hypertropia may be seen in eye contralateral gaze, i.e. left hypertropia on right gaze and right hypertropia on left gaze.
5. There is no head tilt.
6. There is right hyper deviation when the head is tilted to the right shoulder and left hyper deviation when the head is tilted to left shoulder.
7. Esotropia is common.
8. Large excyclotropia specially in down gaze.

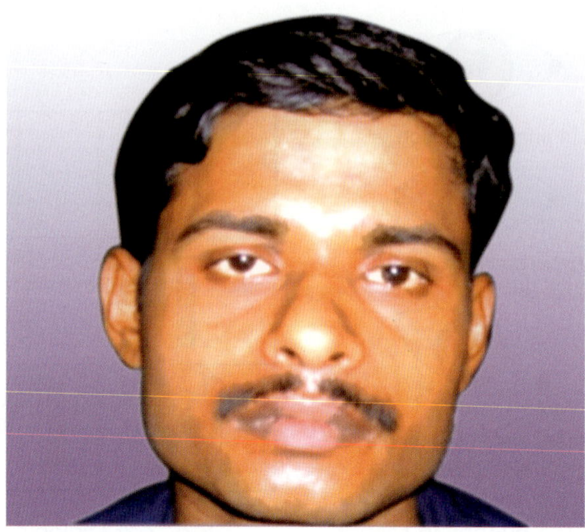

Fig. 7.3: Right superior oblique palsy (*Courtesy:* Dr Santosh Patel)

9. Diplopia is present in all position except up gaze.
10. **Commonest cause of bilateral fourth nerve palsy is head injury.**
11. All patients complaining of diplopia following head injury irrespective of severity should be investigated for bilateral fourth nerve palsy.
12. V pattern is common

Congenital fourth nerve lesion

1. About one third of patients with vertical squint have congenital superior oblique palsy.
2. Person with congenital superior oblique palsy present in two forms:
   i. Childhood palsy
   ii. Adult

I. **The features of congenital superior oblique palsy that present in childhood are:**
   a. Position of one eye is higher than the other either in primary position or in the field of gaze.
   b. Marked head tilt.
   c. A large vertical prism fusion amplitude.
   d. Diplopia on correction of head tilt.
   e. Old photographs betray abnormal head posture.
   f. The condition runs in families.
   g. They may have manifest squint without binocular function.

II. **The adults** may for the first time complain of vertical diplopia in **fifth or sixth decade** for which no cause can be detected. Old photographs may show

Differences between unilateral and bilateral superior oblique palsy

Features	*Unilateral*	*Bilateral*
Head posture	Depressed chin, face turned towards sound side, head tilted towards sound side	Only chin depression
Cover test in primary position	Hyper deviation	Slight or no hyper deviation
Extortion	Mild	Moderate
Lateral version	No reversal of diplopia in lateral version	Reversal of diplopia in lateral version
Bielchowsky test (Fig. 7.1)	Positive when head tilted towards effected side	Positive when head tilted towards any side
Diplopia	Vertical, tortional	Diplopia only when decompensated

abnormal head posture. Rest of the features are same as in childhood oblique palsy.

Bielchowsky test (Fig. 7.1)

1. Prism and cover test is done in all nine positions of gaze to elicit and measure hyper deviation.
2. Maddox double rod test is used to demonstrate and measure extortion.
3. Tortional movements may be observed during direct ophthalmoscopy and slit lamp examination.
4. Perform cover uncover test for hyper deviation (phoria/tropia) say right eye. Measure deviation of the right eye by prism.
5. Ask the patient to look to the non deviated eye, i.e. left. There should be an increase in hyper deviation which is again measured by prism. This deviation causes maximum diplopia.
6. Tilt the eye towards the originally hyper deviated eye, i.e. right eye. Hyper-deviation should increase.

Topical diagnosis of fourth nerve defect

The fourth nerve involvement can be:

1. Unilateral palsy of superior oblique.
2. Bilateral superior oblique palsy:
   i. The nerve may be involved in isolation.
   ii. May be involved with under action of extraocular muscles supplied by third or sixth nerves.
   iii. Sympathetic path is involved in nucleofascicular lesion of fourth nerve.

iv. Multiple extraocular palsies along with superior oblique palsy is seen in lesions of cavernous sinus or orbit.

Localization of fourth nerve lesion

1. Nucleo facial – **It is difficult to separate nuclear lesions from fascicular lesion because:**
   i. The nucleus is small.
   ii. The fascicles are short
   iii. Absence of other neurological signs except Horner's syndrome. All cases of unilateral miosis with contralateral hyper-deviation should be investigated for Horner's syndrome.
2. Sub arachnoid space causes isolated fourth nerve palsy. Commonest cause is trauma, i.e. closed head injury or neurosurgical intervention. Less common causes are tumors.
3. Cavernous sinus – Generally associated with paralysis of paresis of other extraocular muscles supplied by third and sixth nerve. There may be reduced sensation due to involvement of fifth nerve. Horner's syndrome may be added to above features.
4. Orbit – Involvement of second nerve is added to lesions of third, fourth and fifth nerve pathology.

Causes of trochlear nerve palsy

1. **Congenital**, about one-third cases are congenital.
2. **Idiopathic**- In another 20-30% cases no cause can be detected.
3. The remaining may be due to:
   i. **Trauma:**
      a. Accidental
      b. Closed head injury
      c. Frontal bone injury
   ii. **Vascular:**
      a. Ischemia
      b. Infarction
      c. Hemorrhage in the brainstem.
      d. Aneurysm - Rare
   iii. **Infection:**
      a. Meningitis
      b. Herpes zoster
      c. Cysticercosis
   iv. **Inflammation:**
      a. Vasculitis
      b. Tolosa Hunt syndrome
      c. Cavernous sinus lesion
      d. Sinusitis

v. Tumor
vi. Demyelination—Rare.
vii. Congenital vascular malformation

Diabetes is a common cause of transient, unilateral superior oblique palsy that may change side. Closed head trauma is a commonest cause of acquired bilateral superior oblique palsy.

Traumatic fourth nerve palsy

Head injury is one of the **common** acquired causes of fourth nerve palsy. The common injuries that result in superior oblique palsy may be **trivial** or **serious closed cranial injury**. Even patient falling on buttocks or a blow to the **occipital** region may result in fourth nerve palsy. The post head injury fourth nerve palsy is **generally bilateral**.

A patient complaining of vertical diplopia following head injury should be suspected to have bilateral fourth nerve involvement.

The commonest explanation put forward is concussion injury to the nerve in the anterior medullary velum. The nerve can be impinged against the tentorial edge in a counter coupe injury.

Examination of fourth nerve function in presence of third nerve palsy:
Fourth nerve is purely a motor nerve.

Superior oblique is the only muscle supplied by the fourth nerve hence in lesions of fourth nerve there is under action of superior oblique only.

Superior oblique is an intorter, abductor and depressor.

In lesion of the third nerve the eye is abducted and slightly depressed. In associated fourth nerve palsy, the eyeball intorts in an attempt to depress the eye. The intortion can be noted by observing any blood vessel at the superior limbus.

Differential diagnosis of fourth nerve lesion should include—Myasthenia, dysthyroid myopathy, pseudotumor orbit, other cyclovertical palsies especially contralateral superior rectus under action, superior oblique myokymia and Brown's syndrome.

Superior oblique myokymia

Superior oblique myokymia is one of the common causes of vertical and tortional diplopia which is mistaken as superior oblique palsy (Flow chart 7.1). It is a **non-nystagmic oscillation of the eye** due to fine contraction of superior oblique in apparently healthy adult. It may cause **tortional oscillopsia**. The condition is **uniocular**. The patient may or may not be aware of the phenomenon. It may be observed during routine ophthalmoscope or slit lamp examination. The patient may **experience vertical**

Differences between superior oblique and contralateral superior rectus under action

	Feature	*Superior oblique*	*Superior rectus*
1.	Cover test		
	I. Normal eye fixing	Hypertropia/hyperphoria	Hypodeviation
	II. Deviation	More for near	More for distance
2.	Angle of deviation	Increase in down gaze	Increases in up-gaze
3.	Extortion	Common	Rare
4.	Position of chin	Depressed	Elevated
5.	Head tilt test	Positive	Generally negative

Flow chart 7.1: Diagnosis of superior oblique under action

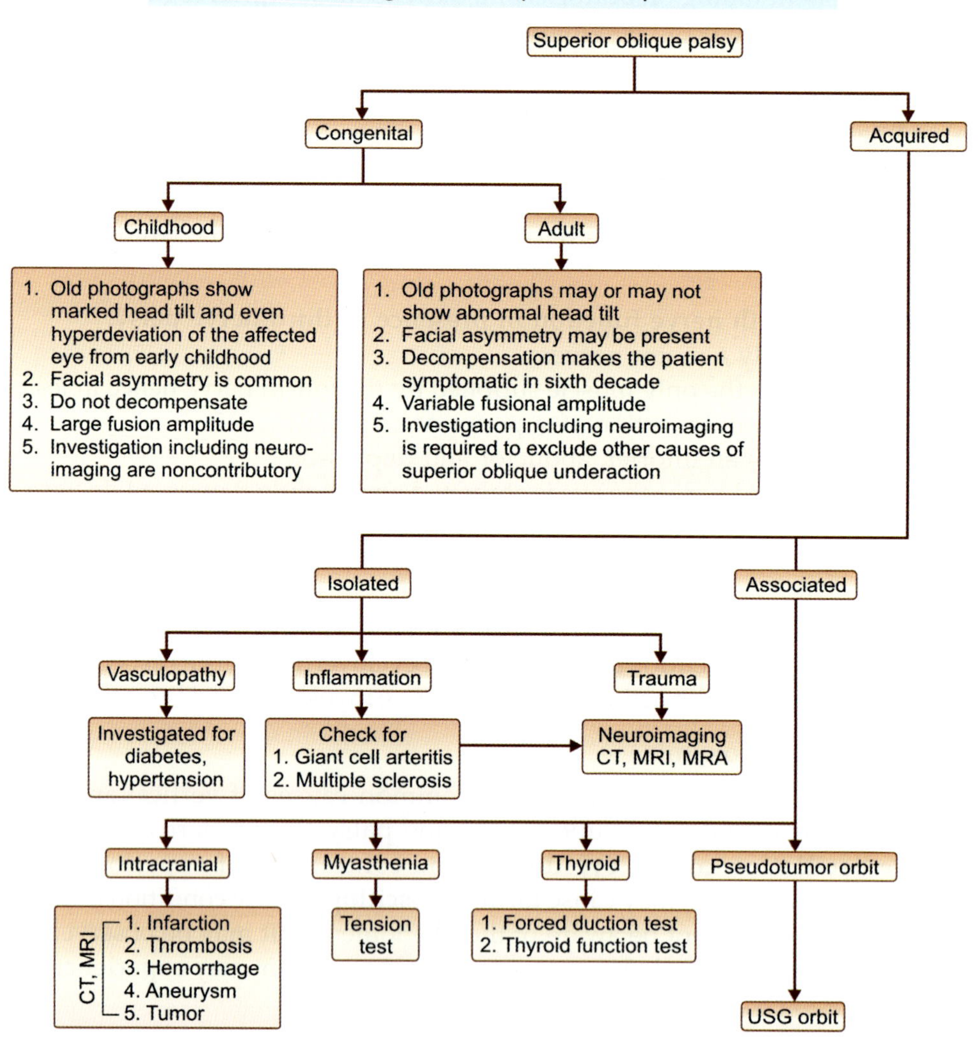

or tortional diplopia and blurred vision. The condition is mostly **benign, non-progressive** without any neuro-ophthalmic sign. Exact cause is not known. Rarely it may be due to **multiple sclerosis** or **posterior fossa growth**, both requiring evaluation and management. The myokymia itself is **self-limited** most of the time. Rarely requiring treatment. The drugs commonly used are tegretol (carbazmazepine), nerontin (gabapenitn) and propranolol.

Superior oblique tenotomy alone or with recession of inferior oblique muscle is rarely required.

Brown syndrome

It is not a neurological disorder. It is a restrictive lesion of superior oblique due to abnormal superior oblique sheath tendon. It could be congenital or acquired.

BIBLIOGRAPHY

1. Astle WF. Rosebaum AL. Familial fourth cranial nerve palsy. Arch Oph 1988;103:532-35.
2. Beck M, Hickling P. Treatment of bilateral superior oblique sheath syndrome. BJO 1980;64:356-60.
3. Bixenman WW. Diagnosis of superior oblique palsy. Jr Cl Neuro Ophth 1981;1:155-208.
4. Brazis PW. Palsies of the trochlear nerve, diagnosis and localization recent concept. May Clinic Proc 1993;68:501-09.
5. Coppeto IR. Superior oblique palsy and contralateral Horner's syndrome. Ann Oph 1983;681-83.
6. Glasser JS, Siatkowski RM. Infranuclear disorders of eye movement in Neuro-ophthalmology 3rd edn. Lippincot William and Wilkins, Philadelphia, 1999;405-60.
7. Hamilton SR. Neuro-ophthalmology of eye movement disorders. Curr Opin Oph 1989;10:405-10.
8. Lee J, Flynn JT. Bilateral superior oblique palsy. BJO 1985;69:508-13.
9. Murray RS. Ajax ET. Bilateral trochlear nerve palsy. Jr Cl Neuro-oph 1989;5:51-58.
10. Park MM. Isolated cyclovertical muscle palsy. Arch Oph 1958;60:1027-35.

8 Neuro-ophthalmic Manifestation of Fifth Nerve

The **trigeminal nerve** is the fifth cranial nerve. It is **motor** as well as **sensory** nerve. It does not contribute any motor neurons to ocular muscles. The motor part innervates the muscles of **mastication**, **masseter**, **pterygoid** and **temporalis**. None of the above are involved in neuro-ophthalmic disorders. It is only the **sensory component** that has ocular involvement. Out of the three sensory branches, i.e. **ophthalmic**, **mandibular** and **maxillary**, the ophthalmic nerve is fully involved in sensory supply of the eye and its adnexa. The **second division** serves a small part of the lower part of orbit and the lower lid. The **maxillary division** does not have any involvement in ocular diseases (Flow chart 8.1).

The sensory component of trigeminal is controlled by three nuclei (see Figs 2.15, 2.22, 2.23, 2.24 and 2.25)

1. Mesencephalic nucleus
2. Main sensory nucleus
3. Spinal nucleus.

The first is involved in **proprioception** from muscles and tendens. The main sensory nucleus is concerned with **light touch** while the spinal nucleus transmits **pain** and **temperature** sensation. The fibers from the three sensory nuclei join to form the trigeminal ganglion (**gasserian ganglion**). The ganglion is situated in **Meckel's cave** ensheathed in the dura, on the lateral side of which lies the **middle meningeal artery**. The medial relation is formed by **cavernous sinus**. The third, fourth, sixth cranial nerves, the internal carotid and the temporal lobe are above the ganglion. The motor root is

Flow chart 8.1: Fifth cranial nerve

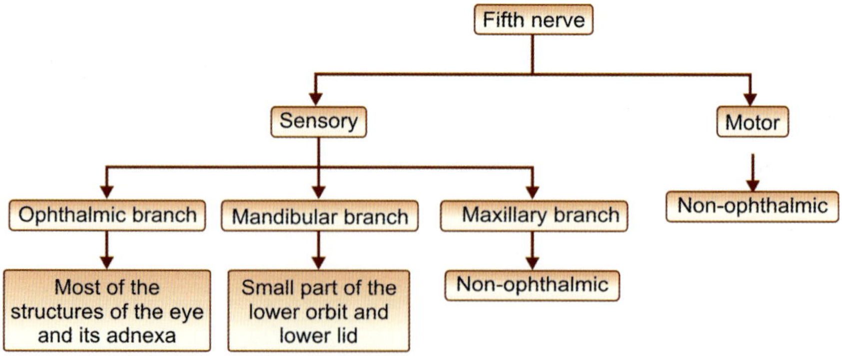

- Fifth nerve
  - Sensory
    - Ophthalmic branch → Most of the structures of the eye and its adnexa
    - Mandibular branch → Small part of the lower orbit and lower lid
    - Maxillary branch → Non-ophthalmic
  - Motor → Non-ophthalmic

inferior to the ganglion. In the cavernous sinus the first and the second division are inferior to oculomotor nerves.

The branches of the ophthalmic division enter the orbit through the **superior orbital fissure**. The two branches, the **lacrimal** and the **frontal** enter outside the **annulus of Zinn** while the **nasociliary** enters within the annulus. The nasociliary gives the sensory twig to the ciliary body.

The trigeminal nerve unlike third and fourth does not decussate, hence the nucleus and the trunk of the nerve supply the ipsilateral eye and its adnexa. The three divisions subserve **well demarcated dermatomes**. There is some overlap in the area of distribution between ophthalmic and mandibular.

The disorders of trigeminal nerve of neuro-ophthalmic interest are:

The lesion of the trigeminal can be:

1. **Central**
   i. **Involving the supranuclear path.**
   The supranuclear lesion can be as follows

Location	Clinical features
1. Precentral	Jaksonian fit, mental changes
2. Internal capsule	Supranuclear seventh nerve palsy, conjugate deviation and hemiplegia
3. Midbrain	Supranuclear seventh, multiple ocular palsy and hemiplegia.

   ii. **Involving single or multiple nuclei of the nerve**.
2. **Peripheral**
   i. Between the pons and the trigeminal ganglion.
   ii. In the gasserian ganglion.
   iii. Distal to the gasserian ganglion.
      a. Between the gasserian ganglion and the cavernous sinus.
      b. In the cavernous sinus.
      c. In the orbit.

The central lesions have some localizing features:

1. A lesion in the medulla and upper part of the spinal cord causes analgesia, loss of thermal sensation with retained light touch sensation.
2. An ascending lesion of the spinal nucleus causes analgesia in the distribution of first division that spreads to second and third division.
3. A pontine lesion retains thermal sensation but loosing sensation of light touch.

The causes of central lesions are:

1. Vascular accidents
2. Neoplasm
3. Infection—tabes, meningitis
4. Syringiomyelia
5. Degenerations.

Peripheral lesions

1. The lesions between the pons and the gasserian ganglion effect all the three division and the motor root.
2. The lesions of the gasserian ganglion also involve all the three divisions.
3. The lesions distal to the ganglion generally involve separate divisions selectively.

The symptoms of trigeminal involvement are:

1. Diminished sensation in the distribution of the trigeminal nerve.
2. Oculo facial pain.
3. Pain with loss of sensation **(Anesthesia dolorosa)**.

A. The causes of diminished sensation in the area of trigeminal distribution are:

I. Corneal:
   a. Leprosy
   b. Herpes zoster ophthalmicus (Fig. 8.1)
   c. Herpes simplex
   d. Cerebello pontine angle tumor
   e. Dysautonomia (Riley day syndrome)
   f. Gradenigo syndrome.

II. Diminished sensation over the skin of the lids, face, ipsilateral skin of forehead.
   a. Leprosy—this is mostly bilateral.
   b. Herpes zoster ophthalmicus—always unilateral (Fig. 8.2).

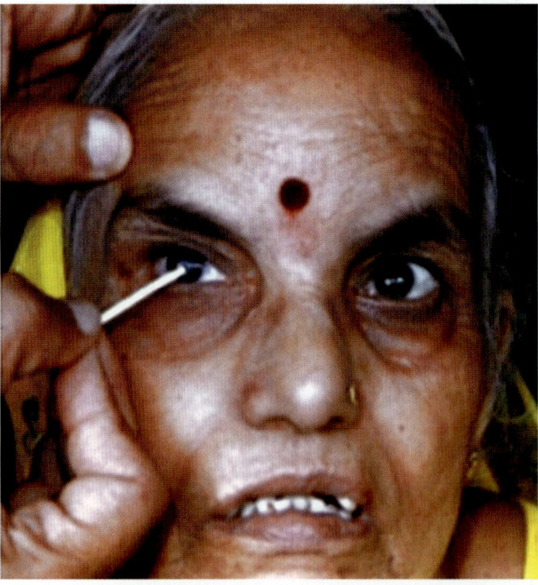

Fig. 8.1: Total loss of corneal sensation in postherpetic neuralgia

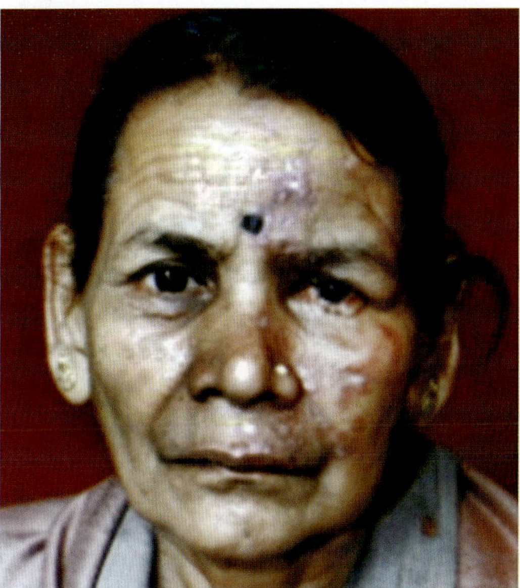

Fig. 8.2: Herpes zoster ophthalmicus involving first and second divison of the fifth nerve causing loss of sensation

c. Neoplasm of any structure between the orbits and middle cranial fossa. The lesion may be bilateral and involve all the divisions.

B. Oculofacial pain

Like oculofacial hyposthesia the pain may be:

i. Due to involvement of the trigeminal nerve.
ii. Referred from the structures supplied by the trigeminal nerve.

The common causes of oculofacial pain are:

1. Trigeminal neuralgia
2. Postherpetic neuroalgia
3. Migraine
4. Painful ophthalmoplegia
5. Raeder's syndrome of paratrigeminal neuralgia.
6. Pain referred from the structures supplied by the trigeminal:
   a. Eye and its adnexia
   b. Paranasal sinuses
   c. Teeth in the upper jaw
   d. Giant cell arteritis
   e. Temporomandibular syndrome
   f. Cervical spine
   g. Irritation of the dura
   h. Nasopharyngeal growth.

Trigeminal neuralgia

This is a **sudden, unilateral, severe pain** in the distribution of the trigeminal nerve that lasts only for **few seconds**. The **second** and the **third** divisions are more frequently involved than the first division but the first division is not totally immune in contrast to post herpetic neuralgia where the first division is mostly involved. Even a particular branch of the ophthalmic division may be involved selectively. The patient almost always has pain in and around the eye during the attack.

The pain has been described variously as sharp, stabbing, excruciating, etc. The first episode happens unexpectedly with sharp pain that passes-off without any treatment only to recur after. The intervening interval may be weeks to months initially, lessening gradually. The duration of pain free period gradually diminishes but never completely disappears. A person may have many attacks in a day. During the period of freedom of typical pain, the patient may have persistent dull ache in the distribution of trigeminal nerve.

The pain is always associated with sudden spasm of ipsilateral facial muscle contorting the face. This imparts the term **tic douloureux** to the condition.

The sensation of skin and cornea are maintained. This is in contrast to post herpetic neuralgia where loss of sensation is the rule.

The pain is invariably precipitated by a **trigger mechanism** that may even be a very soft touch on any part of the skin or mucous membrane supplied by fifth nerve. Remissions are known but are rare.

On rare instances the pain is bilateral, simultaneous or symmetric.

The commonest age of presentation is **fourth decade**, due to some unexplained cause it is more common on the right side and in females.

The exact cause of the condition is not known. It is most probable an episodic irritation of the trigeminal trunk. In case of bilateral involvement **multiple sclerosis** may be present.

Ocular changes

1. The corneal sensation is maintained.
2. There is no loss of ocular motility.
3. The pupil are normal.
4. Ocular findings are restricted to:
   a. Dull ocular pain
   b. Conjunctival congestion
   c. Lacrimation.

Differential diagnosis consists of **migraine, orbital apex syndrome, superior orbital fissure syndrome and postherpetic neuralgia**.

Management

Treatment is difficult and frustrating. Especially if the gap between two episodes are long.

The treatment can be:

1. Medical
2. Surgical

The medical treatment to be effective must be started shortly after the first few episodes.

The commonly used drugs are:

1. Carbamazepine
2. Phenytion
3. Baclofen
4. Gabapentin.

Surgical

Surgical methods are aimed to cut the sensory supply to the trigger zone by trigeminal gangliolysis. This can be achieved by:

1. **Injecting alcohol** in the trigeminal ganglion.
2. **Thermal gangliolysis** by radio frequency.
3. **Microsurgical** decompression of trigeminal root.

Gangliolysis is always followed by anesthesia in the distribution of fifth nerve. Commonest ocular complication being **neuroparalytic keratitis**.

Raeder's paratrigeminal neuralgia

This syndrome is also known by many other names, i.e. **cluster headache, histamine headache**.

The disease is seen mostly in **elderly men** and is a **unilateral disease** which starts as periorbital pain that may involve ipsilateral cranium, **may be episodic like migraine**. The bouts of headache are in clusters with pain free period in between. Gradually the headache persist throughout the day without respite. The headache may occur may times during the day. It is not uncommon for the patient to be awakened at night by the headache (see Chapter 15—Headache).

Sometimes, the headache is associated with **ipsilateral postganglionic Horner's syndrome** which passes off. In some cases the Horner's syndrome may persist.

The ocular features besides periorbital pain are: Conjunctival congestion, and lacrimation. Presence of ptosis or miosis should arouse suspicion of Horner's syndrome.

The exact cause of the condition is not known. Most accepted theory is migrainous dilatation of the internal carotid that may disturb the sympathetic fibers as well.

Differential diagnosis consists of migraine due to its episodic nature, and good response to antimigraine treatment. Other causes should include **trigeminal neuralgia, post herpetic neuralgia, superior orbital fissure syndrome**. If a patient with unilateral headache develops cranial nerve palsy a **parasellar lesion** should be expected and diagnosed by CT and MRI.

Treatment

The pain does not respond to usual analgesics and NSAID.

Satisfactory results are achieved by administering.

1. Ergotamine either as sublingual tablet of 2 mg. Ergotamine is available as nasal spray as well. Ergotamine may be used for prophylaxis also.
2. Sumatriptan is used as nasal spray.
3. Calcium channel blockers can be used as prophylaxis.

BIBLIOGRAPHY

1. Brisman R. Surgical treatment of trigeminal neuralgia. Semin Neurol 1997;17:367-72.
2. Fields HL. Treatment of trigeminal neuralgia. N Eng. Jr Med 1996;334:1125-26.
3. Fromm GH, Sessle BJ. Trigeminal neuralgia. Current concepts regarding pathogenesis and treatment. Butterworth, Boston 1991.
4. Kust RG, Strauss SE, Postherpetic neuralgia: Pathogenesis treatment and prevention. N Eng JM 1996;335:32-42.
5. Mahesh Kumar. Neuro-ophthalmology. 4th edn. Arvind Eye Hospital, Maduri 2007.

9 Neuro-ophthalmic Manifestation of Abducens (Abducent) Lesions

1. Sixth nerve dysfunction is the **commonest** and most **obvious** cause of paralytic squint that is **most difficult to diagnose**.
2. The sixth nerve has a **long intracranial course** next only to the fourth nerve.
3. In contrast to the third and fourth nerves, the sixth nerve **does not decussate** anywhere in its course. The fourth nerve decussates completely in the anterior medullary velum. The third nerve decussates partially in the midbrain.
4. The sixth nerve nucleus lies adjacent to the medial longitudinal fibers that connects the medial rectus nucleus of the other side (Fig. 2.16).
5. It passes through the pyramidal tract.
6. The sixth nerve trunk supplies **ipsilateral single muscle**, i.e. **lateral rectus**.
7. The sixth nerve nucleus sub serves ipsilateral lateral rectus in contrast to fourth nerve where the right fascicles proceed to become left trochlear nerve trunk to supply contralateral superior oblique.
8. There are no aberrant regeneration of sixth nerve in contrast to the third nerve.
9. **Isolated sixth nerve palsy does not have any localizing value**.
10. There are many condition that masquerade as abducens palsy without being so. They may collectively be referred as **pseudo abducens palsy**.
11. Sixth nerve may be involved at any age between newborn to ripe old age.
12. It may be involved on both sides (bilateral) or on one side (unilateral).
13. In contrast to fourth nerve involvement, sixth nerve lesions are more frequently associated with other nerve lesions (facial) or neural tract lesions i.e. dorsal/ ventral pons lesions.
14. It may be associated with oculosympathetic path.

The conditions that masquerade as sixth nerve palsy (Pseudo abducens palsy) are:

- Myasthenia
- Thyroid eye diseases
- Mobius syndrome
- Entrapment of medial rectus in fracture medial wall of orbit
- Infantile esotropia
- Spasm of near reflex

Neuro-ophthalmic features of sixth nerve

Like any other cranial nerve involved with movement of the eyes, the neurological lesions of sixth nerve can be:

1. Nuclear
2. Fasciculus
3. Basal
4. Cavernous sinus
5. Orbital

The nuclear lesion

The nuclear lesions are far less common than infranuclear lesions. **An isolated sixth nerve lesion cannot be a nuclear lesion because a nuclear lesion** is either associated with lesion in horizontal gaze nucleus or lesion of the seventh nerve fascicle.

The lesion can be:

1. Ipsilateral failure of horizontal gaze
2. Ipsilateral abduction defect
3. Ipsilateral seventh nerve palsy.

The fascicular lesion

There are two distinct clinical presentations of fascicular lesion of the sixth nerve that depend on location of the lesion which are in the **pons**. They could be in the **dorsal pons** or in the **ventral pons**. The first is called **Foville's syndrome** or **anterior inferior cerebellar artery syndrome** and the second is called **Millard-Gubler syndrome** (Fig. 9.1).

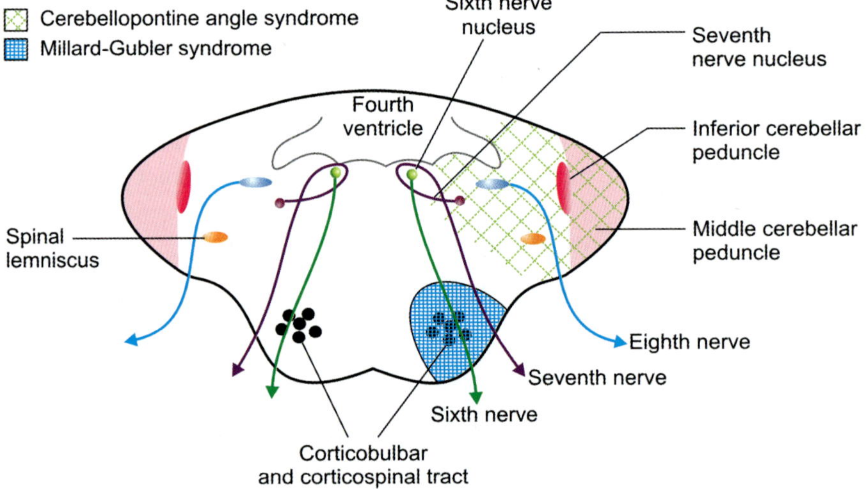

Fig. 9.1: Lesions in the lower pons

Foville's syndrome is produced in fascicle of the sixth nerve as it traverses through the PPRF

It consists of:
- Ipsilateral lateral rectus palsy
- Horizontal gaze palsy
- Ipsilateral facial weakness
- Ipsilateral facial analgesia
- Ipsilateral Horner's syndrome
- Deafness on the same side.

There is no hemiplegia. The lesion besides involving sixth nerve fascicles also involve seventh fascicle, sensory fibers of fifth nerve, eight nerve and central sympathetic path.

Millard-Gubler syndrome—This caused by a lesion more ventral than the former, consists of **ipsilateral sixth** and **seventh nerve palsy** and **contralateral hemiplegia** due to extension of the lesion in corticospinal tract.

Raymond's syndrome consists of ipsilateral sixth nerve palsy and contralateral hemiplegia due to a lesions of the sixth nerve fascicle near the corticospinal tract in the pons.

All the above syndromes are caused by **vascular accident** in the brainstem. The patients are too ill to present to an ophthalmologist. They are mostly seen in emergency rooms or neurology wards.

The basilar lesions

The basilar lesions are **more numerous** than nuclear or fascicular because the course of the sixth nerve is quite long in this space. The sixth nerve in this space does not come in close proximity of any neural tract but comes near the fifth, seventh and eight nerves.

The various lesions could be:
- Cerebellopontine angle syndrome
- Nasopharyngeal tumor extension
- Chordoma of clivus
- Fracture base of the skull
- Raised intracranial pressure
- Gradenigo's syndrome.

1. **Cerebellopontine angle syndrome (Acoustic neuroma syndrome) (Fig. 9.1)**

The syndrome involves **multiple cranial nerves** including the sixth nerve. The course of the sixth nerve and its relations to other structures are important in understanding the clinical features of this syndrome. The sixth nerve comes out of the brain at ponto-medullary junction and passes through the pre pontine basilar space. This is the location when it gets involved in cerebellopontine angle tumors which is a tumor of the **vestibular division of eighth nerve**.

The commonest tumor to involve the vestibular nerve at this site is **Schwannoma**, commonly known, as **acoustic neuroma**. The other tumors of this region are

neurofibroma, meningioma, osteoma and cholesteatoma. The neurofibromas are commonly bilateral.

The tumors are seen between **second to fourth decade**, are generally unilateral unless caused by neurofibroma. Clinical features of cerebellopontine angle tumor may have stigmata of neurofibromatosis.

The symptoms to begin with are due to involvement of the eight nerve which is the primary site. They symptoms are **diminished hearing**. In fact diminished hearing is considered to be the first symptoms of CPAT. The other symptoms are **tinitus, vertigo, vestibular nystagmus**. Rest of the symptoms depend upon spread of the tumor into neighboring structure. They are—**cerebellar ataxia, staggering, tendency to fall on the side of the tumor**.

The neuro-ophthalmic changes are—**Ipsilateral fourth, fifth, sixth, seventh and eighth nerve involvement**. The **fourth** and **sixth nerves** are compressed in the posterior fossa. Sixth nerve involvement is more common than fourth nerve. Involvement of fifth nerve causes **diminished corneal sensation**. Loss of corneal sensation is said to be the first sign of acoustic neuroma.

First symptoms of acoustic, neuroma is hearing loss.
First sign of acoustic neuroma is diminished corneal sensation.

This makes it mandatory to examine corneal sensation and test hearing in all cases of sixth nerve palsy.

Other ocular manifestations of CPAT are

a. Lagophthalmos, exposure keratitis, corneal ulcer.
b. Diminished tearing
c. Gaze palsy
d. Nystagmus
e. Horner's syndrome
f. Papilledema

The nonocular symptoms are—Hyperacusia, tinnitus, vertigo and ataxia. **Other signs of cerebellar dysfunction**—Loss of taste from anterior 2/3rd of the tongue, dysarthria, dysphagia.

Treatment is directed towards the management of the tumor. Lagophthalmos and loss of corneal sensations may require tarsorrhaphy.

2. **Nasopharyngeal tumors**

   The nasopharyngeal tumours that cause extraocular palsy, generally arise in the **roof of the nasopharynx**. They are **highly malignant** and often **radio resistant**. They may be seen at **any age between ten years and sixty years**. They cause neuro-ophthalmic changes when the tumors invade the **paranasal sinuses, orbit, base of the skull, middle cranial fossa** and **pituitary fossa**. They may involve any of the cranial nerves from **third to eleventh**. Involvement of lower cranial nerves are more common than 3rd to 7th. **Fifth cranial nerve is more commonly involved nerve than third and sixth nerve**. Out of third, fourth and sixth, the last is more frequently involved, may be effected alone in its basilar course or with other cranial nerves in cavernous sinus or orbit. The optic nerve is involved either due to extension in the brain or raised intracranial tension leading to loss of vision.

Proptosis is common due to invasion of the orbit by the tumor. **Horner's syndrome** is caused due to compression of the sympathetic chain in the neck by enlarged lymph nodes.

Overall prognosis is poor.

3. **Chordoma of the clivus** are **rare** tumors arising from clivus the **remnants of the notocord**. They are generally in the midline but cause **unilateral sixth nerve palsy**.

   The clivus may be involved in malignancy of nasopharynx and the condition may present as nasopharyngeal growth.

4. **Fracture of the base of the skull**
   The peculiar course of the sixth nerve, i.e. a horizontal course in the posterior fossa and near vertical course in the Dorello's canal makes the sixth nerve vulnerable to closed head injury due either to vertical or horizontal impact that cause fracture of petrous part of the **temporal bone**. It is common for the **seventh nerve** to be involved in fracture of petrous bone because of its long course in the bone. An injury compressing the skull horizontally is likely to cause bilateral sixth and seventh nerve palsy.

   Battle's signs of closed head injury may be present. It consists of **leak of CSF** or **blood** from the **external ear** and **ecchymosis** over the mastoid.

5. **Raised intracranial pressure**
   Any lesion that pushes the **brainstem** down along with the **sixth nerve** can cause stretching of the sixth nerve over the **petrous bone** throttling the nerve. This results in **sixth nerve palsy**. It may be **unilateral** or **bilateral**. The other causes may be **posterior fossa tumors** or **pseudotumor cerebri**. The sixth nerve palsy due to **raised intracranial pressure** is **non-localizing**, gradually developing intracranial tension, may cause insidius sixth nerve palsy that may mimic divergence palsy causing horizontal diplopia for far vision.

6. **Gradenigo's syndrome**
   This used to be a common cause of **unilateral sixth nerve** palsy before advent of antibiotics in children, may still be seen in rural areas where otitis media is either missed or not treated well.

The events are as follows (Flow chart 9.1):

Flow chart 9.1: Manifestations of otitis media

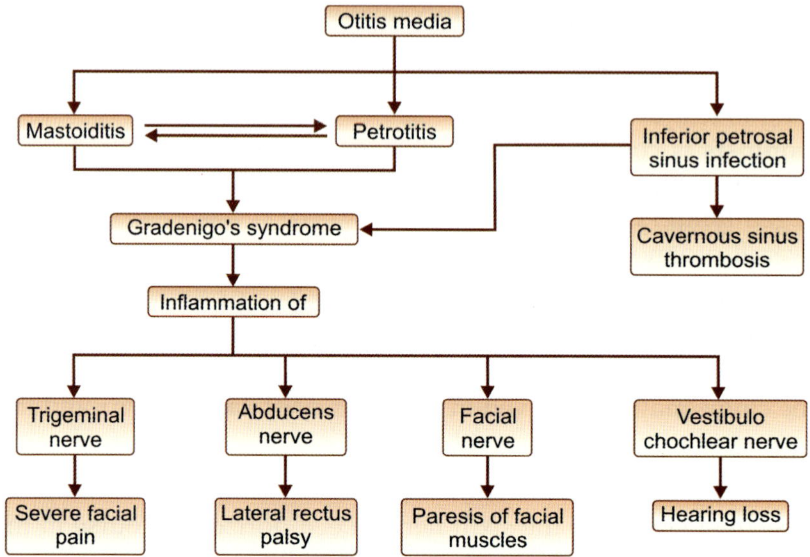

The condition responds well to antibiotics.

Cavernous sinus lesions (see also Fig. 2.8)

The **third**, **fourth** and **fifth cranial nerves** are embedded in the lateral wall of the cavernous sinus. In contrast to this the sixth nerve lies in the substance of the cavernous sinus almost in the middle of the sinus. It is placed at lower level than the above said nerves. The sixth nerve is very near the intracavernous part of the **internal carotid**. The postganglionic fibers of the sympathetic joins the sixth nerve in the cavernous sinus so lesions in cavernous sinus can cause following lesions

1. Isolated sixth nerve palsy due to pressure symptoms of internal carotid artery. This is relatively rare.
2. Sixth nerve palsy with ipsilateral postganglionic Horner's syndrome.
3. Sixth nerve palsy along with third, fourth and fifth nerves defect.
4. A large lesion of cavernous sinus may involve the second nerve, optic chiasma or even the pituitary gland.

The common intracavernous causes of sixth nerve palsy are:
Aneurysm of the intracavernous part of the internal carotid, carotid cavernous fistula, dural shunt, cavernous sinus thrombosis, tumors extending into the cavernous sinus, and trauma.

The orbital lesions

Involvement of sixth nerve in orbit is **rarely isolated**, it is associated with **mild to moderate proptosis**, **chemosis of conjunctiva** and involvement of other nerves related to movement of the eyeball. Involvement of the **fifth nerve is frequent**. Rarely it may be associated with changes in optic nerve.

The condition that may mimic orbital sixth nerve lesions are:
- Myasthenia
- Thyroid eye disease
- Pseudotumor of the orbit.

Diagnosis of sixth nerve palsy

Isolated sixth nerve palsy is a common ocular palsy. It may be associated with brainstem lesion. It has **limited localizing value** requiring consultation with ENT specialist, neurologist, internist and radiologist. To establish neural causes of lateral rectus palsy it is mandatory to exclude lesions of cavernous sinus and orbit.

Diagnosis of unilateral isolated sixth nerve palsy can be reached roughly by symptoms and signs.

Symptoms

1. Diplopia
   (i) Uncrossed
   (ii) Horizontal
   (iii) Worse of distance
   (iv) Worse in the action of affected muscles
   (v) Lessens on face turning towards the affected muscles.
2. Esotropia (Figs 9.2 and 9.3)
3. Head position
   (i) Turn towards the affected muscle
   (ii) No change in position of chin
   (iii) No head tilt

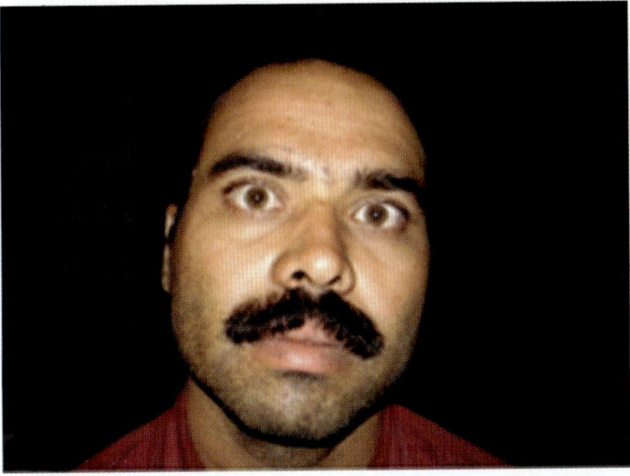
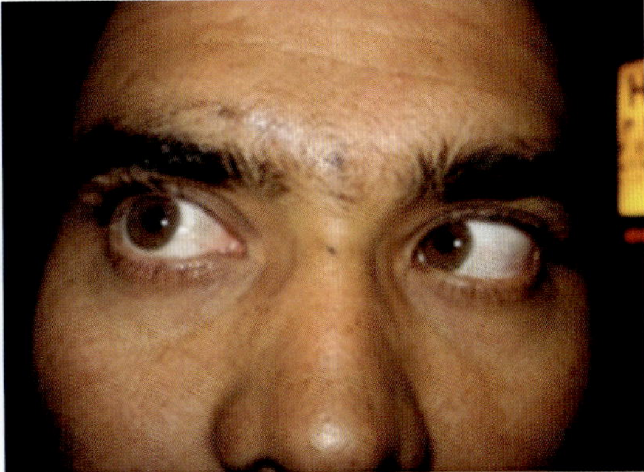

Fig. 9.2: Isolated sixth nerve palsy (*Courtesy:* Dr Santosh Patel)

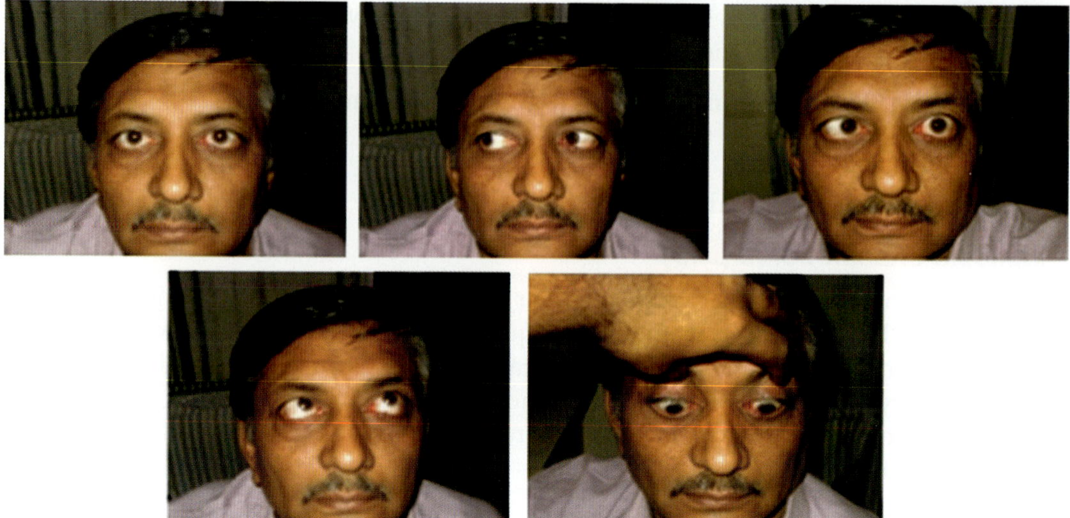

Fig. 9.3: Isolated sixth nerve palsy (*Courtesy:* Dr Sharad Sivasane and Dr Dishant Singh)

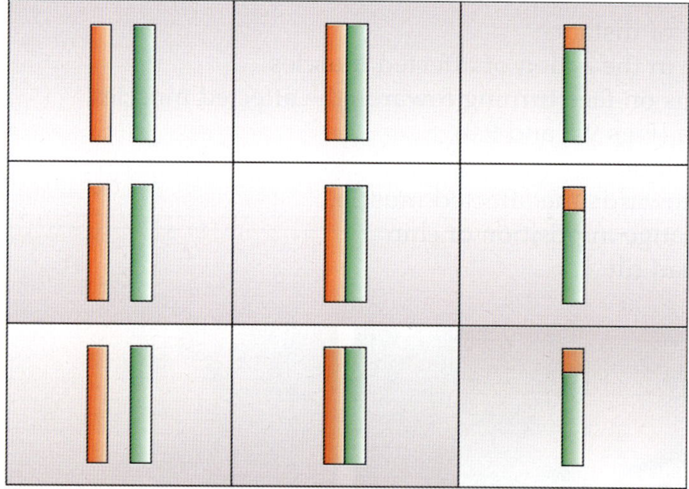

Fig. 9.4: Diplopia chart, sixth nerve palsy, left side left lateral rectus palsy

Sign

1. Esotropia
2. Face turn
3. Movement
   (i) Under-action of (Figs 9.4 and 9.5)
      (a) Affected lateral rectus
      (b) Contralateral lateral rectus

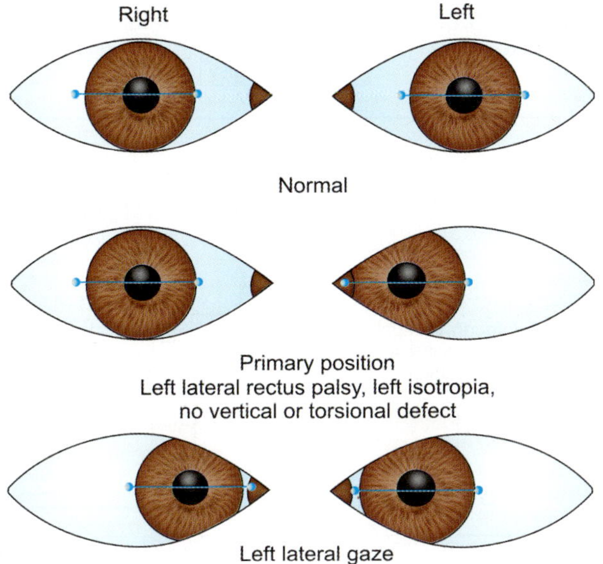

Fig. 9.5: Right eye adducted; left eye no abduction beyond mid-line no torsional or vertical defect

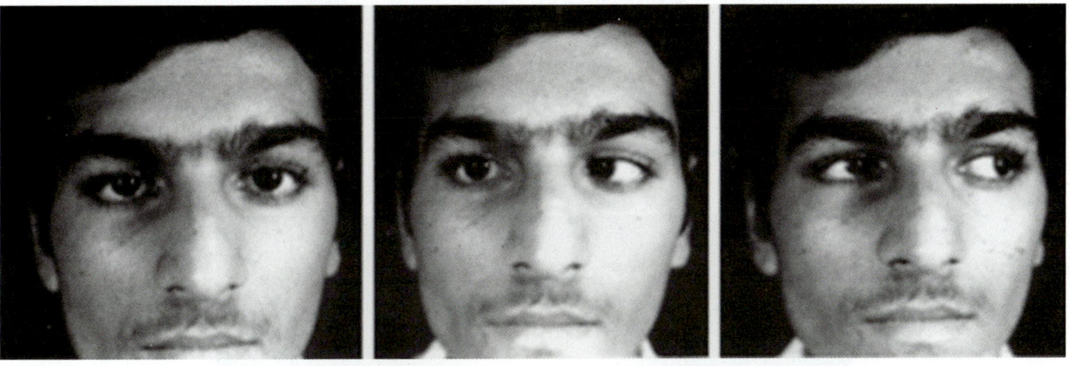

Fig. 9.6: Duane's retraction syndrome (*Courtesy:* Dr ML Garg)

(ii) Overaction of
   (a) Ipsilateral medial rectus
   (b) Contralateral medial rectus

Extraocular muscle palsies in children (Fig. 9.7 and Flow charts 9.2 and 9.3) – (Third, fourth and sixth nerve)

1. Incidence of muscle palsy in children is far less common than in adults that sub serve the extraocular muscle.
2. They may involve isolated nerve or may involve more than one nerve.

Flow chart 9.2: Localization of sixth cranial nerve palsy

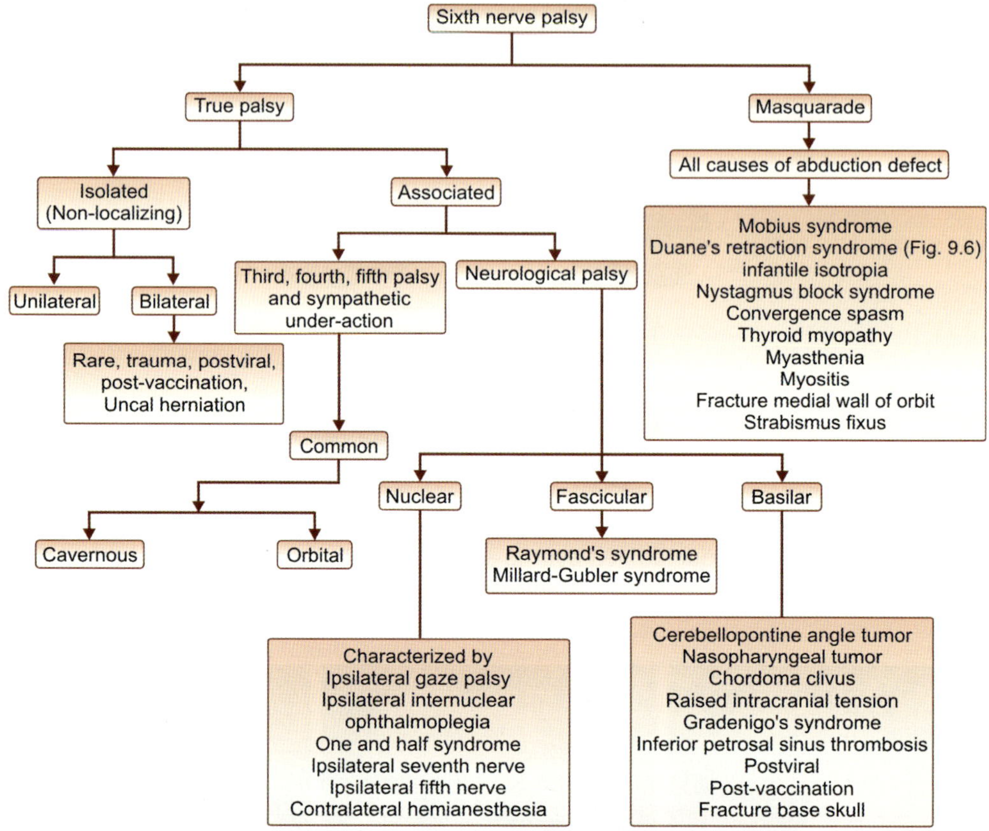

- Sixth nerve palsy
  - True palsy
    - Isolated (Non-localizing)
      - Unilateral
      - Bilateral
        - Rare, trauma, postviral, post-vaccination, Uncal herniation
    - Associated
      - Third, fourth, fifth palsy and sympathetic under-action
        - Common
          - Cavernous
          - Orbital
      - Neurological palsy
        - Nuclear
          - Characterized by
            - Ipsilateral gaze palsy
            - Ipsilateral internuclear ophthalmoplegia
            - One and half syndrome
            - Ipsilateral seventh nerve
            - Ipsilateral fifth nerve
            - Contralateral hemianesthesia
        - Fascicular
          - Raymond's syndrome
          - Millard-Gubler syndrome
        - Basilar
          - Cerebellopontine angle tumor
          - Nasopharyngeal tumor
          - Chordoma clivus
          - Raised intracranial tension
          - Gradenigo's syndrome
          - Inferior petrosal sinus thrombosis
          - Postviral
          - Post-vaccination
          - Fracture base skull
  - Masquarade
    - All causes of abduction defect
      - Mobius syndrome
      - Duane's retraction syndrome (Fig. 9.6)
      - infantile isotropia
      - Nystagmus block syndrome
      - Convergence spasm
      - Thyroid myopathy
      - Myasthenia
      - Myositis
      - Fracture medial wall of orbit
      - Strabismus fixus

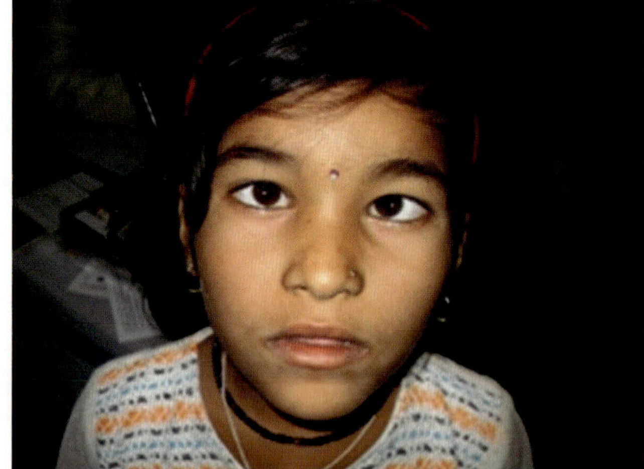

Fig. 9.7: Bilateral sixth nerve palsy in a child (*Courtesy:* Dr Nidhi Pandey)

Flow chart 9.3: Etiology of sixth nerve palsy

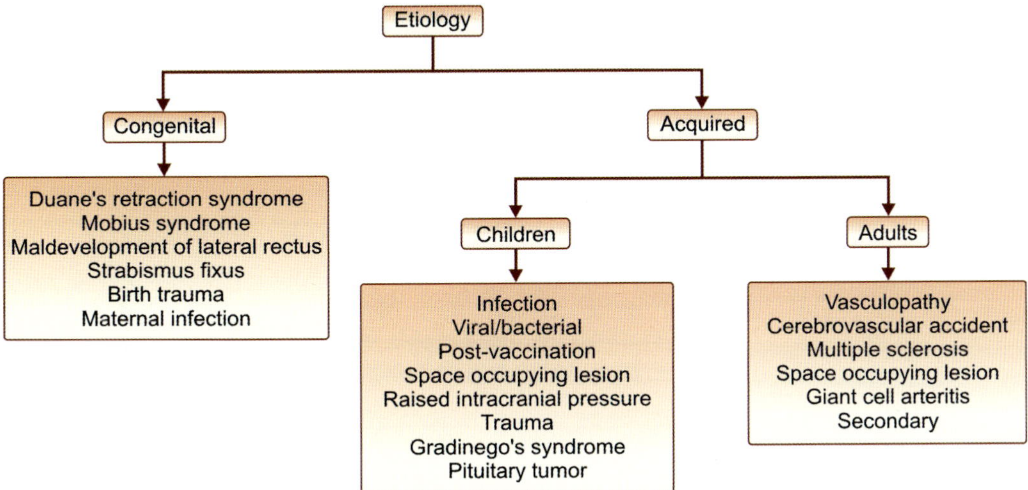

3. Transient sixth nerve palsy in newborn generally passes off without any treatment and is independent of birth trauma.
4. Birth trauma generally cause sixth nerve palsy that is more often bilateral than unilateral and is generally due to trauma by obstetric forceps.
5. Superior oblique is the muscle that suffers congenital anomaly frequently. This is followed by congenital anomaly of sixth nerve.
6. Ophthalmoplegic migraine is seen commonly in first decade.
7. Cyclic oculomotor palsy is seen in early childhood.
8. Postinfection muscle palsy is more common in children.
9. Intracranial space occupying lesions are common causes of sixth nerve palsy they can either be inflammatory or neoplastic.

Investigation

Exclude

(i) Vasculopathy, i.e. diabetes, hypertension, arteriosclerosis
(ii) Compressive lesions by CT, MRI
(iii) Lesions of orbit and cavernous by CT, MRI, USG
(iv) Guarded lumbar puncture to examine CSF.

BIBLIOGRAPHY

1. Afift AK, Bell WF, Menezes AH. Etiology of later rectus palsy in infants and childhood. Jr Child Neuro 1992;7:295-97.
2. Glasser JS, Saitkowski RM. Infranuclear disorders of eye movement in Neuro-ophthalmology. 3rd edn, Glasser J (Eds), Lippincot William and Wilkins, Philadelphia 1989;405-60.

3. Jacobson DM. Progressive ophthalmoplegia with acute ischemic abducens palsy. Am J Oph 1996;122:278-79.
4. Moster ML, Savio PJ, et al. Isolated sixth nerve palsy in young adults. Arch Oph 1964;102:1328-30.
5. Werner DB, Savino PJ, Schatz N. Benign recurrent sixth nerve palsy in Childhood. Arch Oph 1983;101.

10 Neuro-ophthalmic Manifestations of Seventh (Facial) Nerve

Lesions of seventh nerve are more common than third, fourth and sixth nerve and are seen by a long list of medical personnel ranging from family physician to neuro surgeons. The commonest lesion encountered is **Bell's palsy**. The seventh nerve can be involved in **isolation** or in **combination** with other cranial nerves or tract lesions. The former are generally benign and managed with ease, the latter have far reaching systemic manifestation requiring multi disciplinary involvement.

The facial nerve is a **mixed nerve**. It has following components (Table 10.1):

- Motor
- Sensory
- Secretomotor

The lesions of seventh nerve can result in:

I. Facial palsy

II. Facial spasm

The facial palsy can be:

1. **Isolated facial palsy**
   i. Upper motor neuron.
   ii. Lower motor neuron.
2. **Facial nerve lesion with:**
   i. Other cranial nerve lesions
   ii. Tract lesions.
3. **Lacrimal hyposecretion**

To understand the upper motor neuron palsy of seventh nerve, it is essential to revise the supranuclear connections of the seventh nerve.

Table 10.1: Components of facial nerve and their functions

Components	*Functions*
1. Motor (efferent)	Motor supply to muscles developing from mesoderm of second branchial arch, i.e. muscles of facial expression – frontalis, orbicularis oculi, orbicularis oris, risorius, levator angularis, buccinators, nasal muscles, platysma
2. Sensory (afferent)	Sensation from tongue, external ear and soft pallet.
3. Secretomotor (efferent)	Parasympathetic fibers to lacrimal gland, submandibular and sublingual salivary glands.

The outline of supranuclear connections of the seventh nerve are as follows (Flow chart 10.1):

Flow chart 10.1: Supranuclear connections of the seventh nerve

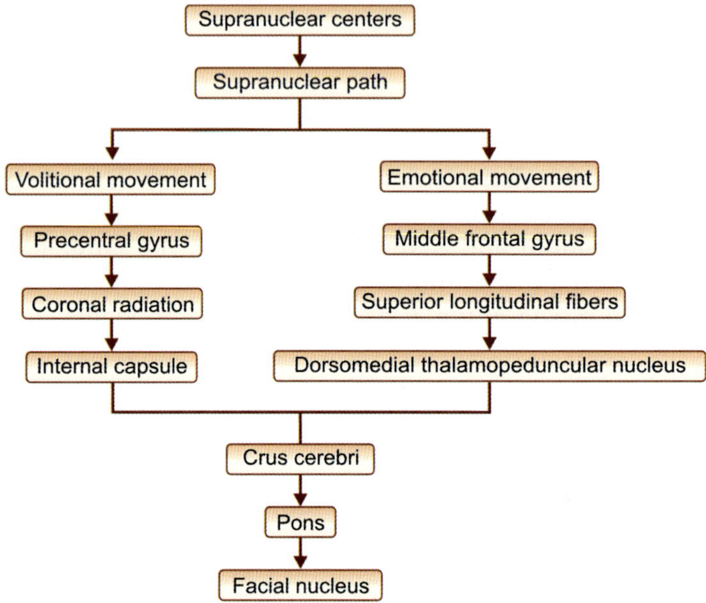

The **supranuclear path** originates in the **frontal lobe** descends through the cortico-bulbar tract and decussates partly (Fig. 10.1). The undecussated fibers go straight to the muscles of the same side and supply the half of face. The decussated fibers reach

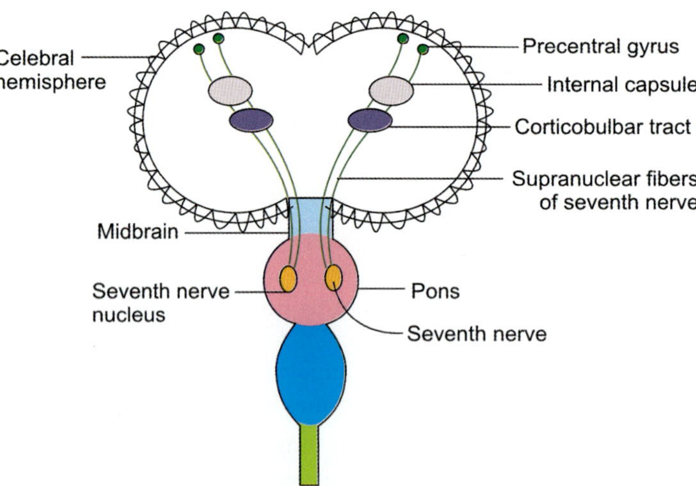

Fig. 10.1: Supranuclear connection of seventh nerve

the facial nucleus on the other side and innervate the lower half of the face. The trunk of the facial nerve carry fibers from both the frontal cortex. The volitional and emotional movement follow different routes from cortex to crus cerebri. There after they pass into the nucleus of seventh nerve in the pons. Both the pyramidal and extrapyramidal systems are said to control the facial nerve.

Difference between the upper motor and lower motor neuron lesions of the facial nerve (Fig. 10.2)

Features	*Upper motor neuron*	*Lower motor neuron*
Part of the face involved	Only contralateral lower face	Ipsilateral whole of the face
Forhead wrinkles	Present	Absent
Closure of eye	Present	Absent - lagophthalmos
Emotional movement	Present	Lost
Hemiplegia (When present)	Ipsilateral	Contralateral
Wasting	Absent	Present
Reaction of degeneration	Absent	Present, starts after 2-3 weeks

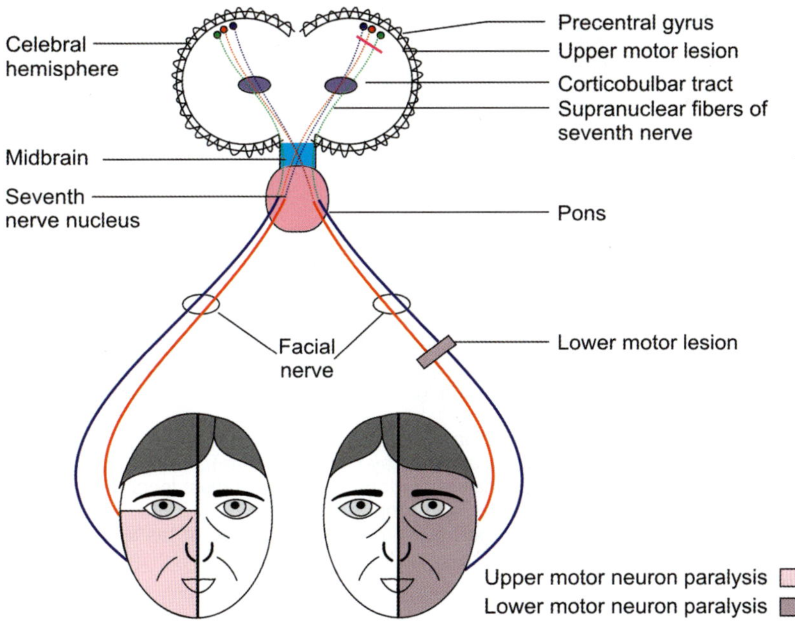

Fig. 10.2: Areas of face involved in upper and lower motor paralysis of seventh nerve

I. Facial palsy

Lower motor neuron facial palsy

The lower motor neuron facial palsies are **more commonly** seen by ophthalmologist than upper motor neuron because the latter hardly has any ocular manifestation.

The various locations, where the seventh nerve can be involved to produce lower motor neuron lesions can be (Fig. 10.3):

1. **Nuclear or nucleofascicular:**
   The lesions are in the **pons** causing (Figs 10.4 and 10.5):
   - Facial palsy
   - Abducence palsy
   - Contralateral hemiplegia
   - Facial anesthesia
2. **Trunk lesion**
   i. In the posterior cranial fossa
   ii. Cerebellopontine angle

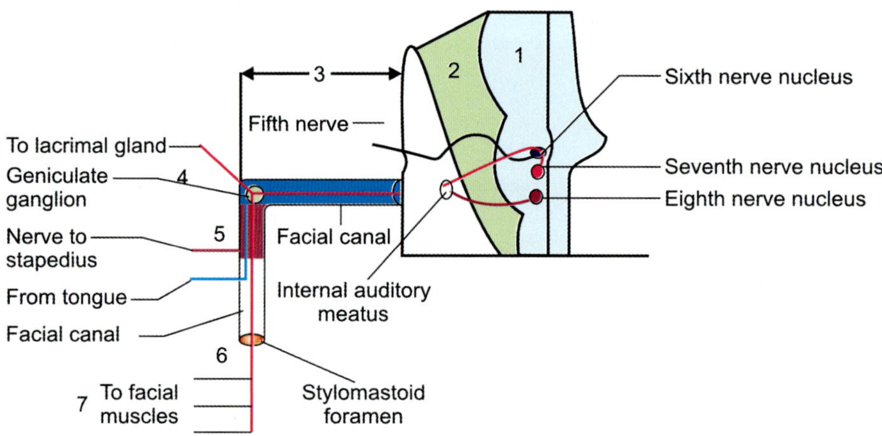

1. Pontine lesion—seventh-sixth nerve palsy, facial anesthesia, (fifth nerve), contralateral hemiplegia.
2. Posterior fossa lesion—facial palsy, facial anesthesia (fifth nerve), deafness tinnitus vertigo (8th nerve), loss of lacrimation, loss of taste from anterior 2/3rd of tongue.
3. Lesion in facial canal above geniculate ganglion—facial palsy, loss of lacrimation, loss of taste from anterior 2/3rd of tongue.
4. Lesion lateral geniculate ganglion—loss of taste from anterior 2/3rd of tongue, hyperacusis and vesicle external ear (Ramsay-Hunt syndrome).
5. Lesion between geniculate ganglion and nerve to stapedius lacrimation preserved hyperacusis loss of taste anterior 2/3rd of tongue.
6. Lesion in the stylomastoid foramen facial palsy without loss of taste and lacrimation, diminished salivation.
7. Intranuclear facial palsy.

Fig. 10.3: Various possible levels of infranuclear seventh nerve palsy

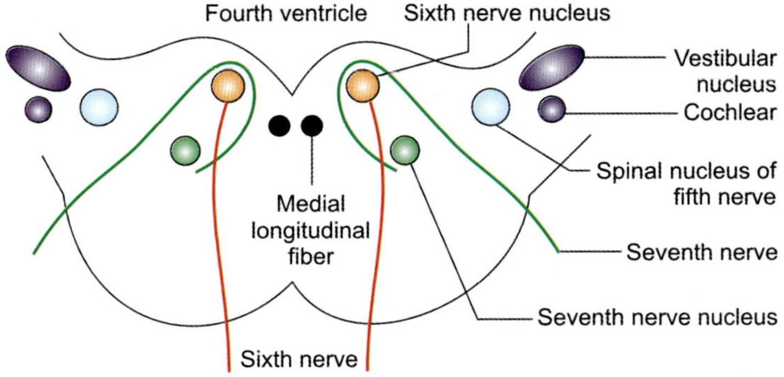

Fig. 10.4: Various cranial nerve nuclei in pons in relation to seventh nerve

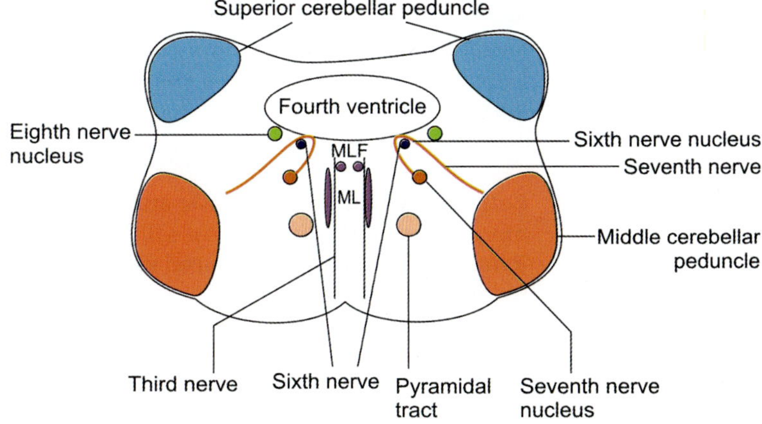

Fig. 10.5: Position of seventh nerve in relation to other neural tract

iii. **Facial canal:**
   a. Above the geniculate ganglion
   b. In the geniculate ganglion
   c. Below the geniculate ganglion.
iv. Stylomastoid foramen.
v. Face.

Unilateral facial palsy

Unilateral facial palsies are more common than bilateral. Out of all unilateral facial palsies, **Bell's palsy** is the commonest palsy.

Following is the list of conditions that cause unilateral facial palsy, they are:

1. Bell's palsy
2. Leprosy (in endemic area)

Chart showing site of lesion, its corresponding features in lesions of seventh nerve (see Figs 9.1, 12.2, 2.16, 2.17, 2.26, 2.27, 2.28)

Site	*Clinical features*
1. **Posterior cranial fossa**	Facial palsy, facial anesthesia, diminished hearing, vertigo and ringing in the ear, diminished lacrimation, loss of taste, sensation from anterior 2/3rd of tongue.
2. **Cerebellopontine angle**	Facial palsy, loss of corneal sensation, paralysis of abducent nerve, nystagmus, cerebellar ataxia, dysphagia, signs of raised intracranial pressure, deafness, tinitus and vertigo (see Fig. 12.2).
3. **Facial canal**	
a. Above the geniculate ganglion.	Facial palsy, diminished lacrimation, loss of taste from anterior 2/3rd of tongue, crocodile tear.
b. In the geniculate ganglion.	Facial palsy, hyperacusia diminished hearing, loss of taste, vesicles on the external ear.
c. Between geniculate ganglion and stylomastoid foramens.	Facial weakness, loss of taste, hypercusia, normal tear.
4. **Stylomastoid foramens**	**Bell's palsy** with retained taste and lacrimation, dryness of month due to hypofunction of salivary secretion.
5. **Face**	Paralysis of orbicularis. Reduced salivation, increased reflex tearing, lagophthalmos

3. Lyme's disease.
4. Ramsay-Hunt syndrome.
5. Trauma – To mastoid–Surgical/accidental
   – Parotid surgery
   – Zygomatic bone fracture
6. Diabetes.
7. Tumors – Cerebellopontine angle tumor, tumors of petrous bone, pontine growth.
8. Vascular – Cerebrovascular accidents
   – Millard-Gubler syndrome
   – Fovilles syndrome
9. Myopathies.

Causes of bilateral facial palsy

1. Congenital – Mobius syndrome
2. Trauma – Birth trauma – Application of forceps
   – Closed head injury
3. Infection – i. Leprosy
   – ii. Syphilitic basal meningitis
   – iii. Postdiphtheretic

Physical findings that lead to localization of the lesion in facial nerve are shown in Flow chart 10.2.

Flow chart 10.2: Physical findings (facial palsy)

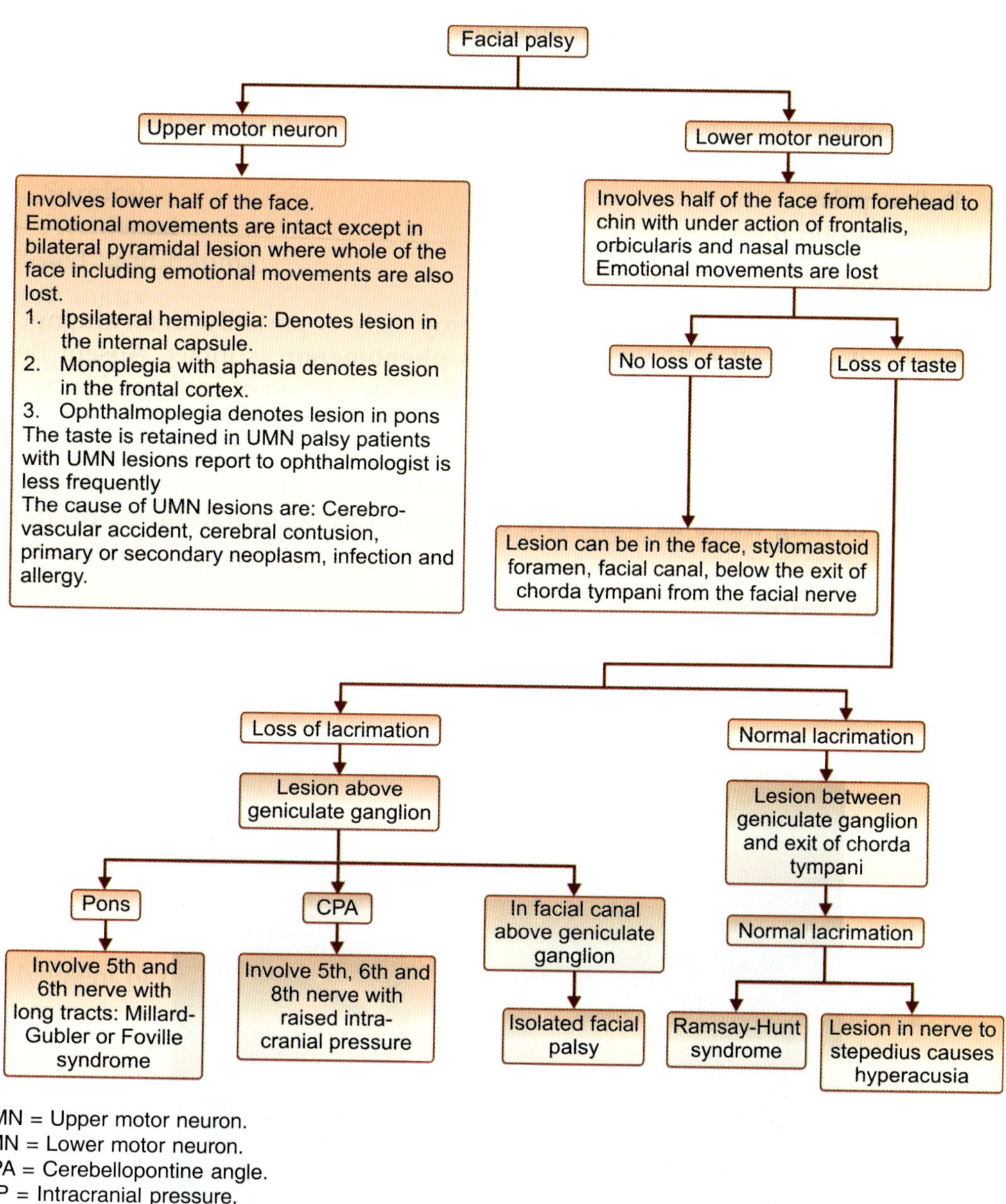

UMN = Upper motor neuron.
LMN = Lower motor neuron.
CPA = Cerebellopontine angle.
ICP = Intracranial pressure.
GG = Geniculate ganglion.

Table 11.1: Differences between congenital ocular palsies and acquired palcies

S.No.	*Features*	*Congenital*	*Acquired*
1.	**Onset**	Noticed at birth or may be missed at birth.	Sudden, may be persistent, recurrent or transient.
2.	**Symptoms**		
	I. Diplopia	Only in the paretic gaze, a small child may not complain.	Sudden onset. Patient is aware of it, may be the symptom for which the patient seeks help.
	II. Deviation of the eye	May or may not be present.	Most of the time the deviation is obvious.
	III. Abnormal head posture	Most of the time present. Patient may not be aware. Old photographs may reveal abnormal head posture.	May or may not be present. Old photographs do not show abnormality.
3.	**Signs**		
	I. Deviation	May or may not be present, abnormal head posture may mask the deviation.	Most of the time present.
	II. Past pointing	Absent	Frequent
	III. Image tilt	Absent	Present and diagnostic
	IV. Secondary muscle changes	May or may not be present	Always present
	V. Forced duction test	May be positive	Absent
	VI. Comitance	Spread of comitance	Incomitant
	VII. Amblyopia	Frequent	Only in children
	VIII. Hess chart	Field equal	Smaller field belongs to affected eye.

Table 11.2: Signs associated with neuro-ophthalmic motility disorder

Sign	*Symptom*
1. **Face**	
i. Obliteration of supraciliary folds	Facial palsy
ii. Obliteration of nasolabial fold	Facial palsy
iii. Deviation of mouth	Facial palsy
iv. Weakness of lower two thirds of face	Supranuclear facial palsy

Contd...

Contd...

2. **Interpalpebral aperture**	
i. Widening of IPA	Infranuclear facial palsy
ii. Narrowing of IPA	Ptosis
3. **Squint**	
i. Divergent	Paralysis of adductors
ii. Convergent	Paralysis of abductors
iii. Hyperdeviation	Paralysis of depressor
iv. Hypodeviation	Paralysis of elevators
4. **Pupillary reaction** – Absent	Use of mydriatic/cycloplegic Internal ophthalmoplegia Blind eye
i. Afferent pupillary reaction	Optic nerve lesion
ii. Argyll-Robertson pupil	Lesion in rostral midbrain
iii. Adeis pupil	Lesion in ciliary ganglion or short ciliary nerve
iv. Hutchinson pupil	Ipsilateral intracranial expanding lesion
v. Miotic pupil	Use of local or systemic miotic drugs Horner's pupil Pontine hemorrhage
5. **Corneal sensation** – Diminished sensation	Recent use of local anesthetic agent Local viral infection Trigeminal neuralgia Involvement of fifth nerve Postherpetic neuralgia Cerebellopontine angle tumor
6. **Hearing**	
i. Deafness	Lesion of eighth nerve
ii. Hyperacusia	Paralysis of stapedius muscle in facial palsy
7. **Ocilopsia**	Nystagmus – Ocular – Labyrinth – Vestibular – Cerebellar – Pontine
8. **Weakness of limbs**	Contralateral hemiplegia
9. **Others**	
i. Loss of taste	Lower motor neuron palsy of seventh nerve
ii. Diminished tearing	Lower motor neuron palsy of seventh nerve

3. **Drooping** of eyelid – Ptosis.
4. **Inability to close the eye** – Lagophthalmos
5. **Widening interpalpebral aperture**
   i. Lid retraction
   ii. Proptosis.
6. **Proptosis**
7. **Diminished vision**
   i. Distant – Optic neuritis
   Optic atrophy
   ii. Near – Cycloplegia
8. **Abnormal color sense** – Optic neuritis.
9. **Field changes** – Patient may be aware of field changes or may not be aware of it.

II. Nonocular

1. **Neurological** – Hemiplegia
   – Tremor
   – Convulsion
   – Unconsciousness
   – Nystagmus
   – Ataxia
2. **Symptoms of raised intracranial tension**
   – Headache
   – Vomiting
   – Diplopia
3. **Headache**
   i. Migraine
   ii. Nonmigraneous
      a. Due to raised intracranial tension
      b. Due to inflammation
      c. Trauma
4. **Symptoms related to systemic infection**
   – Malignancy
   – Diabetes
   – Migraine
   – Hypertension
   – Degenerative condition.

Lesions of supranuclear pathway

The lesions of supranuclear pathway cause **dissociation of various types of eye movement**s both **horizontal** and **vertical**. Any of the following may be involved:

- Saccadic
- Pursuit
- Vestibular movements.

The **horizontal** eye movements are generally initiated in the **pons** and the **vertical** in the **midbrain**. The dissociations result in **gaze palsy**. Any of the two gazes, i.e. **horizontal** or **vertical**, may be involved. The involvement may be **conjugate** or **nonconjugate**. Various other neurological features are also present. The supranuclear lesions maintain parallelism, hence **no diplopia**. All horizontal eye movements are generally in PPRF. From here the output goes to ipsilateral sixth nerve and to contralateral third nerve (see Figs 2.1 to 2.3).

The rule of thumb for conjugate ocular palsies

I. **Central lesion**
   a. Paralytic lesion: The head and the eyes turn towards the side of the lesion.
   b. Irritable lesion: The eyes turn towards the healthy side away from the lesion.

II. **Pontine lesion**
   a. Paralytic – The eyes turn towards the healthy side.
   b. Irritative – The eyes turn away from the healthy side.

The site of the lesions can be at any of the following locations—**Cerebrum, basal ganglion, round the sylvian aqueduct, pons, eighth nerve** or **cerebellum**.

The cerebral lesions are associated with hemiplegia, athetosis and convulsion. It produces gaze palsy to the opposite side.

The basal ganglia lesions produce oculogyric crisis, tremor and rigidity.

The pontine lesions are associated with multiple upper cranial nerve palsy. It produces gaze palsy to the same side.

Horizontal gaze defects

The horizontal gaze defects are:

1. Paralysis of horizontal gaze.
2. Internuclear ophthalmoplegia.
3. One and half syndrome.
4. Tonic deviation of gaze.
5. Locked in syndrome.

Differences between frontal and pontine lesions of horizontal gaze palsy

	Frontal lesion	*Pontine lesion*
Direction	Gaze palsy towards contralateral side.	Gaze palsy towards ipsilateral side.
Deviation	The eyes are deviated to the side of the lesion.	The eyes are deviated away from the side of the lesion.
Hemiparesis	Contralateral	Ipsilateral
Vestibulo-ocular reflex	Normal	Subnormal
Smooth pursuit	Normal	Subnormal

6. Loss of:
   i. Pursuit
   ii. Saccade.

Characteristics of horizontal gaze defects (Table 11.3)

1. There is a conjugate movement of the eyes in an abnormal direction.
2. The patient is unable to move the eye in specific horizontal direction.
3. The patient may not be able to sustain gaze in particular direction.
4. The eyes may move slowly to sustain gaze.
5. Gaze paretic nystagmus is common.

Internuclear ophthalmoplegia (INO)

Inter nuclear ophthalmoplegia is caused due to lesion of medial longitudinal fasciculus (MLF).

The medial longitudinal fasciculi comprise fibers that are situated near the midline of the midbrain on either side. The MLF extends from third ventricle above to the anterior intersegmental tract of the spinal cord.

The MLF joins the nuclei of third, fourth and sixth cranial nerves.

It also receives fibers of **seventh nerve** and some fibers of the eighth nerve.

The internuclear ophthalmoplegia is **mostly unilateral** and is named after the side on which the MLF is involved. Less common is bilateral involvement. It can be **total** or **partial**. It has been divided into two types—**anterior lesion** and **posterior lesion**.

The characteristics of INO are:

1. Subnormal adduction on the side of the lesion.
2. In milder form there may only be slowing of saccade on adduction.
3. Nystagmus on abduction (Fig. 11.1).
4. Retained convergence.
5. Convergence is lost in midbrain lesion.
6. **In bilateral lesions**.
   i. Upbeat nystagmus on looking up
   ii. Both eyes are divergent. This condition is known as **wall-eyed bilateral internuclear ophthalmoplegia** or WEBINO.
   iii. The commonest cause is **multiple sclerosis**.
7. There may be skew deviation in the ipsilateral eye.

The INO is seen in young adults and old age. In young adults, the commonest cause is multiple sclerosis. In old age, the common causes are **vascular** or **neoplastic**. The vascular causes are stroke or arteriovenous malformation. Other causes are **encephalitis** and **encephalopathy**.

One and half syndrome

One and half syndrome is due to lesions more extensive than those that cause INO. The lesions are in **sixth nerve nucleus**, PPRF and **ipsilateral MLF**. The eye moves

Table 11.3: Features of various types of horizontal gaze disorder

Disorder	*Site of lesion*	*Clinical features*
Paralysis of horizontal gaze	PPRF/nucleus of sixth nerve	1. Inability to move the eyes beyond the midline on the side of the lesion. 2. Vestibulo-ocular reflex is intact in lesion of PPRF. 3. Vestibulo-ocular reflex is abolished in lesion of sixth nerve nucleus.
Internuclear ophthalmoplegia	Medial longitudinal fasciculus	1. Subnormal adduction on the same side 2. Nystagmus i. Ataxic ii. Torsional iii. Upbeat 3. Intact convergence. 4. Absent vertical smooth pursuit. 5. Subnormal vestibulo-ocular reflex
One and half syndrome	Medial longitudinal fasciculus /PPRF or nucleus of sixth nerve	1. Gaze palsy on the side of lesion. 2. Contralateral internuclear ophthalmoplegia.
Tonic deviation of gaze	Frontal eye field	1. Eye deviates towards the site of the lesion. 2. Transient deviation to contra lateral side.
Locked eye syndrome	Ventral pons, PPRF, corticospinal path	1. The lid movements are preserved. 2. Vertical eye movements are present. 3. All other movements are lost
Loss of pursuit	Temporal parietooccipital junction	Failure of pursuit on the side of the lesion.
Selective loss of saccade	Diffuse cerebral bilateral frontoparietal	Ocular motor apraxia.

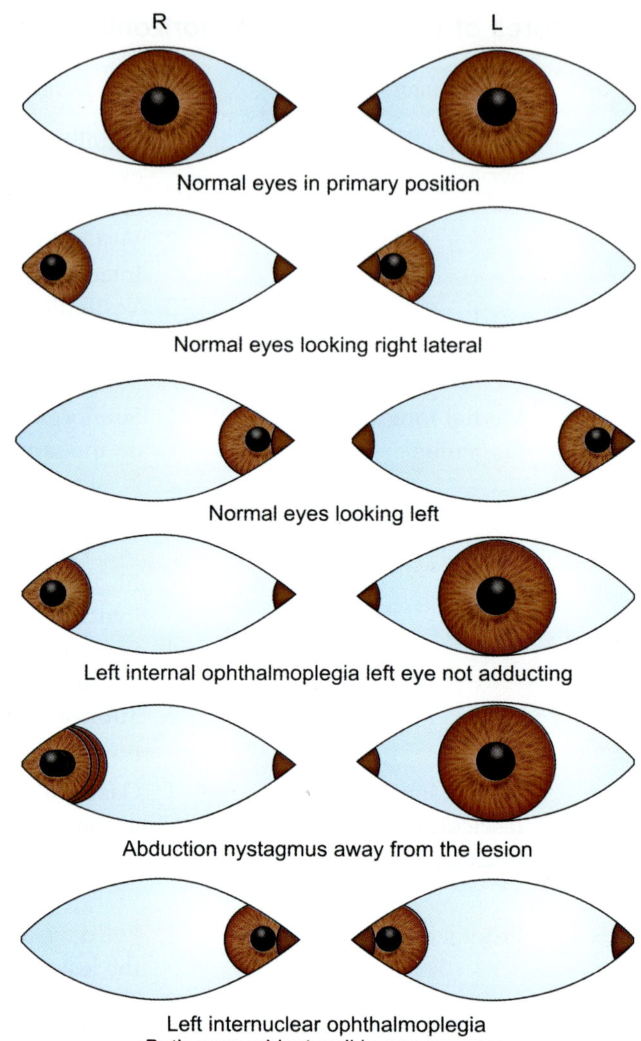

Fig. 11.1: Left internuclear ophthalmoplegia

away from the side of the lesion in the sixth nerve nucleus and PPRF due to associated INO the ipsilateral eye fails to adduct. The condition is also referred to as **pontine exotropia** due to lesion of contralateral MLF lesion.

Vertical gaze defects

The vertical gaze palsies are:

1. Dorsal midbrain syndrome (Parinaud's)
2. Progressive supranuclear palsy

3. Skew deviation
4. Tonic gaze deviation

Parinaud's syndrome of dorsal midbrain lesion (see Fig. 6.1)

This is also known as **pretectal syndrome** or **sylvian aqueduct syndrome** due to site of the lesion. This is not to be confused with nonneuro-ophthalmic Parinaud's ocular glandular syndrome that involves conjunctiva and preauricular glands due to a long list of causes.

The characteristics of the syndrome

1. Vertical gaze palsy or paresis.
2. May be associated with downward gaze palsy (rare)
3. Light near dissociation—Accommodation reflex is retained. Light reflex is sluggish or absent.
4. Convergence deficiency
5. Retraction nystagmus
6. Coller's sign—Bilateral lid retraction due to loss of synkinesis between superior rectus and levator.
7. Spasm of accommodation
8. Spasm of convergence
9. Skew deviation
10. Sunset sign in hydrocephalus

The lesion is in the **pretectal region**. The commonest condition producing the syndrome is a **neoplasm** in the posterior part of the third ventricle. Other causes are **cerebrovascular accident, trauma demyelination, toxins, arteriovenous malformation and hydrocephalus**.

Progressive supranuclear palsy

This is generally seen in **elderly persons** due to **degenerative disease** of central nervous system. In fully developed case there is **supranuclear vertical gaze palsy**. This may be preceded by **down gaze paresis**. Ultimately **horizontal gaze palsy** may be added. The patient is **unable to blink**. **Dementia** is common. Other associated features are **pseudobulbar palsy, Parkinsonism** like features. (The conditions is not to be confused with progressive external ophthalmoplegia). The other conditions that produce supranuclear gaze palsy includes **Wilson's disease** where there is paralysis of up gaze. In contrast to this **Neimann-Pick disease** produces down gaze palsy.

Skew deviation

Skew deviation is caused due to **cerebrovascular accident** involving **pons** or **medulla**. It consists of vertical deviation of the eye with intorsion (not to be confused with cyclo vertical paralysis).

Tonic gaze deviation

Tonic gaze deviation may be seen in **neonates** for a few days without any clinical significance and without any residual effect. In pathological set up it may present as

sunset sign in hydrocephalus otherwise it can be seen in adults secondary to raised intracranial tension or hemorrhage in thalamus.

Nuclear and intranuclear mobility disturbance of the eyes (third, fourth and sixth nerve palsies)

While diagnosing neurological manifestation of third, fourth or sixth nerve palsies the following points should be noted, i.e. where is the lesion, what is the lesion and why is the lesion.

The site of the lesion

1. Supranuclear, nuclear or infranuclear.
2. If nuclear, is it associated with other cranial nerve palsy, i.e. third and fourth, sixth and seventh or more than two nerves?
3. If nuclear, is it associated with tract lesion?
4. Fasciculus lesion – Is it isolated ?
   – Is it associated with tract lesion or other cranial nerve palsy?
5. Basilar – Isolated
   – Associated with other cranial nerves.
6. Cavernous sinus
7. Orbit

Some terms used to denote type of oculomotor palsies

1. **Total ophthalmoplegia**—When all the **extraocular muscles** supplied by third, fourth and sixth nerves are paralysed including **iris** and **ciliary body**. The fifth nerve is frequently involved. The lesion is either in the cavernous sinus or in the orbit. Rarely the condition can be bilateral due to lesion in brainstem or extensive involvement of cavernous sinus. The eyes have total paralyses of levator leading to **complete ptosis**. On lifting the lid the eye lacks all movement, the eye is slightly proptosed, the pupil is dilated and immobile without accommodation (Fig. 11.2).

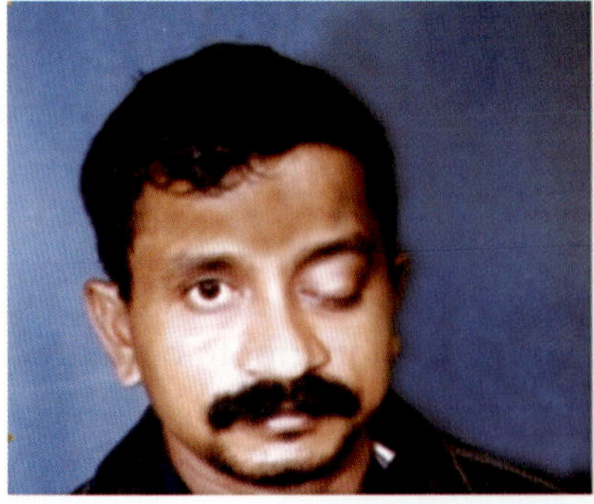
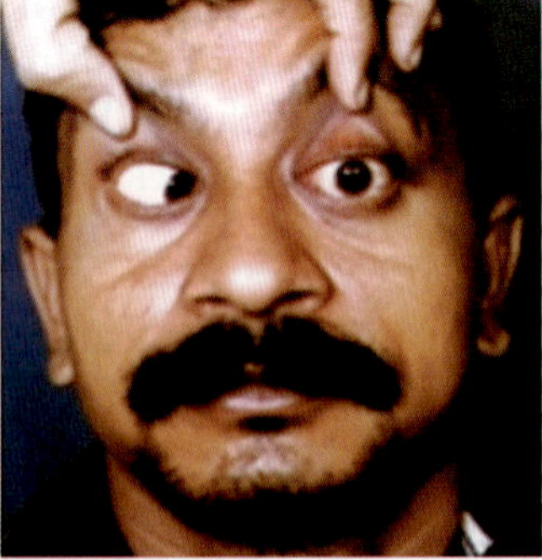

Fig. 11.2: Total ophthalmoplegia

Scheme of ocular palsies as per location is given in Flow chart 11.1.

Flow chart 11.1: Ocular palsies (paralysis of conjugate movement)

- Paralysis of conjugate movement
  - No diplopia
    - Supranuclear
      - Horizontal gaze palsy
      - Vertical gaze palsy
  - Diplopia
    - Nuclear
      - Isolated
        - Third nerve
        - Fourth nerve
        - Sixth nerve
      - Associated with other nuclei
        - Third + fourth nerve
        - Sixth + seventh nerve
    - Infranuclear
      - Fascicular
        - Third nerve
          - Benedict's syndrome, Claude syndrome, Weber's syndrome, Nothnagel syndrome
        - Fourth nerve
          - Difficult to separate from nuclear lesion
        - Sixth nerve
          - Foville's syndrome, Millard Gubler syndrome, Raymond's syndrome
      - Basilar
        - Third nerve
          - Posterior communicating artery Aneurysm, diabetes
        - Fifth, sixth and seventh nerve
          - Gradenigo syndrome
      - Cavernous sinus multiple nerve palsy
      - Orbit multiple cranial nerve palsy

2. **Partial ophthalmoplegia when:**
   i. **Isolated muscle,** i.e. **lateral rectus** or **superior oblique muscle,** is paralysed.
   ii. Muscles supplied by **upper division of third nerve** are paralysed. This does not involve intrinsic muscles of the eye.
   iii. **Lower division of third nerve** is involved. This may involve the intrinsic muscles of the eye.

3. **External ophthalmoplegia**—When only extraocular muscles are involved, may be all or a group of muscles leaving pupillary reaction and accommodation intact. They are nuclear in origin and frequently congenital.
4. **Internal ophthalmoplegia**—When only intrinsic muscles of the eye are involved. It is called **cycloplegia** when ciliary muscles are paralysed and **mydriasis** where iris is paralysed. Isolated mydriasis or cycloplegia due to neurological causes is **extremely rare**. Isolated mydriasis can be produced only by sympatho-mimetic drugs, i.e. adrenaline, phenylpherine, etc. All cycloplegics are parasympatholytic and cause mydriasis along with cycloplegia. There is no known drug that causes cycloplegia without mydriasis. There are many **infections and toxins** that cause selective internal ophthalmoplegia. **Hutchinson's pupil** may be considered as internal ophthalmoplegia. Selective cycloplegia is seen in **diphtheria, herpes zoster and syphilis**.

Characteristics of nuclear palsies of 3rd, 4th and 6th cranial nerves

1. Muscles of both eyes are involved.
2. Muscle palsies may be symmetric or asymmetric.
3. Diplopia is common.
4. Pupil are spared.
5. Nuclear lesion of 4th nerve cannot be differentiated from fasciculus lesion.
6. Nuclear lesion of 6th nerve is never isolated.
7. Unilateral ptosis, external ophthalmoplegia with contralateral normal superior rectus or internal ophthalmoplegia are never nuclear.
8. Bilateral ptosis, bilateral third nerve palsy, unilateral third nerve palsy with contralateral SR palsy are always nuclear.
9. Following bilateral palsies may or may not be nuclear—total third nerve palsy, internal ophthalmoplegia, ptosis.

Outline to localize the level of lesion in neurological defect of extraocular muscle

1. Find out if the diminished action of the muscle/muscles is of neurological origin or restrictive. The symptoms of paralytic lesions are:
   - i. Diplopia
   - ii. Deviation
   - iii. Restricted movement
   - iv. Compensatory head posture
   - v. False orientation
   - vi. Subjective sensation
     - a. Vertigo
     - b. Dizziness
     - c. Headache
2. Exclude supra nuclear lesions

3. Find out facial sensation—subnormal sensation points towards involvement of trigeminal nerve.
4. Normal facial sensation with palsy means involvement of 3rd, 4th and 6th cranial nerves in various combinations, i.e. isolated or multiple cranial nerve palsy. The lesion is either in midbrain or in pons.
5. Isolated nerve palsy is due to lesion:
   a. Either in the interpeduncular space—third nerve, or
   b. In the cerebellopontine angle—sixth nerve.
6. Lesions of midbrain involve 3rd and 4th nerve, which can be-
   a. Nuclear lesion
   b. Lesion in the substance of the midbrain.
      - Nuclear lesion of third nerve is common with distinct feature.
      - Nuclear lesion of fourth nerve is not verified.
      - Lesion of midbrain involves fourth nerve less frequently. Third nerve palsy is associated with ataxia, tremors and contralateral hemiplegia.
7. Lesions of pons involve 6th and 7th nerve which could be
   a. Nuclear
   b. Substance of the pons

   The pontine signs are hemiplegia or quadriplegia with pinpoint pupil, hyper-pyrexa and coma.
8. Multiple cranial nerve palsy with fifth nerve involvement is either due to lesion in cavernous sinus or in superior orbital fissure.

Symptoms of paralytic squint

1. **Diplopia**
   i. This is the first subjective symptom to develop in paralytic squint.
   ii. It can be mild enough to be passed as blurring of vision, which clears on closing the sound eye.
   iii. It can be horizontal, vertical or torsional. Horizontal diplopia is better tolerated than the other two and can be overcome if the fusional amplitude is sufficient to overcome the deviation. Vertical and torsional diplopias cannot be overcome.
   iv. Diplopia develops only in eyes that have fully developed binocular reflex.
   v. Congenital and infantile paralytic squints seldom have diplopia due to lack of binocular reflex.
   vi. The congenital and infantile paralytic squints develop complete suppression of one image with development of abnormal correspondence.
   vii. Diplopia can be overcome either by closing one eye or by compensatory head posture.
   viii. If diplopia is crossed, it increases on looking towards the normal side. The false image in farthest.

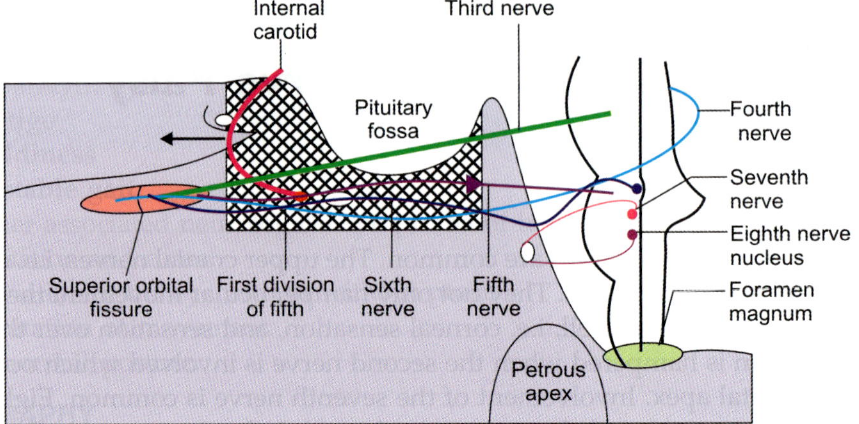

Note: All nerves enters the orbit inside common tendinous ring except the fourth

Fig. 12.2: Relation of cranial nerves in basilar, cavernous and superior orbital fissure. Lesions anywhere in these regions will produce multiple cranial nerve palsies

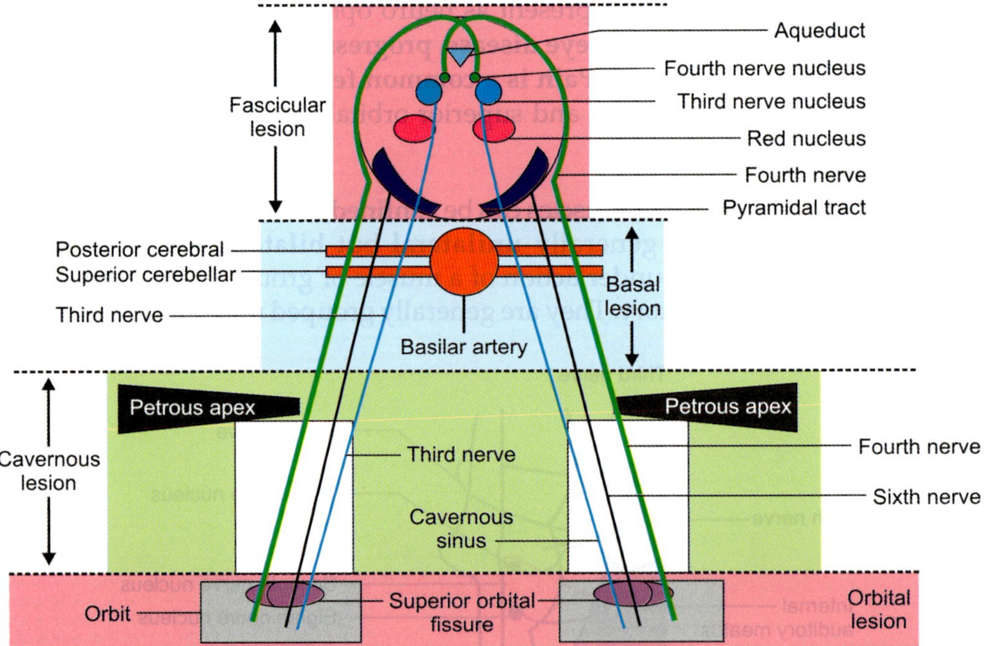

Note:

1. Only fascicular lesions involve neural tracts
2. The third and fourth nerve pass between posterior cerebral and superior cerebellar arteries
3. Sixth nerve passes under anterior inferior cerebellar artery below the third and fourth in the plane of third and fourth nerves

Fig. 12.3: Various possible levels of multiple cranial nerve palsies involving third, fourth and fifth nerve

under action. The common among them are **orbital pseudo tumors, thyroidmyopathy, fracture of orbital wall with entrapment of muscle. Myasthenia** does not fit either under true neurogenic group or restrictive group. This is due to faulty transmission at myoneural junction, may behave as neurogenic palsy and diagnosed as such unless proved otherwise by tensilon test.

The common causes of painful ophthalmoplegia are:

1. **Vascular**
   - i. Ischemic:
     - a. Diabetes
     - b. Hypertension
     - c. Intraneural hemorrhage
   - ii. Compressive
     - a. Aneurysm – Posterior communicating artery (commonest)
       - – Basilar artery (less frequent)
       - – Internal carotid (least)
     - b. Hemorrhage and thrombosis in the midbrain and brainstem.
2. **Tumors**
   - Primary, secondary or extension from neighboring structures. The common examples are meningioma, nasopharyngeal carcinoma, pituitary tumor
3. **Inflammatory**
   - i. Superior orbital fissure syndrome
   - ii. Orbital apex syndrome
   - iii. Cavernous sinus thrombosis
   - iv. Pseudo tumors of orbit
   - v. Osteitis and periosteitis of orbital bones
   - vi. Gradenigo's syndrome.
4. **Infections**
   - i. Herper zoster and postherpetic neuralgia
   - ii. Mucormycosis
5. **Others**
   - i. Ophthalmoplegic migraine
   - ii. Congenital anomalies
   - iii. Trauma

The characteristics of painful ophthalmoplegia are:

1. They generally involve more than one nerve
2. May begin as mono neural palsy.
3. The other nerves invariably get involved.
4. They are mostly unilateral but may become bilateral
   - i. One eye may be more involved.
   - ii. They may change sides.
5. Remissions and exacerbations are known with or without treatment.
6. The commonest inflammatory cause is **delayed cell mediated autoimmune diseases**. The lesion can be **granulomatous** or **nongranulomatous**.

7. The lesions when auto immune in nature are **steroid sensitive**. They require high dose of steroid for long period.
8. Relation of pain with ophthalmoplegic is variable. Pain may **precede, accompany or follow** the onset of ophthalmoplegia.
9. Common nerves involved are **third, fourth and sixth**. The **first division of fifth** is more commonly involved than second. Some times both divisions may be involved simultaneously.
10. If the lesion is in the cavernous sinus there may be involvement of **ocular sympathetic**.
11. The inflammatory lesion in the **orbital apex** involve the **optic nerve**.
12. Difference in clinical presentation depends on location of the lesions. It may be in the **cavernous sinus** and extent to the orbit, may be localized to **superior orbital fissure** with or without involving the **orbital apex**.
13. Various degrees of **exophthalmos** is always present.

II. Bilateral ophthalmoplegia

Bilateral ophthalmoplegia are **less common** than unilateral but not rare. Involvement of both eyes simultaneously is less frequent, generally ophthalmoplegia in one eye is followed by ophthalmoplegia in the other eye. The involvement in two eyes need not be symmetric.

The causes of bilateral ophthalmoplegia can be:

1. Neurogenic
2. Myogenic
3. Inflammatory
4. Dysthyroid status.

A. **Neurogenic**
   i. **Bilateral fourth nerve palsy** is **commonest** type of mono neural ophthalmoplegia that can be:
      a. Congenital
      b. Traumatic
   ii. **Isolated bilateral sixth nerve palsy** is encountered frequently **without any localizing importance**. The common causes are:
      a. Raised intracranial pressure
      b. Viral infection
      c. Trauma.
   iii. Bilateral complete **third nerve palsy** is rare. Partial bilateral palsy of superior rectus and levator denotes nuclear lesion.
   iv. Multiple extraocular muscle palsy with spared pupil is seen in diabetic neuropathy.
   v. Multiple extraocular muscle involvement with pupillary paralysis is more common.
   vi. Bilateral internuclear ophthalmoplegia

vii. One and half syndrome

viii. **Mobius syndrome**—Congenital bilateral sixth and seventh nerve under action with severe restriction of medial rectus.

ix. **Duane's syndrome**—This is congenital co-innervations of lateral rectus and medial rectus by misdirected third nerve fibres. There may be associated hypoplasia of sixth nerve nucleus.

B. **Myogenic causes of bilateral ophthalmoplegia are:**

i. Chronic progressive external ophthalmoplegia and its variations

ii. Ocular myopathies

iii. Myasthenia

iv. Thyroid myopathy

All the above conditions of bilateral progressive loss of ocular movements were considered to be due to changes in the muscle. Later it was found that chronic progressive external ophthalmoplegia has more neurological features than myogenic.

Chronic progressive external ophthalmoplegia

The characteristics of the disease are:

a. The disease is **familial**.
b. There is mutation in mitochondria.
c. It is **chronic in onset** and progresses **relentlessly without pain**.
d. It is **bilateral** and **symmetric**.
e. **Ptosis** is the first feature to develop.
   The ptosis starts as partial ptosis which progresses to become complete covering the pupil requiring the patient to keep the chin elevated initially, throwing the head back and use the frontalis.
f. **The orbicularis** shows weakness.
g. All the **extraocular muscles** are gradually involved.
h. There is no lid retraction.
i. **The pupil is spared**. This imparts the term external ophthalmoplegia to the condition.
j. In spite of paralysis of all the extraocular muscle. **There is no proptosis or diplopia**.

The disease can be broadly divided into two age groups:

1. Adult
2. Infantile/Juvenile

   The adult type—Generally develops between **second to fourth decade**. It has several overlapping variations which are:

   i. Only progressive bilateral ptosis, in fact this may be the initial stage of the disease that involve other extraocular muscle later.

   ii. Ophthalmoplegia with weakness of temporalis.

   iii. Oculopharyngeal form—This includes features of extraocular muscle palsy along with paralysis of pharyngeal muscles.

iv. Ptosis with pharyngeal palsy leaving other extraocular muscles uninvolved.
v. External ophthalmoplegia with weakness of muscles of neck and upper extremity.

Childhood progressive external ophthalmoplegia generally does not have family history. It consist of triad of:

i. Ophthalmoplegia
ii. Cardiopathy
iii. Peripheral retinal pigmentary degeneration

Other changes observed are: Increased protein in CSF, vaculation in cerebrum and brain stem, changes in mitochondria.

Differential diagnosis consists of all conditions of bilateral underaction of extraocular muscle sparing the pupil.

They include:

1. Myasthenia
2. Thyroid myopathy
3. Cerebral and pontine gaze palsy
4. Progressive supra nuclear palsy
5. Bulbar palsy
6. Parkinsonism

None of the condition mentioned above are of sudden on set they can be unilateral or bilateral.

III. Acute ophthalmoplegia

The causes of sudden ophthalmoplegia are:

1. Ischemic—Diabetes, hypertension
2. Brain stem—Vascular accidents
3. Myasthenia crisis
4. Diphtheria
5. Botulinum toxicity
6. Aneurysms of:
   i. Basilar artery
   ii. Posterior communicating artery
   iii. Internal carotid artery
7. Wernicke's encephalopathy
8. Meningitis
9. Bulbar poliomyelitis
10. Trauma (Fig. 12.4)

NON-NEURAL OPHTHALMOPLEGIA

Duane's retraction syndrome (Stilling-Turk-Duane syndrome)

Duane's retraction syndrome is not uncommon, about 1% of children with lateral rectus under action show some degree of the syndrome. The disease is **more common in**

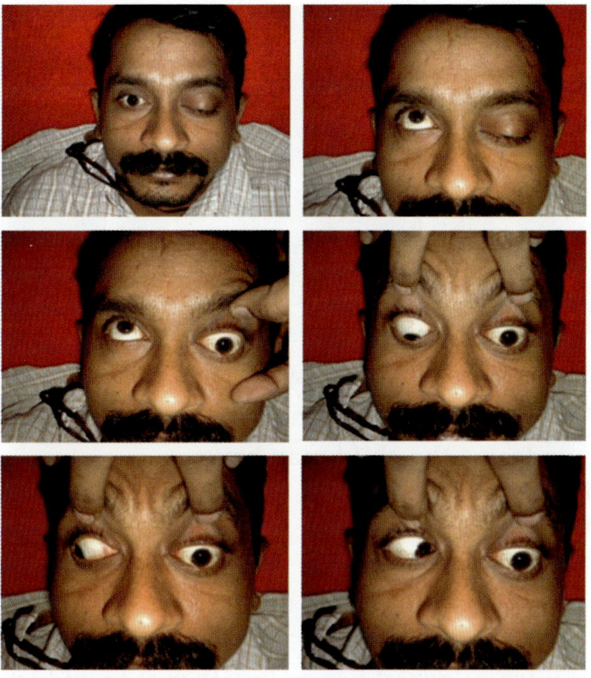

Fig. 12.4: Post-traumatic multiple cranial nerve palsy involving second nerve and internal ophthalmoplegia (*Courtesy:* Dr Santosh Patel)

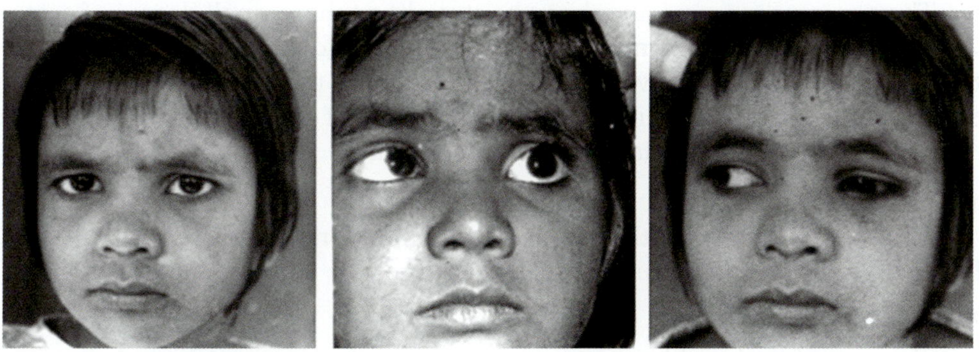

Fig. 12.5: Duanne's retraction syndrome (*Courtesy:* Dr SL Adile)

girls. In about **75% of cases** it is **unilateral. The left eye is more commonly involved** than the right eye. The condition does not follow any fixed hereditary pattern yet **more than one members of the family may show some evidence** of the syndrome. The condition is **congenital** but rarely diagnosed before three years of age. It is nonprogressive (Fig. 12.5).

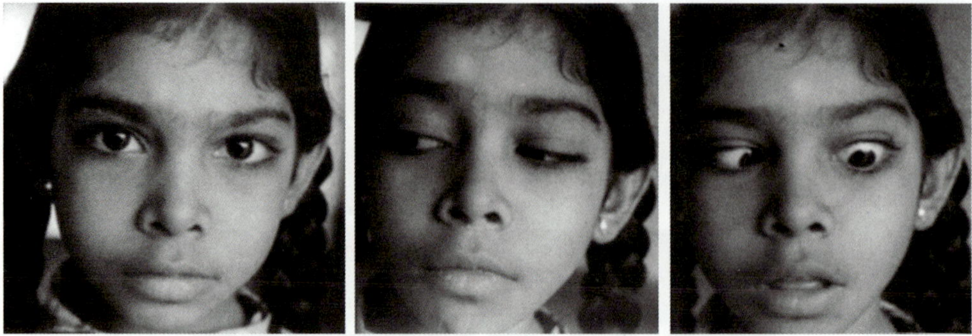

Fig. 12.6: Duanne's retraction syndrome (*Courtesy:* Dr SL Adile)

Besides retraction syndrome the child may have:

1. Other motility disturbances
2. Other ocular lesions
3. Musculo skeletal defects

The typical syndrome consists of:

1. Diminished/absent abduction
2. Narrowing of inter palpebral fissure on attempt to adduct.
3. Retraction of globe on attempt to adduct.
4. Widening of palpebral fissure on abduction.
5. Up shoot/down shoot on adduction (Fig. 12.6).
6. The eye in primary position may be straight or show small degree of esotropia.
7. There may be head turn to overcome abduction defect.
8. About 40% of eyes show anisometropia of more than one Diopter.
9. Binocular vision is maintained hence chance of amblyopia is less and when present is due to associated an anisometropia.

Types of Duanne's retraction syndrome

All cases do not always fit in the characteristics mentioned above.

They fall in three types, which are:

Type 1

This is the **commonest** and have maximum number features mentioned above.

They consist of:

1. Straight eyes, may have small esotropia.
2. Partial or total under action of lateral rectus.
3. Normal or slight defect in adduction.
4. Narrowing of palpebral fissure on adduction.
5. Retraction of globe on adduction.
6. Widening of palpebral fissure on abduction.
7. Up shoot or down shoot on adduction.

Type 2

This is **less common** than the type 1, The features are:

1. Mild to moderate exotropia
2. Partial or total lack of adduction.
3. Narrowing of palpebral fissure on adduction.
4. Retraction of globe on adduction.

Type 3

1. Partial or total absence of both adduction and abduction.
2. Retraction of globe on adduction.
3. There may be narrowing of palpebral fissure on horizontal movement of the eye without retraction. Rarely retraction syndrome similar to Duane's may develop following orbital trauma or secondaries in orbit.

Duane's retraction syndrome may be accompanied by many more ocular defects. They may be motility related or without motility disorder.

The common motility disorders are:

1. Up shoot or down shoot in adduction.
2. Various types of A and V syndrome. Out of the two, V pattern is more common.
3. Marcus Gunn jaw-winking
4. Vertical retraction syndrome
5. Abduction defect with synergestic divergence
6. Nystagmus
7. Ptosis

Other ocular anomalies reported are: Limbal dermoid, anisocoria, coloboma of uvea, coloboma of disc, heterochromia, congenital cataract, crocodile tear.

The nonocular features associated with Duane's retraction syndrome are:

1. Goldenhar syndrome
2. Klippel Feil syndrome

Differential diagnosis

Duane's retraction syndrome is missed because most of the children have straight eyes in primary position, have good vision and no diplopia. While testing binocular movements attention is not paid to changes in palpebral fissure.

The common conditions that are confused with Duane's retraction syndrome are:

1. Infantile esotropia
2. Lateral rectus palsy
3. Simple esotropia.
4. Liberal recession of lateral rectus.
5. Mobius syndrome.
6. Brown syndrome (widening of palpebral aperture in adduction).
7. Orbital blow out fracture.

Mobius syndrome

This is a **congenital** anomaly that has **neuro ophthalmic features** with **musculo skeletal changes**.

1. **The neuro-ophthalmic features consist of:**
   i. **Bilateral sixth nerve palsy** due to **hypoplasia of sixth nerve nucleu**s. The lateral rectus shows under action and the medial rectus is inelastic.
   This leads to:
      a. Inability to move eyeball laterally beyond midline.
      b. The lateral rectus palsy is bilateral but not symmetric. There is **no retraction of globe** or **narrowing of inter palpebral fissure**.
   ii. The medial rectus may shows poor adduction. The medial rectus function is better in convergence than in horizontal gaze.
   iii. Esotropia is common, generally **there is no amblyopia or nystagmus**. In case of asymmetric under action of lateral rectus, the child may assume **abnormal head turn**.
   iv. There is **bilateral infranuclear type of facial palsy** that is not always equal on both sides. The lower facial muscles are involved less. The face is expressionless. There is always some degree of **lagophthalmus** leading to **corneal exposure**.
   v. The Bells phenomenon is retained.
   vi. Rare involvement of third nerve may result in exotropia.
2. **Non-ophthalmic neurological features** consist of hypoplasia of ninth and twelfth cranial nerves leading to difficulty in feeding and atrophy of the tip of the tongue.
3. **Non-neurological features are:** Low IQ, subnormal hearing, dental anomalies, webbed fingers and toes, club feet, hypoplasia of pectoral muscle, generalized hypotony.

Brown syndrome

This is more common than Mobius syndrome.

It has two forms:

1. Congenital
2. Acquired
   i. It is not a **neurological defect**.
   ii. It requires to be differentiated from neurological defect. It is often confused as inferior oblique under action.
   iii. The **pathogeneses** is located in the superior oblique muscle or to be precise the fault is either in the **anterior sheath of the superior oblique** or the **superior oblique tendon is inelastic**. The superior oblique may develop fibrosis and adhesion over the trochlea preventing smooth passage of the tendon of superior oblique.
   iv. Abnormal nerve supply to any of the obliques too have been thought to be the cause.

v. It is **unilateral** in 90% of cases and **bilateral** only in 10%.
vi. The condition becomes obvious in infancy or childhood.
vii. The common presenting features are:
   a. **Abnormal head posture that consist of:**
      - Elevation of chin
      - Ipsilateral head tilt
      - Contra lateral face turn
   b. **Ocular movements**
      - There is defective elevation when the eye is adducted. The elevation improves as the eye abducts and is almost normal in abducted eye.
      - Down shoot of effected eye in adduction.
      - Diplopia in elevation.
      - There is widening of inter palpebral fissure in adduction.
      - AV phenomena is common
   c. **Vision**—Generally there is good vision, amblyopia is less common. The condition is known to resolve without treatment by twelve years of age. It may be intermittent.
   d. **Diplopia**—Children generally do not complain of diplopia. They overcome it by abnormal head posture. Adults with acquired defect notice diplopia and seek help for it.

The two common causes of acquired brown syndrome are rheumatic tenosynovitis and trauma either accidental or surgical. The surgical procedures responsible are neuro surgical, or surgery on superior oblique.

The condition **does not require any treatment**, so long the eye is not grossly hypotropic in primary position or there is significant head tilt. In such cases the surgery is done to restore binocular single vision. The surgical procedure consists of striping the adhesion, leaving the tendon untouched. A complete tenotomy may be needed.

Double elevator palsy

This is mostly **congenital in nature**, rarely may follow **trauma** or **inflammation**. This is one of the frequent causes of **hypo deviation of one eye**. The lesion consists of **absent** or **under action of both the elevators** of the same eye, i.e. the **superior rectus** and **inferior oblique**. Both the elevators are supplied by third nerve, the superior rectus by upper division and inferior rectus by lower division, hence a nuclear or infra nuclear lesion without involvement of other muscles is not possible, a **supranuclear lesion** seems most appropriate.

The condition is seen in **children**. There is **hypotropia** in primary position. When the paretic eye fixes, the contra lateral eye move up and becomes hyper tropic. When the normal eyes fixes, the paretic eye assumes a hypotropic position. This is associated with pseudo ptosis.

The eye can not be elevated in any position of gaze. The child keeps the chin up to counter balance the down ward shift of the eye. This helps in eliminating amblyopia.

Jaw winking may be present.

BIBLIOGRAPHY

1. Karan S, Biswas J, Kumaraswamy, Sharma P, Suniti Solomon. Multiple cranial nerve palsy in HIV positive patients. Ind Jr Oph 2001;49:118-20.
2. Kodsi SR, Young BR. Acquired oculomotor trochlear and abducent cranial nerve palsy in pediatric patients. Am Jr Oph 1992;114:568-74.
3. Lee AG. Ocular myasthenia. Curr Opinion Oph 1996;7:39-41.
4. Sieb JP. Myasthenia gravis emerging new therapy. Curr Op Oph 2005;15:303-7.
5. Trobe JD. Managing oculomotor nerve palsy. Arch Oph 1988;116.

13 Conditions Masquerading as Neuro-ophthalmic Disorders

There are many diseases that are **myogenic** in nature but present **as neuro-ophthalmic diseases**. Some of them are **congenital** others are **acquired**.

The conditions of mimic neuro-ophthalmic disorders are:

1. **Neuromuscular junction disorders**
   i. Myasthenia gravis
   ii. Myasthenia like syndromes
      a. Lambert-Eaton syndrome
      b. Toxic
2. **Myopathies**
   i. Chronic progressive external ophthalmoplegia (CPEO)
   ii. Variants of progressive myopathies
      a. Kearns–Sayer syndrome.
      b. MELAS syndrome (**M**itochrondrial **E**ncephalopathy, **L**actic **A**cidosis, **S**troke like syndrome)
3. **Dystrophies**
   i. Oculopharyngeal dystrophy
   ii. Myotonic dystrophy
4. **Dysthyroid myopathy**
5. **Retraction syndrome**
   i. Duane's retraction syndrome
   ii. Vertical retraction syndrome.
6. Miscellaneous conditions
   i. Brown syndrome
   ii. Strabismus fixus
   iii. Blow out fracture
   iv. Adherence syndrome
   v. Conjunctival shortening syndrome
   vi. General fibrosis syndrome
   vii. Orbital myositis

All the above condition have

1. **Squint** that may be variable or fixed, may alternate between the eyes, may be stationary or progress.
2. **Diplopia**—Many of the condition, i.e. myasthenia, dysthyroid, myopathy, blow out fracture and orbital myositis have diplopia.

3. **Restricted movements**.
4. Abnormal head posture.
5. **Amblyopia is generally absent**.
6. No ocular or neurological deficit are produced by the conditions *per se*.
7. May have non neurological features and complications.
8. Some may have hereditary predisposition.
9. Some are congenital and stationary, others are congenital and progressive.

Myasthenia gravis

Myasthenia gravis is a **chronic** disorder of **neuromuscular junction** of striated muscles. It does not involve plain muscles, both pre and post synapses may be involved. The disease does not have any neurological features but may be mistaken as a neurological disorder. It has been called a **great mimic** and may **masquerade** as paralysis of any of the striated muscles including the ocular muscles hence **ptosis** and **diplopia** are very common and early presentation.

The disease has a **world-wide** distribution, **all races** are equally involved. The disease can manifest at **any age** from newborn to old age**. It can rarely be congenital**. Though no age group is immune from the disease it is commonly seen between 20 and 60 years of age. The incidence of typical myasthenia falls sharply in and after seventh decade when **atypical myasthenia** becomes more common, which may involve plain muscles resulting in paralysis of iris and ciliary body.

The disease is seen more in **women** as compared to men in a ratio of 3:2. A **pregnant** woman may pass the antibodies responsible for the disease to the unborn child who may show the features of the disease soon after birth. Though myasthenia is not a true hereditary disorder, **family history** is positive in as much as 5% patients.

The disease is chronic disease generally progressive or intermittent. In some patients, the disease is **self limiting** and the clinical features disappear without treatment. Rarely the disease may pass into **crisis**. The chronic cases may become **fixed,** i.e. not responding to treatment, which should alert the physician to think of other conditions as well i.e. chronic progressive external ophthalmoplegia.

The disease can broadly be divided into two distinct groups:

1. Primary myasthenia where antibodies against **synaptic acetylcholine receptors** are present and the disease inflicts striated muscles only.
2. Secondary due to systemic disease, drugs, and toxins.

As per age myasthenia gravis can be divided into:

1. Myasthenia of children
2. Myasthenia of adults

Out of all the types of myasthenic conditions listed above, **primary myasthenia of adults** which may otherwise be called **typical myasthenia** is the commonest form.

All the myasthenic condition irrespective of causes are clinically divided into two forms:

1. Ocular
2. General.

Ocular myasthenia may pass into general myasthenia and vice versa.

Ocular myasthenia (see Chapter 5)

A myasthenic patient is said to be suffering from ocular myasthenia when the striated muscles involved are restricted to extraocular muscles including the orbicularis. The internal muscles remain normal. The vision is unaffected.

1. Only 20% of cases of myasthenia belong to category of pure ocular myasthenia.
2. In case of systemic myasthenia about 90% of cases develop ocular involvement.
3. In 75% of cases with **generalized myasthenia**, the initial symptoms are ocular i.e. ptosis and diplopia.
4. About 80% of cases of ocular myasthenia will be converted to generalized myasthenia in about two years.

The two common complaints of ocular myasthenia are **ptosis** and **diplopia**. The hallmarks of myasthenia are—fatigability that may last for few minutes to few days followed by improvement. The period of remission may also vary between hours and weeks.

Ptosis

The ptosis is the commonest feature, the ranges of ptosis vary between few millimeters to complete ptosis, fortunately the latter is rare. The ptosis may be **unilateral** and **shift** to the other eye, the first eye involved returning to normal position or **both the eyes may be involved**. Involvement of two eyes is seldom symmetric.

Onset of ptosis forces the patient to use the frontalis, the head is thrown back and the chin is elevated. This may be associated with head tilt and turn that is due to involvement of cyclo vertical muscle and not related to ptosis.

The amount of ptosis may be offset by **paralysis of the orbicularis**. Paralysis of orbicularis is very common. It may cause ectropion of lower lid.

In case of unilateral ptosis, the contralateral lid is lifted up resulting in lid retraction. If the ptotic lid is lifted the retracted lid falls to its normal position.

The myasthenic ptosis is worsened

1. In the evening.
2. If the patient undergo moderate exertion.

Tests for ptosis

1. In **Cogan lid twitch sign**

   This consists of

   a. The patient is asked to fix a distant object, the position of the lid in relation to the pupil is noted.

3. Positive Cogan lid twitch test.
4. Give positive tensilon test
5. Improves with neostigmine or pyridostigmine.

Tensilon test is said to be the gold standard of diagnosis, however it is not an infallible test. There may be both **false positive and negative results**, about which the clinician should be well aware of.

The tensilon test

Tensilon is **edrophonium hydrochloride**, which is a **short acing anti choline esterase drug**. It is used as **intravenous injection**. Due to its short action **it has no therapeutic value**. The short action is utilised for diagnosis.

The procedure is as follows:

1. The patient is explained the procedure. It is better to obtain written consent for the test.
2. The ptosis and diplopia are evaluated.
   It is better to have-
   i. Photographic record of the ptosis before start of the test.
   ii. A diplopia charting done before starting of the test.
3. 0.4 mg of atropine is injected intramuscular 15 minutes before the procedure is started to counter act the cholinergic side effect of tensilon.
4. Injection of tensilon
   i. A vein in the dorsal arm is punctured by a scalp vein needle.
   ii. 1 ml of saline is injected in the scalp vein and the patient is observed for one minute. This should not produce any change in ptosis or squint.
   iii. If no change is observed, 0.2 ml of Tensilon is injected in the tube that is flushed with 1 ml of normal saline
      a. Prompt improvement in ptosis/squint is highly suggestive of myasthenia.
      b. No change in ptosis and squint. Denotes negative test.
   iv. Inject remaining 0.8 ml and observe.
5. Observation
   A positive result consists of improvement of ptosis, improvement in squint, return of movement. These should be photographed for record.

There are three types of responses

1. Improvement of ptosis and tropia
2. Worsening of ptosis and tropia
3. Reversal—A left hypertropia is changed to right hypertropia.

The responses 2 and 3 are seen in non-myasthenic conditions.

Neostigmine test

Neostigmine test is equally effective but takes more time to show response. It is generally employed in children or non cooperative adults.

The procedure is:

i. Inject 0.4 mg atropine 1 m, 15 minutes before.
ii. Inject 0.5 mg of neostigmine methyl sulphate intramuscular.
iii. Examine the child after half an hour and one hour.

The positive results are similar to Tensilon test (Fig. 13.1).

The next one, which is less effective than injection of **prostigmine**, (neostigmine) is oral administration of **pyridostigmine** tablet in a dose of 30 to 60 mg BD × 3 days. In a case of myasthenia the condition should improve, if the condition improves the drug is continued.

Other Investigations

1. X-ray, CT and MRI of chest for presence of thymoma.
2. Tests to exclude thyroid myopathy.
3. Presence of acetylcholine antibodies.
4. Electromyography.
5. Forced duction test.

The conditions that mimic myasthenia gravis are:

1. **Lambert-Eaton syndrome**—The disorder is seen in persons in **sixth decade** who suffer either from **autoimmune disease** or **small cell carcinoma of lung**. The cause is disturbed presynaptic **calcium channel** resulting in decreased acetylcholine at the neuromuscular junction.

   The ocular features differ from myasthenia. They consist of tonic pupil, decreased lacrimation both of which are not met within myasthenia gravis. Ocular muscle and bulbar muscle may be spared. Tendon reflexes are diminished. Anticholine esterase drugs have little effect on the condition.
2. **Drugs**—There is a long list of therapeutic agents including commonly used antibiotic that cause myasthenia like disorders

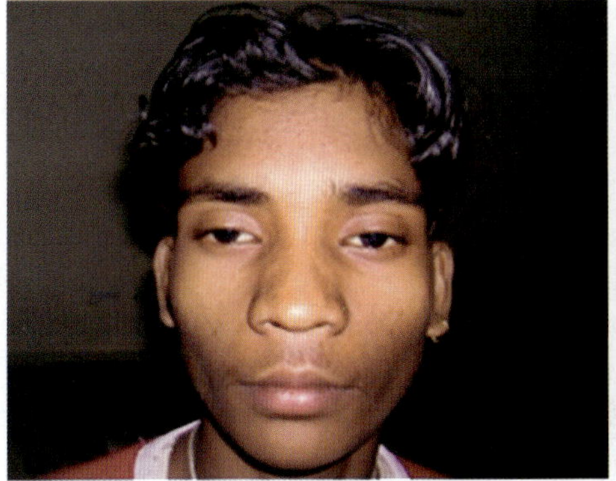
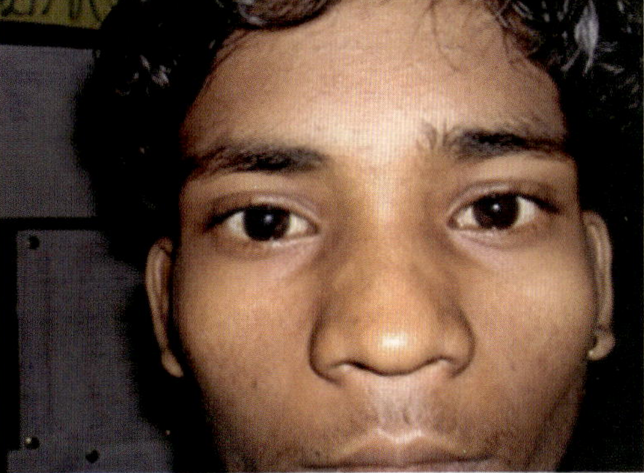

Fig. 13.1: Positive prostigmine test in a case of myasthenia (*Courtesy:* Dr Santosh Patel)

The drugs are:

- **Antibiotics**—Aminoglycosides are most commonly blamed antibiotic to cause myasthenia. They are streptomycin, neomycin, kanamycin, polymixin.
- **Antineoplastic**—Vincristine, vinblastin.
- **Other drugs** are quinidine, lithium, penicillamine, propranolol, barbiturates and alcohol.
- **Chemicals**—Organophosphates

Treatment

1. **Anticholinesterase drugs**
   In an established case of myasthenia gravis the first line of treatment is administration of anticholine esterase drugs. The anticholine esterase drugs should be long acting.
   The commonest drug used is **pyridostigmine (mestinon)**. The drug is administered **orally**. The dose is calculated empirically depending upon its response, weighing against side effects.
   Pyridostigmine is started in a dose of 30-60 mg oral two times a day and result noted after two-three days. In case of poor response the dose is gradually increased upto to 450 mg/day.
   The commonly used therapeutic dose in adults is **60 mg every four hourly**. The action starts within 30 minutes, reaches peak in two hours and starts declining. The other drug used is **neostigmine** (prostigmine) orally in a dose of 15 mg tablet every four hourly.
   Less commonly used drug is Ambemonium chloride. This is more potent than neostigmine or pyridostigmine.
2. **Steroids**
   Steroids are indicated in cases refractory to anticholine esterase or in case of intolerance to anticholine esterase drugs either along with anticholine esterase or separately. Generally 10 mg to 20 mg of prednisone is given, in divided doses and gradually increased to reach the best result. Once the best response has been reached, the total dose is given in single daily dose, which is changed to alternate day dose and gradually tapered over weeks to months.
3. **Immunosuppressive drugs**
   Many immunosuppressive drugs are used in cases refractive to anticholine esterase drugs and steroid. The drugs take longer time than the anticholine esterase drugs or steroid. They are potential hemotoxic and hepatotoxic, hence it is mandatory to monitor blood picture and liver function regularly. The commonly used drugs are: **Azathioprine** (Imuran**), cyclosporine** and **cyclophosphamide**.
4. **Other therapeutic methods used are Plasmapheresis** and **immunoglobulin**. The former is used in acute myasthenia and myasthenia crisis, the latter is used in refractory cases as intravenous injection.

Myasthenia crisis

Crisis in myasthenia gravis are rare.

They can either be

1. Myasthenic crises
2. Cholinergic crisis

Myasthenic crises: This is **acute** exacerbation of symptoms due to **infection, emotional disturbance** or precipitated by many drugs that include antibiotic, sedatives. They are commonly met in patients with inadequate medical treatment. The myasthenia crisis improves with increased dose of neostigmine.

Cholinergic crisis: This represents **overdose of anticholine esterase** and worsens with IV Tensilon or IV prostigmine. The condition is more common when steroids are added to anti choline esterase drugs or following thymectomy. The symptoms are similar to over dose of cholinergic drugs i.e. bradycardia, miosis, increased secretions, respiratory distress. The condition is treaded by stopping anticholine esterase drugs and administering IV atropine.

Management of ocular myasthenia

The ocular signs and symptoms are abolished by medical treatment that may take few days to few weeks to be effective. In the mean time diplopia may incapacitate the person to lead normal life. The patient learns to close one eye to avoid diplopia in unilateral case. In these patients, patching of one eye may be other alternative.

In some cases, prism may give some relief but as diplopia is variable the strength of prism and position of the base may require adjustment. This makes use of prism less popular. Surgery for squint and ptosis are restricted to cases that have stable muscular imbalance for at least one year with medical treatment.

Ocular myopathies

Ocular myopathies are difficult to classify (Flow chart 13.1). Various classifications have been put forward from time to time, none of which is suitable. The best classification should be on the basis of cause. The etiology itself is elusive. Most commonly used classification is based on systems involved. If the condition is localized to ocular muscles only, it is called chronic progressive external ophthalmoplegia.

Chronic progressive external ophthalmoplegia

This is a **rare** disease of **unknown etiology**. There are **two schools of thoughts**, one consider it to be **primary myopathy** the other consider it of **neurogenic origin**. The recent theory is that it is associated with mitochondrial DNA. The disease is seen in two forms, i.e **adult** and **juvenile**.

The juvenile form is more likely to develop systemic manifestation.

The characteristic of the conditions comprise of: Bilateral progressive almost **symmetric ptosis** and extraocular **muscle under action** without remission and fluctuation. The **orbicularis** is also involved. The **iris and ciliary muscles are always**

Flow chart 13.1: Ocular myopathy

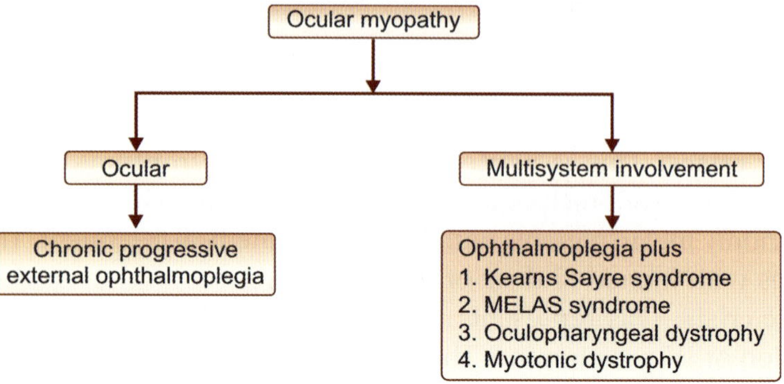

spared. The vision is within normal limit. There is no lid retraction or proptosis. The condition is **painless**. There is **no sensory loss**.

The **ptosis** is often the first feature to appear and progress, the muscle palsy is invariably a late manifestation. On rare occasions the ptosis may follow extraocular muscle palsy. The ptosis progresses over years to become total and cover the pupil causing loss of vision. Patient learns to lift the lid to have better vision. The patient initially uses the frontalis, elevates the chin and throws the head back to overcome ptosis.

Extraocular muscle palsies are slow to develop. There is no fixed pattern of ocular palsy. The ocular palsies do not change side like in myasthenia. The palsies are symmetric. Ultimately the eyes get fixed for all distances. In spite of muscle palsies the patients **do not complain of diplopia**.

Absence of diplopia is explained on the basis of following points:

1. The ptotic lids cover the pupillary area.
2. The muscle palsies are slow to develop.
3. The palsies are symmetric.
4. The eye is fixed in one position.

There may be some **exposure keratitis** due to **under action of orbicularis** and **absence of Bell's phenomenon**.

The ocular palsies are not effected by caloric stimulation and doll's head, movement.

The palsies give negative tensilon test.

Differential diagnosis consist of:

1. Dysthyroid myopathy (Fig. 13.2).
2. Bilateral pseudotumor of orbit.
3. Progressive supranuclear palsy.
4. Cerebral gaze palsy.
5. Pontine gaze palsy.
6. Parkinsonism.
7. Bilateral pupillary sparing third nerve palsy.

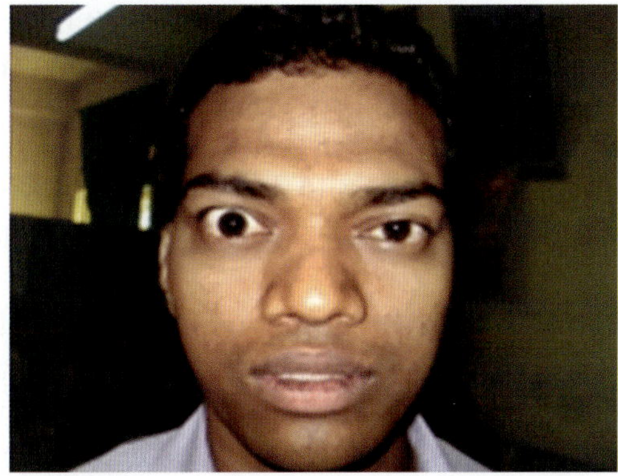

Fig. 13.2: Dysthyroid myopathy (*Courtesy:* Dr Santosh Patel)

8. Myasthenia.
9. Myotonic dystrophy.

Management

There is no known specific treatment. The ptosis and ocular palsies are treated symptomatically. **Ptosis crutches** are often prescribed to improve vision. They are not always accepted by the patient.

Surgery—Orbicularis palsy and absence of Bell's phenomenon are two points that require attention before ptosis surgery is contemplated.

The type of surgery depends upon available levator function. Good to moderate levator function may be corrected by **levator resection**. Absent or poor levator function in managed by **bilateral sling operation**.

Other progressive ocular myopathies

1. **Kearns-Sayre Syndrom**e is generally seen to inflict person in **early twenties, infantile** and **juvenile** forms are also known.
   The condition has triad **of:**
   - Progressive external ophthalmoplegia
   - **Pigmentary change in retina**
   - **Variable heart block** that may be managed by cardiac pace maker or may prove to be fatal.

   Besides the triad other systemic features are:
   i. Weakness of facial muscles, trunk and limbs.
   ii. Nystagmus
   iii. Vertigo, hearing defect.
   iv. Cerebellar ataxia.

   The condition is caused by mutation in DNA mitochondria.
2. **MELAS syndrome** consists of **chronic, progressive external ophthalmoplegia**. The other ocular features are **cortical blindness** and **hemianopia**. The systemic features are encephalopathy and lactic acidosis.

3. **Oculopharyngeal dystrophy**—This is a hereditary disorder seen in some families developing in the sixth decade. It is not a **DNA mitochondrial disorder**. The most prominent feature is **progressive external ophthalmoplegia** and **ptosis**. The systemic features are difficulty in swallowing, first solid and then liquid as well due to paralysis of pharyngeal muscles. The condition is most probably a type of **myotonia** where relaxation of muscle after contraction in delayed.
4. **Myotonic dystrophy**—This is an autosomal dominant disease of muscles. **This involves pupil as well**. Basically this in a muscular dystrophy that is myotonic.

The ophthalmic features are: Mask like mourning face, bilateral ptosis, bilateral progressive ophthalmoplegia, miosis, weakness of orbicularis, posterior polar cataract, poly chromatic congenital lens opacities, Christmas tree cataract, retinal dystrophy.

The systemic features are: Myotonia, diminished intelligence, baldness, dysphasia, dysphagia, cardiac myopathy, heart block and testicular atrophy

Dysthyroid myopathy

The dysthyroid oculopathy is part of **systemic dysthyroid status**. However, it may be present in **euthyroid** persons also, who may develop systemic dysthyroid status later. Thus dysthyroid ocular myopathy can be seen in **hyperthyroid** in (Grave's disease**)** **hypothyroidism** (Hashimoto's diseases) or in euthyroid persons.

Myopathy is the first ocular manifestation of dysthyroid eye disease that includes restrictive myopathy of extra ocular muscles and changes in the lid. Other ocular manifestations are conjunctival congestion over the attachment of horizontal muscle, scanty tear, proptosis.

The lid changes are:

Many eponyms have been used in the past to describe ocular changes in dysthyroid myopathy including lid changes. They are no more *in vogue* in clinical practice. The two important lid signs are **lid retraction** and **lid lag**.

The lid retraction is due to sympathetic over activity.

It can be unmasked in apparently normal lid of dysthyroid patient, following instillation of sympathomimetic drug like phenylephrine.

Lid lag is due to fibrosis of the levator.

Extraocular muscle changes

The orbicularis is not involved. The extraocular muscle changes consist of variable restrictive extraocular muscle palsy that is generally bilateral, may be simultaneous or one side may be involved more than the other. Less common is uniocular involvement. The first sign is poor elevation due to fibrosis of inferior rectus, the next muscle commonly involved is lateral rectus. Various combinations of paralysis may result between the two eyes.

The iris and ciliary body are not affected.

The sensations are normal.

Other common ocular involvement is thyroid optic neuropathy. That may precede or may be concurrent with myopathy. It is due to throttling of the optic nerve at the apex of the orbit either by exophthalmos producing substance or swollen muscle.

Proptosis which is generally referred to as **exophthalmos** is common in Grave's disease. Here the bulging eye develops exposure keratitis, corneal ulcer that may perforate.

Other ocular manifestations are **conjunctival congestion, ocular surface disorder, shift of refraction towards hypermetropia, puffiness of lids**.

Diagnosis

Diagnosis of dysthyroid myopathy is not difficult in Grave's disease and hypothyroidism where systemic manifestations and thyroid functions results confirm the diagnosis. Difficulty arises in euthyroid status.

Forced duction test is single important test. Negative Tensilon test excludes myasthenia.

Myasthenia is very frequently associated with dysthyroid myopathy.

X-ray orbit does not contribute much to the diagnosis. **Ultrasonography** of the orbit reveals enlarged swollen extraocular muscles. **CT** confirms the muscle changes and unmasks bone changes at the apex of the orbit. In CT both the coronal and axial cuts are taken. **MRI** is less useful than CT in myopathy but superior to CT in optic neuropathy. The orbital bones are not visible on MRI.

The differential diagnosis consist of: Myasthenia gravis, myasthenia like condition, orbital pseudotumors, myositis of extraocular muscle, secondaries in the orbit, chronic lymphoma of orbit.

Management

Ocular Graves disease is a self-limiting disease which resolves in few months without treatment. At the most the eyes require local lubricants. The lid retraction is treated by resection of Muller's muscle alone or with advancement of levator. This is done only when the lid retraction has been stable at least for one year.

Extraocular muscle surgeries may be required to correct restrictive myopathy.

High dose of systemic steroid is required in acute phase. It improves motility and reduces exophthalmos, this protects cornea. However it does not influence long-term restrictive problem.

BIBLIOGRAPHY

1. Bartley B. The differential diagnoses of eyelid retraction. Ophthalmology 1996;103:168-76.
2. Bartley GB, Fatourechiv Kadrmas EF. The chronology of Grave's ophthalmopathy in an incidence cohort. Am Jr Oph 1996;121:426-34.
3. Cogan DG. Myasthenia gravis in a review of disease and description of lid twitch a characteristic sign. Arch Oph 1965;74:217-21.
4. Drachman DK. Myasthenia gravis. Nu Eng Jr Med 1994;330:1797-1810.

5. Gorelic PB, Pena R, et al. An ice text for diagnosis of myasthenia gravis. Oph 1999;106: 1282-96.
6. Kazim M, Gold berg RA, Smith TJ. Insight into pathogeneses of thyroid associated orbitopathy. Arch Oph 2002;60:280-89.
7. Kumar SN. Myasthenia gravis in neuro-ophthalmology, 4th edn, Arvind Eye Hospital, Maduri 2007.
8. Kuncl RW, Hoffman PN. Myopathies and disorders of neuromuscular transmission in clinical neuro-ophthalmology. Vol I. 5th edn, William and Wilkins, Baltimore 1998;1351-1460.
9. Lisak RP, Barchi RL. Myasthenia gravis and myasthenic syndromes. Marcel Dekkor, New York, 1994.
10. Odel JG, Winter Korn JMS, Behrensmon. The sleep test for myasthenia gravis. J Cl New Oph 1991;11:288-92.
11. Sprunger DT, Helveston EM. Thyroid extraocular muscle disorder in current ocular therapy, 5th edn. Fraunfelder FT and Roy FH (Eds), WB saunders Company, Philadelphia 2000;411-16.
12. Van Dyk, HJ. Orbital Grave's disease. A modification of the no specs classification. Ophthalmology 1981;88:479-83.
13. Yonger DS, Worrall BB, Penn AS. Myasthenia gravis historical perspective and overview. Neurology 1997;48:51-57.

14 Vascular Lesions of Neuro-ophthalmic Interest

To understand the vascular anomalies of neuro-ophthalmic structures, it is essential to know in brief the blood supply to these structures and their venous drainage. Each of which has distinct clinical features.

Blood supply to structures of neuro-ophthalmic interest

The visual path and other neural paths associated with neuro-ophthalmic features are supplied by **two systems** of arteries with elaborate venous drainage. The venous drainage does not correspond to arterial supply always.

The two systems of arteries are:

1. The internal carotid
2. Vertebrobasilar

The carotid system

The branches arising from the carotid system of neuro-ophthalmic interest comprise of:

I. Ophthalmic artery
II. Posterior communicating artery
III. Anterior cerebral artery
IV. Middle cerebral artery
V. Small arterioles of internal carotid

The vertebrobasilar artery are:

I. Cortical
II. Central
III. Choroidal

All of which arise from **posterior cerebral arteries** which are the terminal branches of **basilar artery**.

The two systems are joined by a complicated system of connections to form an **irregular polygon** that is commonly known as **circle of Willis**. All the limbs of the vascular polygon are neither equal in shape and size nor in caliber (Fig. 14.1).

The function of the circle is to regulate the blood flow to various parts of the brain and act as efficient collateral when one of the systems fails.

The circle is situated in the interpeduncular space in the interpeduncular fossa.

The two internal carotid after they emerge from the roof of the cavernous sinus lie on either side of the optic chiasma and divide into two branches — the **anterior cerebral**

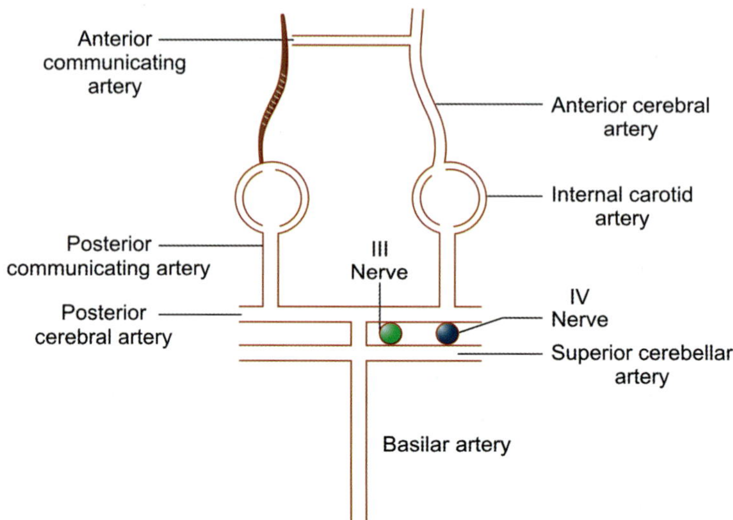

Fig. 14.1: Diagrammatic representation of circle of Willis

and **middle cerebral arteries** and give rise to **posterior communicating artery** that joins the carotid system with the vertebrobasilar system through posterior communicating artery that joins the posterior cerebral artery.

The two anterior cerebral arteries are joined to each other by a small artery called **anterior communicating artery** to complete the polygon.

The basilar artery is formed by confluence of **two vertebral arteries** at the lower border of the pons. The basilar artery lies in the midline, ventral to the pons. It divides in the two **posterior cerebral arteries** at the upper border of the pons (Figs 14.2 to 14.4).

Thus, it will be summarized that the so called circle of Willis is formed by:

1. Anteriorly by anterior communicating artery which is the smallest and most slender of all the arms of the polygon.
2. Anteriolaterally by anterior cerebral artery.
3. Posteriolaterally by the posterior communicating artery.
4. The anterior cerebral and posterior communicating arteries do not communicate with each other directly. They join the internal carotid at different levels.
5. The **middle cerebral artery** does not take part in formation of circle of Willis. It gives a branch called deep optic branch of middle cerebral artery. This supplies the optic radiation. The middle cerebral artery communicates with calcarine artery that is a branch of posterior cerebral artery to supply the visual cortex.
6. Posteriorly, the basilar artery divides into two posterior cerebral arteries completing the polygon.

   There are two types of branches that arise from the circle of Willis. They are:

   i. Central (Rupture or occlusion of which leads to cerebral vascular accidents)
   ii. Cortical

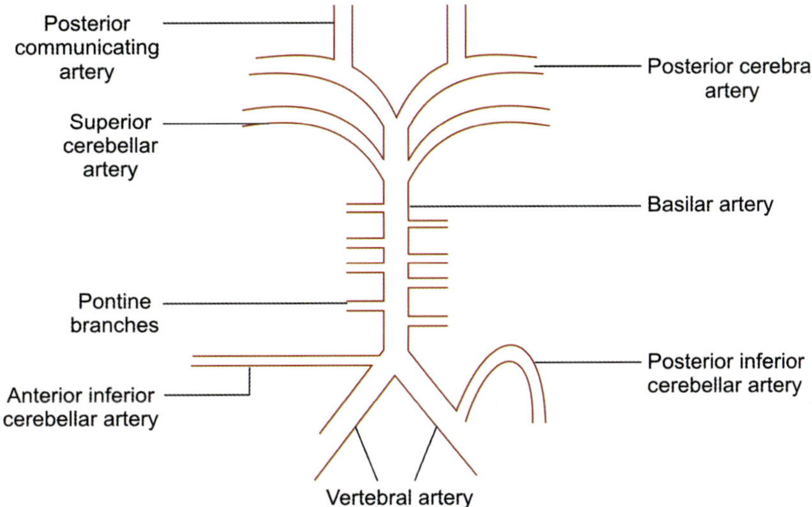

Fig. 14.2: Vertebrobasilar artery systems

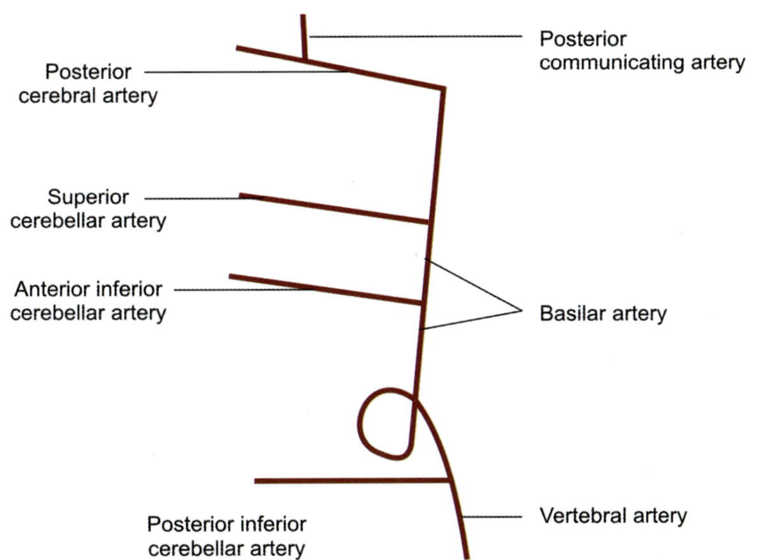

Fig. 14.3: Diagrammatic representation of vertebrobasilar system

The central branches are end arteries. They supply deeper structures of the cerebral hemisphere. They are arranged in six sets.

The cortical branches ramify on the surface and supply the cortex.

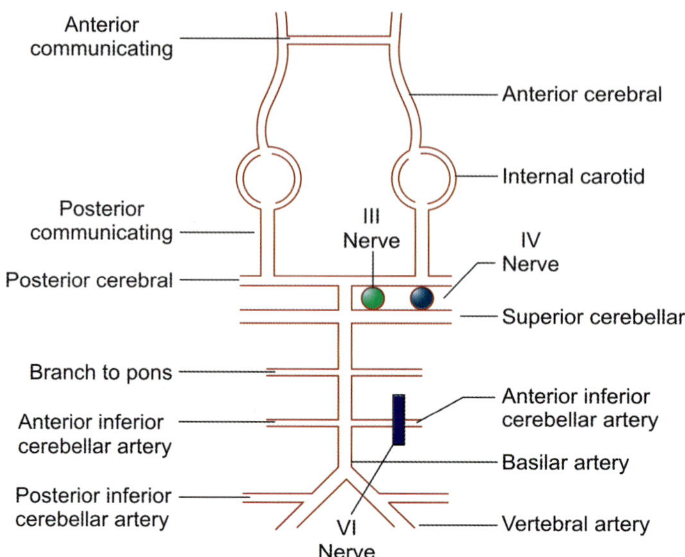

Fig. 14.4: Diagrammatic representation of vertebrobasilar and carotid system in relation to third, fourth and sixth nerves

Blood supply to individual parts of visual path

The various parts of the visual path have specialized blood supply, they are:

1. The optic nerve
2. The chiasma
3. The optic tract
4. The optic radiation
5. The visual cortex. Each visual cortex has its own blood supply with some overlap between adjoing parts.

Blood supply of the optic nerve

The blood supply of the optic nerve can be divided into two parts (Figs 14.5 and 14.6):

I. Blood supply to the optic nerve head
II. Blood supply to the optic nerve proper.

Blood supply to the optic nerve head

The optic papilla has an **elaborate multilayered blood supply** from both the **central retinal** as well **ciliary circulation**. Both the systems are branches of **ophthalmic artery**, which is the main artery of the orbit, and it's contents.

The central retinal artery extends from the apex of the orbit to the optic nerve head. In the orbit, it travels under the optic nerve. The nerve enters the substance of the nerve, 12.5 mm behind the globe, passing through the subarachnoid and subdural space.

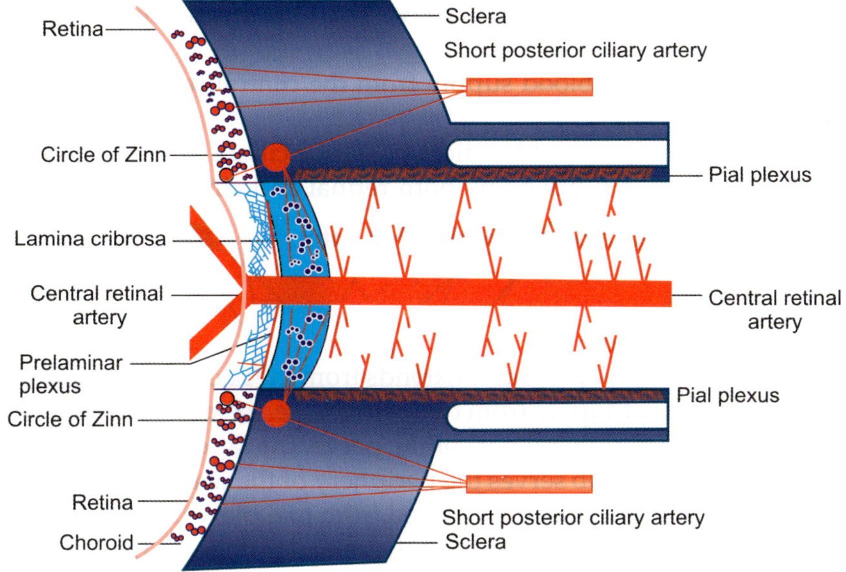

Fig. 14.5: Blood supply to the optic nerve head

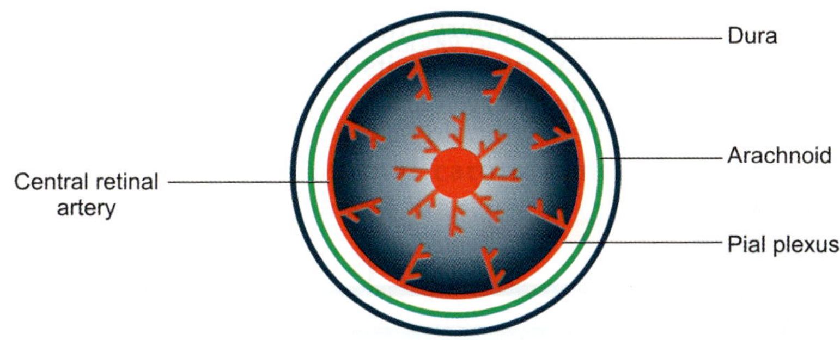

Fig. 14.6: Transverse section of optic nerve showing arrangement of blood vessels

Just before entering the optic nerve, it gives following branches:

1. Pial plexus
2. Central collateral retinal artery
3. Central artery of optic nerve
4. Interneural branches.

The ciliary circulation

The ciliary circulation is derived from the **short and long posterior ciliary arteries** which anastomose to form the circle of Zinn in the substance of the sclera near the optic nerve head all round the head. It sends branches to the choroids, the optic nerve and to the pial plexus.

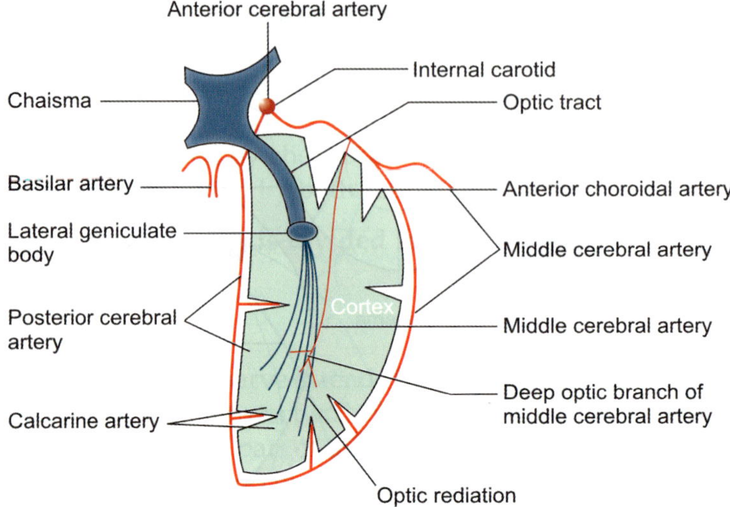

Fig. 14.9: Blood supply of posterior visual path

remaining part gets its blood supply from posterior communicating and anterior choroidal arteries.

Blood supply to the lateral geniculate body (Fig.14.9)

The lateral geniculate body is a compact mass of visual fibers, has a rich blood supply from posterior cerebral artery through posterior choroidal artery, which supplies the area concerned with superior homonymous field. The anterior choroidal artery supplies the part of lateral geniculate body concerned with inferior homonymous fibers.

Blood supply to optic radiation (Fig. 14.9)

The optic radiation is spread over a large area. It gets its blood supply from **middle cerebral** and **posterior cerebral arteries**. The blood supply to the optic radiation is divided into three parts, i.e. **anterior, middle** and **posterior**. The anterior blood supply comes from anterior and posterior choroidal and middle cerebral arteries. The middle part is supplied by deep optic artery which is a branch of middle cerebral artery. The posterior part is supplied by calcarine artery, which is a branch of posterior cerebral artery.

Blood supply to the visual cortex (Fig. 14.9)

The **posterior cerebral artery and the middle cerebral artery** are the main source of blood supply to the visual cortex. The branches of the **posterior cerebral artery** that supply the visual cortex are — calcarine, posterior temporal and parieto occipital arteries. The lateral part of the visual cortex is supplied by terminal branches of middle cerebral artery.

The macular area of the cortex gets its blood supply from both the arteries, i.e. the posterior cerebral and the middle cerebral. Hence, in occlusion of one, the macula is spared.

Blood supply to various part of the brain that are related to neuro-ophthalmic lesions are:

Part	*Arterial supply*
I. Cerebrum	Anterior, middle and posterior cerebral arteries.
II. Midbrain	Posterior cerebral, posterior communicating and superior cerebellar arteries.
III. Pons	Basilar artery by long and short pontine branches.
IV. Medulla	Posterior inferior cerebellar artery which is a branches of vertebral artery.
V. Cerebellum	Superior cerebellar, anterior inferior cerebellar and posterior inferior cerebellar artery.

The important arterial connections of neuro-ophthalmic importance are:

Anastomosis	*Arteries jointed*
1. External carotid to internal carotid.	Maxillary branches of external carotid to ophthalmic artery branches.
2. Internal carotids to internal carotids.	Anterior communicating arteries.
3. Internal carotid to vertebrobasilar system.	Posterior communicating arteries.
4. Among anterior middle and posterior cerebral arteries.	Leptomeningial anastomosis on surface of brain.

Intracranial vascular lesions are frequent causes of neuro-ophthalmic disorders. The vascular lesions can be **congenital** or **acquired**. The congenital lesions need not produce symptoms at birth, they generally manifest after few years or in adult age. The vascular lesion in all ages may either have ocular features in the form of **field defect, motility disorder** and **fundus changes** only or have associated systemic features of **loss of motility and sensation, altered consciousness, convulsion, headache, speech disorder, coma** and **signs of raised intracranial pressure**.

The neuro-ophthalmic features can be:

1. Related to arterial diseases
2. Related to venous diseases.

The neuro-ophthalmic features of vascular lesion can either be that of:

1. A mass lesion, i.e. aneurysm, hematoma
2. Changes in the vessels in the form of embolism, thrombosis or hemorrhagic episodes.

1. **The arterial diseases are:**
   I. Aneurysm
      a. Saccular
      b. Fusiform

II. Occlusion
   a. Embolism
   b. Thromboembolic
III. Hemorrhage
IV. Malfomation
V. Inflammation and trauma may also cause arterial disorders
VI. Trauma

2. **The venous diseases are:**
   I. Thrombosis
   II. Inflammation
   III. Malformation

Arterial lesions of neuro-ophthalmic interest

Intracranial aneurysm

About 2%-3% of persons have intracranial aneurysms, all of which do not produce clinical features. The symptomatic aneurysm are the commonest cause of spontaneous nontraumatic intracranial bleeding in the form of **subarachnoid hemorrhage**.

Aneurysms according to **age** of manifestation can be **congenital** or **acquired**. The aneurysms are also classified according to their **shape**, i.e. **saccular (berry)** and **fusiform**. The former are more frequent in carotid system while the latter are mostly seen in vertebrobasilar system. Only 5% of aneurysms of vertebrobasilar system are saccular. The saccular aneurysms when bilateral are generally mirror image in shape and site of the contralateral lesion.

The predisposing factors in producing aneurysms are:
1. Congenital malformation
2. Hypertension
3. Atherosclerosis (fusiform basilar)
4. Elastic tissue defect (Ehlers-Danlos)
5. Degeneration

The **Pressure effect** of the aneurysms are slow, progressive and chronic. **Acute signs** and symptoms occurs only when the aneurysms rupture. The effect of rupture can either be a leak or large bleeding.

The bleeding can occur as:
1. Subarachnoid hemorrhage
2. Intraventricular hemorrhage
3. Intracerebral hemorrhage

The common sites of saccular aneurysm are:
I. **Internal carotid** (Figs 14.10 and 14.11)
   a. Intracavernous (subclinoid)
   b. Supraclinoid
   c. Carotid
   d. Ophthalmic

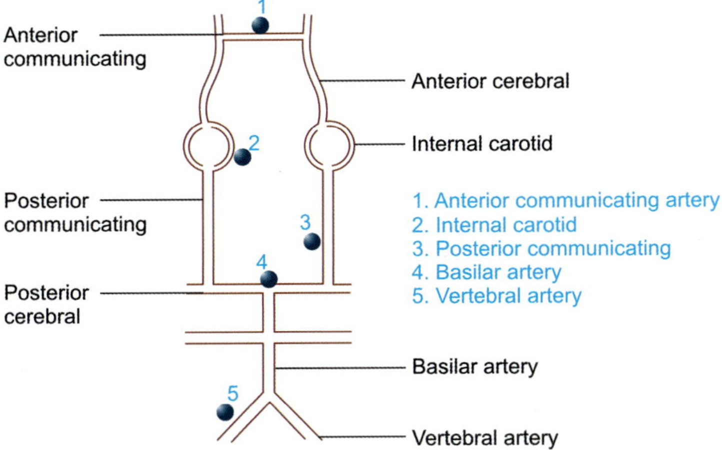

Fig. 14.10: Various aneurysms related to circle of Willis

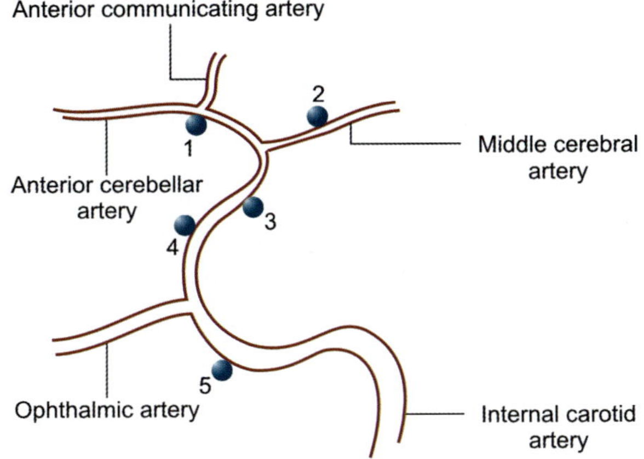

Fig. 14.11: Common sites of saccular aneurysm in carotid system

II. Posterior communicating artery
III. Middle cerebral artery
IV. Anterior communicating artery

Vertebrobasilar system

I. Basilar artery
II. Posterior cerebral artery

Common sites of fusiform aneurysms are:

1. **Carotid system**
   i. Internal carotid
      a. Intracavernous
      b. Intracerebral
2. **Vertebrobasilar system**—main trunk of basilar artery.

Characteristics of saccular aneurysms

Their **spherical shapes** impart the name saccular aneurysms to this type of intracranial aneurysms. For the same reason, they are also called berry aneurysms. The size of the aneurysms varies from **pinhead** to **half a centimeter across**. Aneurysms smaller than 5 mm do not rupture. Only aneurysms larger than 2.5 cm produce **symptoms of mass lesion**. They are caused by **congenital weakness in the arterial wall** and worsened by hypertension, atherosclerosis and elastic tissue deficiency. The aneurysms develop only in arteries. **95% of saccular aneurysms develop in carotid**. They vary in number, 20% persons have multiple aneurysms. When multiple, they develop at the corresponding site on the opposite side, i.e. mirror image. **The aneurysms manifest after puberty**. They are more common among **women**. Most of the saccular aneurysms remain **asymptomatic** throughout the life.

Fourth to mid sixth decades are the common decades when the saccular aneurysms rupture.

Due to some unexplained factors, men are more likely to develop rupture in anterior communicating artery and women are more prone to develop rupture at the junction of internal carotid and posterior communicating artery.

Mortality varies between 20% to 40% following rupture.

Commonest neuro-ophthalmic feature of unruptured saccular aneurysms is cranial nerve palsy that may involve any of the nerves from second to sixth. Out of all cranial nerves **third nerve** is more likely to be involved in mass effect of aneurysms. Commonest aneurysm causing third nerve palsy is **posterior communicating artery aneurysms** followed by internal carotid artery aneurysm.

Characteristics of fusiform aneurysms are:

- They are less common than saccular aneurysms.
- As atherosclerosis is the main cause, they are seen in elderly person.
- They are fusiform in shape, which are infact tortuous dilatation of atherosclerotic arteries along the long-axis.
- Common site is at the bifurcation of basilar artery at a level of exit of third nerve from brainstem. This makes third nerve more vulnerable to palsy than other cranial nerves in case of basilar artery aneurysm.
- Vertebrobasilar system is more frequently involved than carotid system.
- They are more likely to develop pressure symptoms and thrombosis than rupture.

Fusiform aneurysms of the carotid system can either be intracavernous or intracranial. They may press either the optic nerve or the chiasma resulting in corresponding field defect and optic atrophy.

Fusiform aneurysms of the vertebrobasilar system are mostly seen in elderly males with hypertension and atherosclerosis. They act as mass lesion in the posterior fossa causing features of corticospinal and spinothalmic tract involvement, cranial nerve palsy, hydrocephalus. They may be associated with fusiform aneurysms of abdominal aorta as well.

Neuro-ophthalmic features of aneurysms of carotid system

Neuro-ophthalmic features depend on location size of the aneurysm.

Intracavernous carotid aneurysms (Subclinoid)

These aneurysms are **mostly saccular**. They are **relatively infrequent**, mostly **unilateral, do not involve neural tracts**.

They produces two types of lesions are:

1. **Mass lesions** due to expansion of the aneurysm and its pressure effect. The mass effect depends upon location and size of the aneurysm.
2. **Rupture** of the aneurysm resulting in carotid cavernous fistula.

Gradual enlargement of the aneurysm acts as a mass on the floor of the middle cranial fossa where many anatomical structures are crowed resulting in multiple cranial nerve palsy and erosion of adjoining bony structure depending on its extension in surrounding.

Extension	*Clinical features*
Anterior extension	Produces unilateral loss of vision, proptosis and multiple cranial nerve palsy due to erosion of anterior clinoid process, apex of orbit or superior orbital fissure.
Medial extension	Produces signs simulating pituitary tumor due to destruction of sella turcica.
Posterior extension	Produces seventh nerve palsy and deafness, due to erosion of petrous bone. There may be involvement of fifth nerve.
Inferior extension	Erodes sphenoidal sinus and may reach nasopharynx as well.

The growth may have extension in more than one direction

The clinical features

The features develop slowly either with **diplopia** or **pain in the distribution of the fifth nerve**. The **sixth nerve** is commonest and earliest to be involved. The fourth nerve is least affected. The third nerve involvements may be in between. **Multiple cranial nerve** involvement is frequent that includes **optic nerve**. The **seventh** and **eighth nerves** are involved only when petrous bone is involved.

monoocular loss of vision and optic atrophy due to involvement of optic nerve. They may involve the chiasma as well with associated field changes.

Posterior communicating artery aneurysms

Aneurysm at this site is a **common cause of unilateral isolated pupillary involving third nerve palsy**, seen commonly in **elderly persons**. The aneurysms are **saccular**. They arises mostly at the junction of posterior communicating artery and internal carotid. The aneurysms are slow to grow. Initially, it is symptomless, as the size increases it compresses the third nerve and gets adherent to it. Later the aneurysm ruptures.

The common symptoms are gradually increasing **headache, ptosis** and **diplopia**. The symptoms are acute in case of rupture of the aneurysms. The third nerve palsy is complete which includes all the muscles supplied by it, mydriasis and cycloplegia.

Presence of mydriasis is so consistent with posterior communicating artery aneurysm that it almost always excludes diabetic third nerve palsy but not diabetes.

There is no loss of sensation because the fifth nerve is not involved in contrast to intracavernous aneurysm which is commonly associated with loss of sensation.

Once the aneurysm ruptures, the CSF shows frank blood. Some recovery of movements is common. **Aberrant regeneration** is frequent.

Differential diagnosis consists **diabetic** and **compressive third nerve palsy**.

Middle cerebral artery aneurysm

These aneurysms **do not have neuro-ophthalmic manifestation unless they rupture**. On rupture, they cause intracerebral hematoma that result in homonymous field defects of varied shape and size. There may be contralateral hemiplegia and sensory loss.

Anterior communicating artery aneurysm

In spite of proximity to the anterior visual path and it being **commonest intracranial aneurysm, neuro-ophthalmic features are absent unless the aneurysm ruptures**.

A ruptured aneurysms causes unilateral loss of vision. Occasionally, it may cause compressive lesion of optic nerve that lies above the artery, this may result in para central temporal scotoma. In ipsilateral loss of vision, the other side may show temporal field defect.

Neuro-ophthalmic manifestation of aneurysms of vertebrobasilar artery (see Fig. 14.10)

Anatomy of vertebrobasilar arterial system—The basilar artery is formed by junction of two vertebral arteries on each side of the midline. They enter the cranium through foramen magnum and go upwards and medially in front of the medulla and unite to form basilar artery in the midline at the lower border of the pons. The basilar artery ascends up to upper border of the pons and divides into two posterior cerebral arteries one on each side of the midline. The posterior cerebral arteries are the terminal branches of the basilar artery. The posterior cerebral arteries are connected to the internal carotid via posterior communicating arteries. The superior cerebellar artery arises from the vertebral artery below the posterior cerebral artery. The third nerve passes between the two arteries. The other arteries of vertebrobasilar system are posterior inferior cerebellar and anterior inferior cerebellar artery. They supply the medulla, pons and cerebellum.

Vertebrobasilar system aneurysm

About 5% of intracranial aneurysms are found in the **posterior fossa**, arising from vertebrobasilar arterial system. Incidence is distributed almost equally among **fusiform** and **saccular aneurysms**.

The aneurysms of neuro-ophthalmic interest can be broadly divided into:

1. Basilar artery aneurysm
2. Posterior cerebral artery aneurysm

1. Basilar artery aneurysms

The commonest site for the aneurysm to develop is at the **bifurcation of the basilar artery**. Less commonly they arise near the origin of the superior cerebellar artery.

The exit of the third nerve from the midbrain is very close to the bifurcation of the basilar artery. Hence, it is expected that the third nerve palsy should be very common but this does not happen unless the aneurysm ruptures. An expanding aneurysm causes pressure symptom on **chiasma** with corresponding field defect. It may invade the third ventricle and behave like a **parasellar growth**. The aneurysms may present with **dorsal midbrain signs** and **subarachnoid hemorrhage**.

The third nerve palsy when present may be isolated or associated with hemi-paresis, homonymous hemianopia, cerebellar ataxia, nystagmus, malfunction of trigeminal nerve and sixth nerve palsy.

An aneurysm near the origin of superior cerebellar artery impinges the third nerve against the posterior cerebral artery.

2. Posterior cerebral artery aneurysm

Posterior cerebral artery aneurysms are rare. The commonest neuro-ophthalmic feature **is third nerve palsy**. When the aneurysm ruptures, it cause visual symptom due to involvement of occipital cortex.

Neuro-ophthalmic manifestation of cerebrovascular disorders

They are generally referred to as **cerebrovascular accidents** or **stroke**. The causes of which are **thrombosis, embolism, intracerebral bleeding** and **subarachnoid hemorrhage**.

They can be seen at **any age** but are more common after fifth decade. The incidence rises with age. They are **equally common in two sexes** and all races.

They can be broadly divided into:

- Occlusive disorder
- Hemorrhagic disorder

The occlusive disorders can either be

- Arterial, which are mostly embolic or thrombotic
- Venous mostly thrombotic

Arterial obstructive disorders

Arterial obstructive diseases can involve either:

1. Carotid system
2. Vertebrobasilar system

Each has its distinct characteristics. The two common features of arterial occlusive disease are:

1. Transient ischemic attack (TIA)
2. Cerebral infarction

The transient ischemic attack (TIA)

The TIA is an episode of **short duration**, **localized**, deficiency of cerebral functions due to block in its arterial supply. The attacks are precursor of cerebral stroke that may follow within weeks to months.

The duration of an attack may vary between two minutes to fifteen minutes. The attack passes off without any residual effect. The gap between the two attacks varies. They may be as frequent as ten to fifteen in twenty four hours. One or two episodes in a week is common frequency.

The episodes may be localized either to **carotid or vertebrobasilar system**.

The characteristics of carotid system TIA are:

1. Amaurosis fugax
2. Homonymous hemianopia
3. Unilateral sensory loss
4. Unilateral motor weakness
5. Aphasia
6. Combination

The characteristics of vertebrobasilar system TIA are:

1. Diminished vision
2. Variable homonymous field defects
3. Bilateral altitudinal field defects
4. Ataxia
5. Vertigo
6. Variable degree of motor weakness which may change side and involve all the limbs may cause quadriplegia.
7. Variable sensory loss.

Neuro-ophthalmic manifestation of cerebral infarction

Cerebral infarctions are **common** vascular disorder of the nervous system, mostly seen in **elderly** persons. **They rarely report to ophthalmologists**. They are referred by neurologist.

The infarction can be brought about by

1. Atheromatous thrombous that initially narrows the lumen of the artery but latter may completely obliterate the lumen.
2. Embolism

The features of cerebral infarction at various levels are as follows:

Location of occlusion	*Ophthalmic features*	*Neurological features*
1. Internal carotid artery	I. Symptomless. II. Homonymous hemianopia.	I. Contralateral hemiplegia. II. Contralateralloss of sensation. III. Aphasia, agraphia, ataxia.
2. Middle cerebral artery	I. Homonymous hemianopia.	I. Contralateral hemiplegia. II. Contralateral hemianesthesia.
3. Vertebral artery	I. Nystagmus. II. Horner's syndrome.	I. Dysphagia, dysarthria. II. Altered pain and temperature sensation of ipsilateral face. III. Contralateral impaired pain.
4. Posterior inferior cerebellar artery	-do-	-do-
5. Anterior inferior cerebellar artery.	I. Facial palsy. II. Horner's syndrome.	I. Loss of pain and temperature on the contralateral side.
6. Basilar artery		
a. Main trunk	Bilateral or unilateral paralysis of third, fourth and sixth nerves, paralysis of horizontal gaze. Horner's syndrome, cortical blindness.	Paralysis of face, tongue, dysarthria, quadriparesis.
b. Penetrating branch	Foville's, Weber's, Benedict's and Claude's syndrome.	Ipsilateral paralysis of tongue, contralateral hemiplegia.
7. Posterior cerebral artery	Visual agnosia and palinopia	Hemiplegia hemianesthesia

Occlusive vascular diseases of neuro-ophthalmic interest

The occlusive disease can either involve the **arterial systems** or **venous systems**. The arterial occlusive disease can involve either the **internal carotid system** or the **vertebro-basilar system**. The **carotid occlusive diseases** mostly produce features of cerebral involvement in the form of:

1. Disorder of visual path causing diminished vision and field changes
2. Supranuclear gaze disturbance

3. Extraocular palsies are less common and transient due to development of collateral in short period.

The occlusive diseases of the **vertebrobasilar system** causes mostly **brainstem syndromes** without involving the visual path unless associated with raised intracranial pressure.

Occlusive diseases of the carotid system

The neuro-ophthalmic conditions produced by carotid occlusive diseases are:

1. **Amaurosis fugax**
2. **Supranuclear gaze anomaly**
   i. Horizontal gaze palsy
   ii. Spastic conjugate gaze
3. **Ischemic syndrome**
   i. Venous stasis retinopathy
   ii. Chronic ocular hypoxia
   iii. Chiasmal syndrome

1. Amaurosis fugax

Most of the times, it is the **first symptoms** of carotid insufficiency. It is **transient monocular loss of vision.** A typical attack lasts from two to five minutes with complete recovery. The loss of vision may involve, whole of the field or part of it. The typical loss of vision is ascending or descending of a dark curtain in front of the eye. The curtain passes off in the reverse order, i.e. if it has descended from above, it will ascend from below to resolve. The density of the curtain is referred by various terms ranging from dark black to translucent film. Though amaurosis fugax is a major manifestation of carotid insufficiency, it is never associated with transient ischemic attack of the hemisphere at the same time. The condition is generally seen in persons with **hypertension and atherosclerosis**, other associated condition may be **coronary artery disease, hypercholesterolemia, diabetes, valvular diseases, arrhythmia, prolapse of mitral valve, giant call arteritis, other congenital heart diseases** and **carotid artery stenosis**.

The mechanisms of amaurosis is **microembolization of the retinal circulation** or **ophthalmic artery**. Association of arterio spasm is common. There may be sudden transient fall of arterial blood flow with lowered perfusion.

The emboli may be **cholesterol, platelet** or **fibrin**.

Externally, the eyes are normal during the episode except **dilated pupil**. Fundus examined during and soon after may have evidence of **retinal vasculopathies** like diabetes or hypertension. There may be visible emboli in the retinal vessels or there may be signs of **retinal ischemia** in the form of **retinal edema** and **retinal hemorrhage**. The fundus may not have any evidence of embolism after few hours.

Though the predisposing factors that cause amaurosis fugax are also shared by cerebral infarction, the exact incidence of cerebral infarction following amaurosis fugax is not known.

The differential diagnosis consists of other causes of transient uniocular loss of vision.

They include **Migraine, hypotension, papilledema**.

Investigation should include exclusion of hypertension, diabetes, and coronary heart disease. The specific investigation includes **doppler ultrasonography, carotid phonoangiography, B scans, ultrasound, angiography**.

Management of amaurosis is outside the domain of ophthalmologist. In fact they should be investigated and treated by neuroradiologist and neurosurgeons.

2. Supranuclear gaze anomaly

i. **Abnormality of horizontal gaze**—These features depend upon the location and extent of the lesion generally caused by **hemorrhage** in frontal or parietal lobe rather than **infarction**. It produces **contralateral gaze palsy**. The eyes and the head are turned towards the lesion due to unopposed action of contralateral frontal eye field. During doll's eye movement and caloric test, the eyes move away from the lesion due to **intact vestibular path**. After the test is over, the eye deviate towards the lesion. After a week, the eye regains voluntary eye movements away from the lesion. The patients are generally **comatose** hence are seen in neurological wards.

ii. **Spasticity of conjugate gaze**—During forced closure of the eyes, the eyes should move up and laterally due to Bell's phenomenon. In vascular lesions of parietal or temporal lesions, the eyes move up and away from the lesion. **This has no localizing value**, can only lateralize the lesion.

3. Ischemic syndromes associated with carotid arterial system

i. **Venous stasis syndrome**—The syndrome is also known as **slow flow retinopathy** and **partial central retinal vein occlusion** (which it is not) and **confused as diabetic retinopathy**. The disease is caused **due to reduced perfusion pressure** in internal carotid secondary due to atheromatous changes in the internal carotid. It is **generally monocular** with diminished vision. The fundus picture is similar to diabetic retinopathy. The most important difference is that diabetic retinopathy generally develops in the posterior pole and spreads to periphery. The venous stasis syndrome starts on the periphery and spreads to the posterior pole. The picture consists of **venous dilatation, increased tortuosity of veins, superficial hemorrhages**, and **exudates**. **Neovascularization** is a late common feature. Neovascularization may extend in the iris and cause neovascular glaucoma that requires pan retinal photocoagulation. Venous stasis syndrome may be followed by chronic ocular hypoxia syndrome.

ii. **Chronic ocular hypoxia**—**Internal carotid artery** is the sole source of blood supply of the eye. Obstruction of internal carotid of one side is generally partially compensated by development of collateral from the other side. This prevents infraction of the eye but a state of chronic hypoxia persists that initiates changes

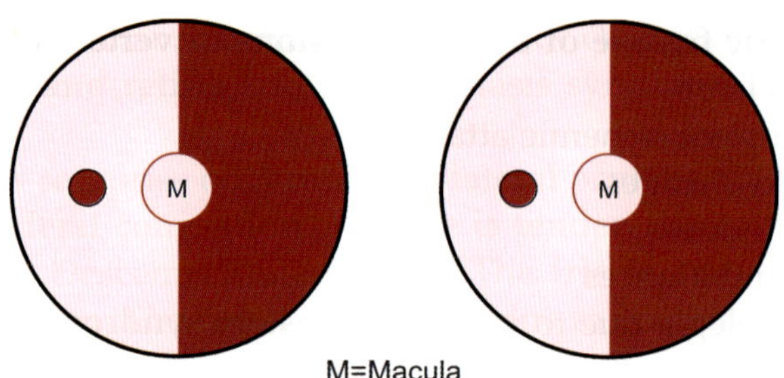

Fig. 14.12: Field changes in macular sparing

almost normal central vision but have difficulty in reading, locating objects placed in front of them and even walking (Fig. 14.12).

The value of field changes should be corroborated with neurological signs.

Only lesions of occipital lobes have typical homonymous hemianopia with macular sparing and no neurological signs.

iii. Cortical blindness

Cortical blindness is **sudden, painless loss of vision in both eyes** in a person with apparently normal vision.

The triad of the condition consists of:

a. Sudden diminished vision
b. Normal pupillary reaction
c. Normal fundus, excluding pre-existing fundus changes.
   i. The loss of vision is **sudden** and **symmetric**. The patient complains that the lights of the room have been dimmed suddenly. This may be associated with **photopsia**. The patient is known to **deny blindness (Anton's syndrome).** The loss of vision is generally not less than of 3/60. The patient may have unformed hallucinations. Denial of blindness and hallucination are associated with other **neuropsychiatric disorders**. The vision starts improving after some days to weeks mostly following trauma and occlusive vascular diseases. The patient first regains brightness, this is followed by form and color. The patients who do not regain vision pass into more severe brainstem disorders. The movements of the eyes are not affected by lesions of occipital cortex per se. The movements are affected by brainstem lesions only.

2. Oculomotor imbalances

i. Ophthalmoplegia associated with various forms of brainstem lesion in occlusive disorders are:

Involvement			*Signs*	*Eponym of syndrome*
Cranial nerve	*Site*	*Tract and/or nuclei*		
Third	1. Base of the midbrain	Corticospinal tract	Third nerve palsy and crossed hemiplegia	Weber's syndrome
	2. Tegmentum of midbrain	Red nucleus and corticospinal tract	Third nerve palsy, contralateral tremor, ataxia, hemiplegia	Benedickt's syndrome
	3. Tegmentum of midbrain	Red nucleus	Third nerve palsy with contralateral ataxia and tremors	Claude's syndrome
Sixth and seventh	Base of pons	Cortiospinal tract	Ipsilateral seventh and sixth nerve palsy, contralateral hemiplegia	Millard-Gubler syndrome
Fifth, sixth, seventh and eighth	Dorsolateral tegmentum of pons	Sensory tract of fifth nerve, sympathetic chain	Ipsilateral facial hypothesia, sixth, seventh nerve palsy with Horner's syndrome	Foville syndrome

ii. Gaze palsy

Occlusive diseases of the vertebrobasilar arterial system can cause both **horizontal and vertical gaze palsy** due to lesion at different levels. Each type is accompanied by different sets of clinical features.

a. **Horizontal gaze palsy** is caused due to involvement of **pontine paramedian reticular formation (PPRF).** The horizontal gaze palsy can either be bilateral or unilateral. The former is caused due to occlusion of main trunk of basilar artery. It causes coma, bilateral gaze palsy, bilateral lesions of corticospinal tract with miotic pupil that reacts to light.

   Unilateral lesions can either be complete or incomplete.

   Complete unilateral lesion of PPRF result is permanent conjugate horizontal gaze palsy. The eye is deviated away from the lesion. Ipsilateral facial palsy with contralateral paralysis of limbs and diminished sensation.

   Incomplete lesion of PPRF cause ipsilateral gaze paresis. There may be **gaze paretic nystagmus**. The eyes remain in mid position.

   Conjugate horizontal gaze palsy may be seen in internuclear ophthalmoplegia.

b. **Vertical gaze palsy** is caused due to infarction of rostral midbrain. Paralysis of up gaze is more common than down gaze. It is associated with lid lag, lid retraction, retraction nystagmus, convergence palsy and large pupil with light near dissociation.

iii. **Horner's syndrome**

Incidence of Horner's syndrome in occlusive diseases of vertebrobasilar system is variable. It is most frequently seen in infarction of lateral part of medulla and commonly associated with brainstem syndrome of Wallenberg that consist of:

1. Ipsilateral 9th, 10th and 11th nerve lesion along with Horner's syndrome.
2. Cerebral ataxia, facial hypesthesia and facial pain.
3. Contralateral loss of pain and temperature in the limbs

iv. Nystagmus

Nystagmus are common feature of brainstem ischemia, lesion of PPRF

Part involved	*Nystagmus*
Vestibular nucleus, PPRF	Horizontal gaze paretic
Rostral midbrain tegmentum	Convergence retraction
Brainstem	Pendular vertical alternate
Cerebellum	Pendular vertical alternate

For details of nystagmus see Chapter 16

Other abnormal involuntary movements of the eye due to occlusive diseases are **ocular bobbing, ocular flutter** and **dysmetria**.

3. Ocular pain

Ocular pain in case of occipital lobe infarction is felt on the **same side** as the infracted lobe. This is thought to be referred from the dural cover of the occipital lobe via ophthalmic branch of trigeminal nerve.

Occlusive venous disorders of neuro-ophthalmic interest

The venous drainage of the brain differs from its arterial supply. The venous drainage is through the dural sinuses (venous sinuses). The dural sinuses do not correspond with the arterial supply. The function of the dural sinuses are — (1) draining venous blood from brain and its covering, (2) absorbs CSF, (3) equalize pressure between the intracranial venous pressure and venous pressure in the scalp through emissary veins. The walls of the venous sinuses are formed by splitting of the dura which is two layered, i.e. endosteal and meningeal. The dural sinuses are lined by endothelium, they are irregular in shape and caliber. They do not have smooth muscles in their walls and lack valves making them vulnerable to infection both ways.

Anatomical venous sinuses can be divided into:

1. **Paired sinuses**
   a. Cavernous sinus
   b. Superior and inferior petrosal sinuses
   c. Transverse sinus
   d. Sigmoid sinus
   e. Sphenoparietal sinus
   f. Pterosquamous sinus
   g. Middle meningeal sinus

2. **Unpaired sinuses**
   a. Superior and inferior sagittal sinus
   b. Straight sinus
   c. Occipital sinus
   d. Anterior and posterior intracavernous sinus
   e. Basilar plexus

The lesions of all the venous sinuses do not have neuro-ophthalmic manifestation. Only a few cause neuro-ophthalmic features.

The lesions include:

1. Infection, and inflammation of the wall of the sinus.
2. Formation of thrombus in the sinus obliterating the sinus.
3. The obliterated sinuses impede venous drainage. This leads to stagnation of the blood in the draining area.
4. Rupture of the sinus secondary to thrombus formation.
5. Deposition of neoplasm in sinus and trauma.
6. The venous channels do not develop embolism like arterial channel.

Cavernous sinus (Figs 14.13 to 14.15)

Out of all the venous channels, the lesions of the cavernous sinus have maximum number of neuro-ophthalmic features. The cavernous sinus lies in the middle cranial fossa on either side of the sphenoid body. It extends from the medial end of the superior orbital fissure to the tip of the petrous bone. The sinus is divided into small pockets that communicate freely with each other. Thus, an infection of one side quickly spreads to the other side.

The cavernous sinus is joined anteriorly by superior and inferior ophthalmic veins, tributaries from sphenoparietal sinuses. The superficial middle cerebral vein opens above. The inferior cerebral vein and middle sinuses communicate from the lateral sinus.

The relation of the cavernous sinus on each side of the midline have great clinical significance (Fig. 14.15).

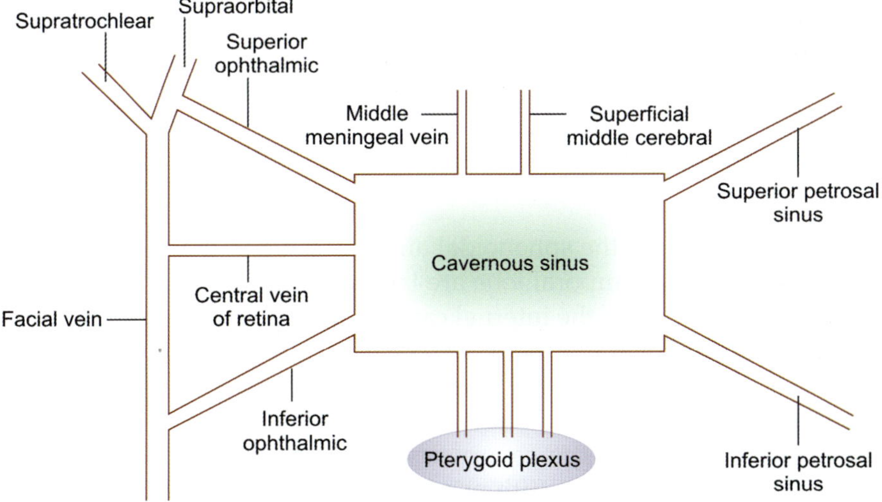

Fig. 14.13: Connection of cavernous sinus

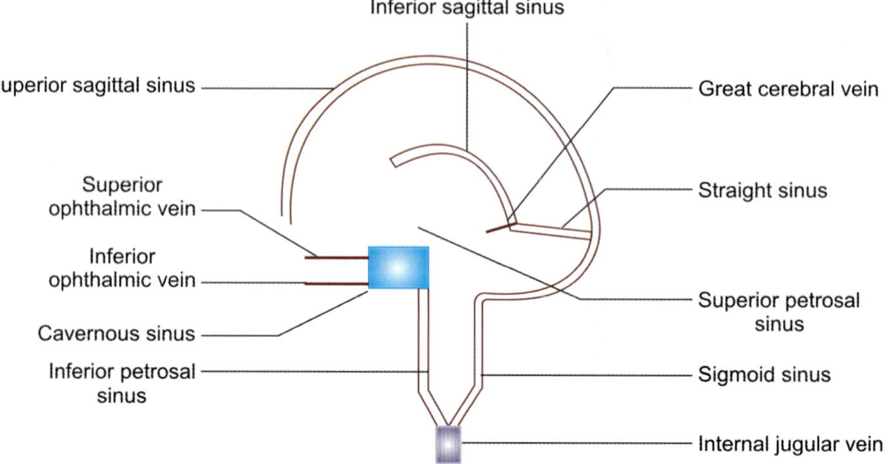

Fig. 14.14: Dural venous sinuses

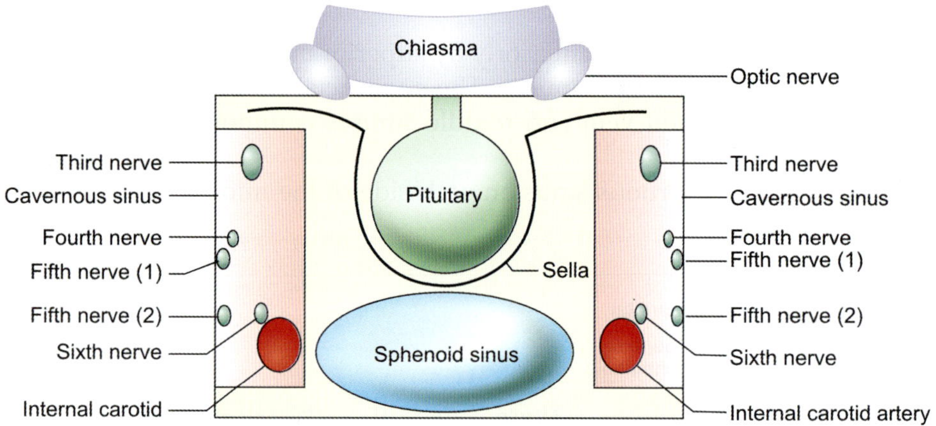

Fig. 14.15: Relation of cavernous sinus to other structures

1. The sella turcisa and the sphenoidal air sinuses lie in the middle of the sinus.
2. The uncus and the temporal lobe are lateral to the sinus.
3. Extracavernous part of the internal carotid, the posterior communicating artery and the optic tract are above the sinus.
4. The intracavernous part of the internal carotid along with its sympathetic chain lies in the substance of the cavernous sinus.
5. The other contents of the cavernous sinus are third and fourth nerve, the ophthalmic division of the fifth nerve, and the sixth nerve.
6. The sixth nerve lies in the substance of the cavernous sinus lateral to the internal carotid.

7. The third, fourth and fifth nerves are embedded in the lateral wall of the sinus.
8. The floor is the narrowest part formed by confluence of the lateral and the medial walls.

The cavernous sinus drains passively due to the pulsation of the internal carotid artery. The blood is drained via superior and inferior petrosal sinus into the jugular system. The emissary veins drain into pterygoid plexus, some of the blood drain in the vertebral plexus as well.

The venous drainage of neuro-ophthalmic interest can clinically be divided into:

1. Those related to cavernous sinus (see Figs 14.13 and 14.14)
2. Those not related to cavernous sinus

The lesions of cavernous sinus of neuro-ophthalmic interest are:

1. Cavernous sinus thrombosis
2. Cavernous sinus syndromes

Cavernous sinus thrombosis

This is an infective/inflammatory process of the wall of the sinus and intrasinus trabeculum while cavernous sinus syndrome is noninfective/noninflammatory in nature caused by:

1. Vascular lesions
   (a) Intracavernous carotid aneurysm
   (b) Posterior cerebral aneurysm
   (c) Carotid cavernous fistula
2. Neoplasm
   (a) Extension from primary growth in the neighboring structures
      i. Pituitary tumor
      ii. Meningioma
      iii. Neurofibroma
      iv. Neuroma
      v. Craniopharyngioma
      vi. Nasopharyngeal tumors
   (b) Extension from distant organs
3. Trauma

The cavernous sinus thrombosis can either be **aseptic thrombosis** following trauma that may be accidental or surgical, both of which may get infected and result in a infective process. More common is spread of acute or chronic infection from the area drained by the sinus **mostly by bacteria**. The bacterial infection can be **acute** due to pyogenic organism or **chronic** due to granuloma forming organism. The former is more common. **Herpes zoster ophthalmicus** may occasionally cause cavernous sinus inflammation. Fungal infections are rare but can prove to be fatal.

The infection to begin with is unilateral, starting with pain in and around the eye, ipsilateral headache, malaise, and fever. It is seen in all ages and equally in two sexes.

The ocular signs are conjunctival congestion, conjunctival chemosis, edema of the lids, fast growing proptosis. In fully developed cases, the signs comprise of loss of movement due to involvement of various cranial nerves in different combination, loss of corneal sensation due to involvement of fifth nerve. The later features are internal ophthalmoplegia and edema of the disc.

Tenderness over the ipsilateral mastoid is an ominous sign that denotes involvement of the contralateral cavernous sinus. The early signs of contralateral involvement is paralysis of the lateral rectus.

A chronic inflammation of the anterior cavernous sinus may present as **superior orbital fissure syndrome** or **orbital apex syndrome** while a posteriorly placed lesion may mimic infection of the petrous apex.

A cavernous sinus thrombosis is a medical emergency that require urgent neuro-ophthalmic evaluation and management by fast acting broad spectrum antibiotic.

The differential diagnosis consist of orbital cellulitis, endophthalmitis and panophthalmitis.

The venous channels are incapable of developing embolism. They are occluded by thrombosis formation.

The effect of occlusive diseases of the intracranial venous and dural sinuses are:

1. Dilatation of proximal part of the vein.
2. Rise of intravenous pressure.
3. Diminished venous drainage of the intracranial tissues.
4. Intracortical edema, ischemia and hemorrhage.
5. Diminished absorption of CSF resulting in raised intracranial pressure.

The result of venous occlusive diseases are:

1. Motor and sensory loss in limbs
2. Paralysis of extraocular muscles
3. Papilledema
4. Homonymous hemianopia
5. Convulsion
6. Speech disturbance.

The common occlusive venous diseases are:

1. Cavernous sinus thrombosis (see above)
2. Superior sagittal sinus thrombosis
3. Lateral sinus thrombosis
4. Inferior petrosal sinus thrombosis
5. Thrombosis of small venous channels
6. Central retinal vein thrombosis

Superior sagittal sinus thrombosis

It is one of the large dural sinuses of the brain that not only receives venous blood and transmits it to jugular system, **it also absorbs CSF**. It is one sinus that is more frequently occluded than others. Commonest cause of occlusion being **aseptic thrombosis**. Infective thrombosis when present is due to spread of infection from transverse sinuses.

The clinical features commonly met with are **bilateral nonlocalizing sixth nerve palsy** and **papilledema.**

The diagnosis is best confirmed by cerebral angiography and CT.

Lateral sinus thrombosis

Thrombosis of lateral sinus is more **frequently septic** due to spread of infection from **mastoid** and **middle ear**. The thrombus may extend to the cavernous sinus causing signs and symptoms of **cavernous sinus thrombosis**. It is a frequent cause of **brain abscess**. Extension of infection in inferior petrosal sinus causes ipsilateral isolated sixth nerve palsy.

Inferior petrosal sinus thrombosis

Inferior petrosal sinus thrombosis is a common cause of **Gradenigo's syndrome**, causing unilateral sixth nerve palsy, facial pain and weakness on the same side due to extension of infection into the petrous bone. The commonest cause is **otitis media**.

Hemorrhagic disorders of neuro-ophthalmic interest

The hemorrhagic lesions responsible for neuro-ophthalmic features are all intracranial.

They can be:

1. Intracerebral (parenchymatous)
2. Extracerebral
   - i. Subdural
   - ii. Subarachnoid
   - iii. Intraventricular

The causes of hemorrhages can be:

1. **Microangiopathy**
   - i. Hypertensive
   - ii. Diabetes
2. **Rupture of**
   - i. Aneurysms
   - ii. Venous/dural sinus
   - iii. Congenital malformation
3. **Trauma**
4. **Bleeding due to**
   - i. Blood dyscrasia
   - ii. Malignancy
   - iii. Anticoagulant therapy

        d. Ophthalmoplegic
        e. Retinal
        f. Familial hemiplegic
        g. Acephalic
        h. With prolonged aura
        i. With acute aura
    ii. Without aura
        – Common migraine

2. **Nonmigraineous**
    i. Vascular
        a. Intracranial aneurysm
        b. Angioma
        c. AV malformation
        d. Hypertension
        e. Diabetes
        f. Febrile
        g. Subarachnoid hemorrhage
        h. Subdural hematoma
    ii. Head injury
        a. Localized intracranial/extracranial
        b. Intracranial stretching of blood vessels or nerve
        c. Raised intracranial tension.
        d. Post concussion
    iii. Nontraumatic raised intracranial tension.
    iv. Infection
        a. Meningitis
        b. Encephalitis
        c. Venous sinus thrombosis
        d. Orbital infection
        e. Ocular infection
        f. Otitis
        g. Infections of mouth, teeth, and nasal mucosa.
    v. Inflamation
        a. Temporal arteritis
        b. Tolosa Hunt syndrome
        c. Cranial neuritis
    vi. Intracranial space occupying lesions.
    vii. Referred
    viii. Cranial bone deformity
    ix. Systemic infection
    x. Drugs
    xi. Psychogenic

xii. Malingering
xiii. Ocular headache

Some of the causes of headache cause acute pain of short duration. Others causes chronic headache of longer duration.

Causes of acute headache are:

1. **Infection**
   i. Local – Periostitis, osteomyelitis, acute sinusitis, acute iridocyclitis, acute glaucoma, orbital cellulites
   ii. Systemic – Acute infection with fever
   – Meningitis, encephalitis
   – Secondary and tertiary syphilis
2. **Head injury**
3. **Vascular** – Subarachnoid hemorrhage
   – Cerebral hemorrhage
   – Cerebral thrombosis.
   – Hypertension
   – Diabetes
4. **Spinal** – Trauma to cervical spine
   – Lumbar puncture
   – Spinal anesthesia.
   – Myelography
5. **Drugs** – Vasodilators.
6. **Toxins** – Alcohol, carbon monoxide, quinine, lead
7. **Miscellaneous** – Uremia
   – Sunstroke

Cause of chronic headache are:

1. **Infection** – Meningovascular syphilis.
   – Chronic intracranial granuloma
   – Intracranial parasitic cysts
   – Herpes zoster ophthalmicus
2. **Trauma** – Post head injury headache
   – Post lumbar puncture
   – Spinal anesthesia
   – Myelography
3. **Intracranial space occupying tension**
   – Intracranial tumors
   – Intracranial cysts
4. **Benign intracranial hypertension**

5. **Inflammation** – Cervical spondylitis
   – Temporal arteritis
   – Trigeminal neuralgia
   – Sphenopalatine neuralgia
   – Occipital neuralgia
6. Ocular – Errors of refraction
   – Muscle imbalance
7. Coronary dilators, oral contraceptives, vitamin A are some of the commonly used drugs that cause chronic headache.
8. Others - Hypertension, hypotension, diabetes, chronic sinusitis, food and drug allergy, alcohol withdrawal.
9. Migraines

Diagnosis

Headache is not a disease it is a symptom complex. What is required in a case of headache is to find out its cause on which depends its management.

1. **History**—A detailed history helps in differentiating between migraine and other headaches. Some of the rules generally followed are:
   i. Aura—Points towards migraine.
   ii. Acute severe persistent headache with neck rigidity and fever means meningitis.
   iii. The above findings without fever is most probably subarachnoid hemorrhage, both require lumbar puncture.
   iv. An acute persistent headache of few days with body ache and fever is due to systemic febrile infection.
   v. A headache of increasing frequency, duration and severity over months is most probably due to intracranial mass.
   vi. Projectile vomiting with diplopia, blurred vision should also arouse suspicion of intracranial space occupying lesion.
   vii. An elderly person with severe localized headache of few days or weeks is most probably a case of temporal arteritis. Presence of thickened tender temporal artery is highly suggestive. Raised ESR in such cases is almost diagnostic which is confirmed by biopsy.
   viii. A frontal dull ache after prolonged near work is most probably of ocular origin.
   ix. Time of headache may give some clues regarding etiology of headache.

Time of headache	*Probable cause*
Morning	Hypertension, migraine, sinusitis, cervical spondylitis, space occupying lesion
Evening	Ocular headache
Night	Space occupying lesion, meningitis, cluster headache, migraine

2. Investigations:
   i. Recording of blood pressure—Diastolic pressure more than 110 mm is most of the time associated with morning headache that lessens as day passes.
   ii. Exclude diabetes.
   iii. Raised ESR is suggestive of temporal arteritis
   iv. X-ray skull used to be most frequently ordered investigation before advent of CT, MRI and Doppler have mostly replaced X-ray skull. X-ray has limited role only in fracture skull, congenital anomalies of skull and raised intracranial pressure.
   v. CT is a more precise method of evaluating intra cranial structures in congenital anomalies, infection, neoplasm, parasitic cysts, and vascular malformations.
   vi. MRI is more accurate than CT especially lesions of posterior fossa, para pituitary area, pituitary fossa and temporal lobe. It delineates many lesions not visible on CT, i.e. vascular pattern, white matter changes, neoplasm and congenital anomalies.

Ocular headache

Ocular examination is the most often ordered investigation for most of causes of headache, without realizing that ocular disorders are relatively infrequent causes of headache.

The causes of ocular headaches are divided into two broad groups:
1. Headache with congested eyes (Red eyes)
2. Headache without congested eyes (White eye)

Headaches with congested eyes are generally:
i. Acute or acute on chronic in nature.
ii. Unilateral
iii. The pain radiates on the distribution of ipsilateral trigeminal nerve.
iv. Commonly seen in — Inflammation
— Trauma
— Acute glaucoma

Inflammatory cause of ocular headaches are:
Uvea
Uveitis:
- Acute and chronic anterior uveitis and endophthalmic.
- The pain is worse at night.
- Posterior uveitis, retinitis and vasculitis do not cause pain.

Cornea: Foreign bodies, keratitis, corneal ulcer.
Sclera: Scleritis, episcleritis.
Orbit: Orbital cellulites, cavernous sinus thrombosis, panophthalmitis
Vascular: Ocular hypoxia.

Headaches without congested eyes

The headache is mild and dull in natures, worse in the evening or after prolonged near work. It never causes neurological deficits though may be associated with transient diplopia. The pain is localized in forehead, temple, orbit or periorbital area. It may be bilateral. Ocular headache is generally associated with asthenopia.

The common causes are:

1. **Errors of retraction:**
   i. Uncorrected hypermetropia
   ii. Astigmatism
   iii. Over corrected myopia
   iv. Uncorrected presbyopia
   v. Wrong alignment of axis of astigmatism
2. **Muscle in balance:** Vertical and torsional phorias and tropias cause more headache than horizontal deviation.
3. **Muscle palsy:** Trochlear palsy causes more headache than other palsies.
4. **Convergence insufficiency**
5. There may be a **combination** of error of retraction and muscle imbalance.

Most of the above factors cause sustained contraction of extraocular muscles, frontal muscles, neck and occipital muscles. **Uncorrected myopia rarely causes headache. Uncorrected astigmatism is the main cause of headache. Faulty angle of axis** causes more discomfort than uncorrected astigmatism.

Though eyestrain is not a frequent cause of headache, all cases with headache should be:

1. Refracted under suitable cycloplegic especially in children.
2. Undergo orthoptic work up.
3. Fundus should be examined for:
   i. Papilledema
   ii. Hypertension
4. Migraine should be excluded.

Migraine

Migraine is a **common, nonfatal, non-blinding** disease for which ophthalmic consultation is sought. Though ophthalmic disorders are infrequent cause of headache and are rarely known to trigger migraine yet ophthalmic check up is the first investigation ordered by physicians and pediatricians.

> Migraine is better managed by physician than ophthalmologist

About **15% of population** suffers from some type of migraine some times in life. They are more common in developed countries than in non-developed, may be sufferers in nondeveloped countries do not seek medical help as frequently as in developed countries. **High strung intellectuals are more prone** to develop migraine.

There is striking difference in sex. **Females out number males in 2:1 ratio**. Migraine is disease of **children and young adults.** It is not seen after fourth decade. It is rare for an individual to develop first episode of migraine after thirty years of age. After thirty the frequency of attacks as well severity gradually diminish.

Most of the adults have their first attack in childhood. The disease has **strong hereditary tendency**. Most of the patients have **positive family history.** An offspring of a migraineous mother is more predisposed to develop migraine than migraineous father. It is not uncommon to find **many members** of the same family to suffer from migraine.

The four Ps of migraine
Migraines is a protean, periodic disorders, that is **poly symptomatic** and appears in **paroxysms**.

Predisposing factors

Besides family history there are some factors that predispose migraine-

1. Migraine is common in premenstrual period and may pass off after the periods.
2. Migraine does not occur during pregnancy.
3. Oral contraceptives increase intensity of migraine.
4. Some foods like chocolate, cheese, red wine, nuts, citrus fruits, tea, coffee monosodium glutamate (Ajinomoto).

   Many other foods are known to trigger migraine. Alcohol and tobacco too have been blamed to cause migraine. Hunger may also initiate an episode of migraine. Role of allergens have not been evaluated fully. The migraineous attack may be precipitated by bright light, loud sound or unpleasant smell.
5. Drugs: Nitrates, nitroglycerine, reserpine, cemitidine, antihypertensive, estrogen, and surprisingly some analgesics like indomethacin are known to cause migraine.

Pathogeneses of migraine

The pathogenesis is **ill understood**, though it has been studied extensively. The most widely accepted theory is that it is a **microvascular phenomenon** associated and triggered by chemical mediators. Migraine is most probably caused by **vasodilatation** of cerebral blood vessels. Dural blood vessels are most commonly involved. Vasodilatation in migraine is preceded by **vasoconstriction**. This causes **aura**. The vascular changes activate the **trigeminovascular complex**. There is release of vasoactive neuropeptides from perivascular trigeminal axons. There is growing evidence that **5-hydroxytriptamine** is the cause of the vascular changes. The 5-HT starts the vasoconstriction. It also initiates release of prostaglandin and bradykinin that cause vasodilatation and headache.

Classification of migraine

A disorder with so many variables is difficult to classify. The most widely used division is to put migraine in two broad groups i.e.

1. Neurological
2. Non-neurological

The former is now referred to as **migraine with aura** and latter as **migraine without aura** or **common migraine** (Flow chart 15.2).

Aura too has been categorized as **simple, acute aura** and **prolonged aura**. Aura is mostly **visual**; it is less **frequently motor**. There may be other sensations also associated with aura.

Migraine with aura is again divided into two broad classes i.e. classic (classical) migraine and complicated migraine. There is a paradoxical situation were there is migraine, aura but no headache. Headache is replaced by other neurological symptoms. This is called **acephalgic migraine**.

Common migraine

The migraine **without aura** is **the commonest form** of migraine. The malady most often starts in **childhood**. There is **positive family history**, in about 75% of cases.

The common migraine has following features

1. **Prodromes:** Though there are **no auras**, common migraine is generally preceded by prodromes which may occur hours before the on set of headache. This may be depression, gastrointestinal disturbance. This leads to cerebral ischemia which triggers chemical changes.

Flow chart 15.2: Classification of migraine

- Migraine
  - Migraine without aura
    - Common migraine
  - Migraine with aura
    - Classic migraine
      - Acute aura
      - Prolonged aura
    - Complicated migraine
      - Ophthalmoplegic migraine.
      - Retinal migraine
      - Basilar migraine
      - A cephalic migraine
      - Cluster headache.
      - Familial hemiplegic migraine
      - Sporadic hemiplegia migraine
      - Abdominal migraine
      - Posthypoglycemic migraine

2. **Headache:** This is the **primary symptom**, which is **unilateral**. The pain may shift to the other half of the head or may involve whole of the head later. The pain is r**ecurrent**, severe and may be **throbbing**. The duration of headache is variable. It may subside within few hours or may persist for days. The precipitating factors are bright light (photophobia), loud sound (phonophobia), motion sickness, foods and drugs, too much of sleep and surprisingly beginning of holiday.
3. **Autonomic disturbance:** The commonest symptom is **nausea**. This may be followed by **vomiting**. Vomiting generally occurs during peak of headache. Vomiting generally gives some relief to the headache.
   I. At least five attacks.
   II. At least **two** of the following:
      i. Unilateral
      ii. Moderate to severe
      iii. Throbbing
      iv. Worsened by movement.
   III. At least **one** of the following:
      i. Nausea
      ii. Photophobia
      iii. Phonophobia.
4. **Ocular manifestation:** There may be redness of the eyes with or without watering, foreign body sensation, photophobia, puffiness of periorbital tissue.
5. **Relation to classic migraine:** Some of the case of common migraine may pass into classic migraine later.

To be designated as migraine, the headache should have:

Classic migraine

This type of migraine is **less common** than common migraine. **Only one fifth** of all migraines come under this category. This has some similarities with common migraine i.e. age, sex, family history, predisposing factors and prdrome. In fact some of the cases of classic migraine may initially present as common migraine.

Presence of **aura** and **neurological features** differentiates classic migraine from common migraine. It has strong family history than common migraine.

The syndrome consists of:

1. Prodrome
2. Aura
3. Headache
4. Resolution phase
5. Recovery period.

The **aura** is most striking and constant feature. **The aura is mostly visual**, which often brings the patient to the ophthalmologist. The aura may be motor or sensory.

The visual aura is the main feature of migraine. Its presence is almost diagnostic. The visual aura generally **precedes** the headache. In some patients, it may sometimes **accompany** the headache. The aura is **generally unilateral**. It starts at a point slightly eccentric to the point of fixation as a grey area with diffuse borders. The grey area than expands slowly towards the periphery. There may be wave like lines radiating from the grey spot and the figure shows **scintillation** and fortification. Sometimes **flashes of light** (photopsia) may accompany. There may be **metamorphopsia**, stationary objects seen to be moving. The auras are not fully ocular in origin. **They are central phenomenon**, hence have been reported in blind eyes also. Patient may have **polyopia** as well as **diplopia** without motor palsy. Other visual presentations are **obscuration, homonymous hemianopia**, and **altitudinal field loss**, even **uniocular loss of vision**. Extraocular motor components are aphasia, agraphia and hemiplegia.

Other sensory phenomenon are vertigo, paresthesis, hyposthesia and analgesia.

Headache

Headache is never the sole symptom of migraine.

There may be migraine without headache. It is caused due to vasodilatation. The headache is intense, unilateral and is preceded by aura. There may be tenderness over few points on the scalp. Headache may be intense enough to cause loss of sleep. The patient may wake up from sleep due to pain. The headache may put the person off from usual domestic or professional job.

The headache has been divided into follows phases:

1. **Prodromal phase**—This is seen only in few patients. It generally sets in about a day before the aura or headache. The symptoms are mostly **changes in mood** that may result in either **euphoria** or **depression**. There may be increased hunger or thirst. Drowsiness is common.
2. **The second phase** consists of neurological symptoms of aura and sensory changes.
3. **The headache phase** is due to vascular dilation of mostly branches of **external carotids**. Other arteries involved are **middle meningeal**, **temporal** and **occipital**. The neurological symptoms gradually clear and the headache sets in, which is characteristically unilateral generally developing contralateral to neurological features. The headache generally last for 4-6 hours in severe case. It may last for twenty-four hours at a stretch. The headache when lasts more than six to eight hours becomes bilateral and may creep to the neck and shoulder. The headache generally subsides by vomiting or sleep. The headache is generally associated with redness of eyes, watering from the eyes, photophobia and phonophobia.
4. **Postheadache phase** consists of exhaustion, tenderness over the scalp. The patient may go to sleep.

Systemic complication of migraine

1. **Status migraineous**—This is a rare conditions. The term denotes a migraine headache that lasts for more than 72 hours. The headache need not be of same severity all through, there may be relief of pain for few hours in between. It is seen both in **common as well as classic migraine**.
2. **Migraineous infarction**—This is still rarely diagnosed it requires advanced neuro-imaging, seen in both types of migraine, i.e. with or without aura.
3. **Neurological defect**, which are paroxysmal and transient, may become permanent, which includes hemiplegia, homonymous field defect, speech disorders, alexia, amnesia, transient loss of color vision, inability to recognize familiar persons.

Ocular complications are

Ocular complications comprise of retinal artery occlusion, ischemic optic atrophy, mydriasis, Adies pupil, **retinal migraine** and **ophthalmoplegic migraine**. Persons with migraines are more prone to develop low tension glaucoma

Other types of migraine

Migraineous headache other than in common and classic migraine are generally referred to by various confusing terms. Some of them are: **Complicated migraine, migraine equivalent, migraine accompagnae, migraine associea**.

Ophthalmoplegic migraine is a definite clinical condition.
Term **ophthalmic migraine** is used to denote ocular symptoms of classic migraine.

Cerebral migraine

This is an ill defined condition dominated by neurological features that could be **motor** or **sensory** including **visual symptoms**. The condition is most probably an exaggerated form of classic migraine. The sensory symptoms last for 15-30 minutes that may precede or accompany headache that lasts for 6 to 12 hours. The visual symptoms are **scintillating scotomas, transient hemianopia, bilateral upper quadrantic field change, permanent hemianopia**.

Ophthalmoplegic migraine (Trigeminoophthalmoplegic syndrome)

This is a **rare** but well defined condition though it is listed under complicated migraine. Physicians differ in pronouncing the exact cause of it.

The characteristics of the condition are:

a. It starts before ten years of age.
b. There is no differences in sex ratio.
c. Most of the patients give history of migraineous headache without family history which is unilateral throbbing.
d. The intensity of headache increase gradually in crescendo.

e. The most striking feature of the disease is ophthalmoplegia which is generally ipsilateral to hemicrania but may alternate.
f. Timing of onset of ophthalmoplegia is variable.
g. The commonest onset is after the headache has subsided.
h. There is generally a gap of few days between cessation of headache and onset of ophthalmoplegia.
i. Rarely ophthalmoplegia may be simultaneous with headache. In very rare instance ophthalmoplegia may be followed by headache.

The commonest nerve to be involved is **oculomotor** followed by **sixth**. Involvement of third nerve is ten times more frequent than sixth nerve. The fourth nerve involvement is still less. Seventh nerve involvement is least. The third nerve may be involved **totally** or **partially**. **Iridoplegia** and **cycloplegia** are constant features. **The ophthalmoplegia is self limiting.** The recovery may take days to weeks. Repeated attacks are common. Recovery from ophthalmoplegia is prolonged following repeated attacks.

Differential diagnosis should consist of all the causes of fluctuating unilateral ophthalmoplegia in children and young adults.

They include—Myasthenia gravis, sphenoidal mucocele, Tolosa Hunt syndrome, intracranial tumors, and congenital intracranial vascular malformation. In adults possibility of diabetes and intracranial aneurysm should be excluded.

The exact cause is not known. Most accepted theory is **swelling of some of the intracranial vessels**, **pituitary**, or the **intracranial nerve trunks**. However, the above factors have not been proved on angiograms, MRI may show swelling of the oculomotor nerve.

Retinal migraine (Anterior visual pathway migraine)

Retinal migraine is a migraine **with visual aura** seen in **young adults**. There is a positive history of migraineous headache. The retinal migraine manifests as **unilateral**, temporary or permanent **loss of vision** with or without headache. The episode is generally preceded by **aura**. When visual loss is temporary the state of diminished vision does not last more than one hour. It may be as short as ten minutes only to be followed by subsequent attacks. The interval between two attacks is variable so are the number of attacks. The permanent loss of vision may be total loss or may be a localized scotoma. The exact cause of the disease is not known. Most commonly accepted theory is that it is caused due to spread of migraineous vascular changes in retinal vascular system.

The differential diagnosis should consist of **retinal artery spasm, amaurosis fugax, non arteritic anterior ischemic neuropathy** in elder patients, central retinal artery embolism, **papillitis, central serous retinopathy.** None of the conditions mentioned above have history of aura and are rarely associated with migraineous headache. Absence ophthalmoplegia distinguishes it from ophthalmoplegic migraine while basilar migraine is a bilateral condition.

Basilar migraine (Bicker staff migraine, basilar artery migraine, posterior fossa migraine)

This is a **rare** form of migraine with **aura**, seen in **children**, has **good prognosis**. **Complete recovery is common**. There is a history migraine in the family. Girls are affected more than boys. There is definite aura and migraineous headache followed by **transient neurological changes** which are similar to **vertebrobasilar insufficiency** in elderly. The lesions are caused due to insufficiency of blood supply by basilar artery, its branches and posterior cerebral arteries leading to brainstem, cerebellar and occipital lobe dysfunction. Involvement of brainstem, reticular formation is the cause of impaired consciousness. The occipital lobe involvement is bilateral. This results in bilateral field loss. Diplopia when present is due to brainstem involvement. Dysarthria and ataxia are of cerebellar origin. Due to brainstem involvement multiple cranial nerves may be involved. There may be epileptic fits, vertigo and tinitus.

The headache is brief. The symptoms last for two minutes to about forty minutes. The condition has benign prognosis. The child may pass into classic migraine following recovery of basilar migraine.

Cluster headache (Horton's syndrome, histamine headache)

Due to its onset at night in paroxysm, this is also called **paroxysmal nocturnal cephalgia** as well.

It is seen mostly in men, the ratio between **men and women is 5:1**. The **attack awakes** the patient during the rapid eye movement or two to three hours after falling asleep. The pain is so intense that the patient paces in the room. The pain is **unilateral**, localized in the orbit or paraocular structure. It has pronounced ocular manifestation that can be divided into two groups:

1. Those similar to histamine reaction i.e. ipsilateral edema of the conjunctiva, conjunctival congestion, lacrimation, para orbital edema, nasal congestion, flushing of face.
2. Those due to involvement of oculo sympathetic system leading to pictures of ipsilateral transient Horner's syndrome, i.e. ptosis, miosis. Rarely there may be involvement of other cranial nerves.

The pain comes in bunches (clusters) and last one to two hours. The pain tends to recur almost every night for several weeks to months. The patient goes to bed with fear of being awakened by attack.

The pain subsides as dramatically as it has started leaving no trace of the disease.

There may be variable pain free period lasting for months to years. There are some unconfirmed predisposing factors, commonest among them is past history of ipsilateral trauma. Others are alcohol, nitroglycerine and tyramine.

The exact mechanism of the disease is not known. It is thought to be periodic narrowing of extradural part of internal carotid on the same side.

Acephalgic migraine

Acephalgic migraine is difficult to diagnose because there is only aura without headache. There is generally positive family history of migraine.

Pediatric migraine

There is a widespread misconception that migraine does not occur in childhood. The fact is far from this, most of the migraines develop in childhood or adolescence except for cluster headache. **Ophthalmoplegic migraine** and **retinal migraine** are very common in childhood. **Basilar migraine** starts in adolescent girls. History of head injury is generally present in sizable patients.

The migraineous attacks are more frequent than expected, **associated abdominal discomfort** is common. The child may occasionally be labelled wrongly as functional.

The visual symptoms are common. They include transient loss of vision that may be unilateral or binocular with various types of field defect, macropsia and metamorphopsia. There may be visual hallucination. Management of childhood migraine is same as in adults, it requires co-operation of parents, teachers and the patient.

Diagnosis of migraine

Diagnosis of a case of migraine that has both **aura** and **headache** is not difficult. Difficulty arises when aura is absent, i.e. **common migraine** or there is aura without headache i.e. **acephalgic migraine**. The former should be differentiated from other causes of headache i.e. **intracranial aneurysms, subdural hematoma, subarachnoid hemorrhage, meningitis, encephalitis, space occupying lesions, benign intracranial hypertension, temporal arteritis, purulent sinusitis.**

The acephalgic migraines are less common, may be mistakes as gastrointestinal disturbance, premenstrual disturbance, hypoglycemia, diabetes or even functional.

Migraine, is mostly diagnosed by typical history. Presence of neurological signs and symptoms require evaluation of each case by complete neurological evaluation, CT, MRI, X-ray skull, paranasal sinuses and fundus examination.

Management

Management of migraine is difficult and frustrating. All the drugs used are mostly symptomatic in nature. The drugs relieve the symptoms, may prevent attack but do not cure migraine. All patients do not require treatment.

Many of the patients are able to continue with migraine without treatment.

The treatment of migraine is broadly divided into:

1. Prevention
2. Management of attack
3. Reduction in frequency and severity

The best treatment of migraine is to prevent the attack. It is easy said than done. Prevention can be divided into **two groups**:

1. Nontherapeutic methods
2. Therapeutic methods.

Nontherapeutic methods consist of:

1. Avoiding provocative factors like food, beverage, allergen, offending sound, bright light, fasting, etc.
2. Stress management training.
3. Adjusting chrono-biological relationship.

The therapeutic methods consist of administering many drugs of diverse action for 3 to 6 months after the last attack.

They are:

1. Calcium channel blockers.
2. $5HT_2$ receptor antagonist.
3. Beta adrenergic receptor antagonist
4. Tricyclic antidepressant.

Management of acute attack consists:

1. Analgesic
2. Antiemetics
3. 5HT receptor agonist
4. Ergotamine.

The drugs may have to be in combination.

Migraine is better managed by an internist or a neurophysician.

BIBLIOGRAPHY

1. Adams RD. Headache in principles of internal medicine. 9th edn, Isselbacher KJ, Adams RD, Braunwald E, Petersdrof RG Wilson JD. McGraw-Hill, Kogakusha Tokyo 1980;18-27.
2. AMA Adhoc committee on classification of headache 1962;179:717.
3. Bhattacharya SK, Sen P, Ray A. Drugs in migraine in pharmacology second. Elsevier, New Delhi, 2003.
4. Campbell JK. Diagnosis and treatment of cluster headache. Jr Pain Symp, Manage 1993;8: 155-64.
5. Duke Elders. Ophthalmoplegic migraine in system of ophthalmology. Vol XII, Duke Elders and Scott GI (Eds). Henry Kimpton, London 1971;782-85.
6. Duke Elders, Scott GI. Migraine in system of ophthalmology. Vol XII, Henry Kimpton, London 1971;550-88.
7. Ekbom K, Olivarius B. Chronic migranious neuralgia diagnostic and therapeutic aspect Headache, 97-101.
8. Foster RW. Migraine in basic pharmacology. 4th edn, Arnold London 500-502.

9. Gami NK. Investigation of a case of headache in bedside approach to clinical neurology. 1st edn. Current books international, Kolkata 1983;160-64.
10. Hupp SL. Migraine in Walsh and Hoyts clinical neuro-ophthalmology. Vol 3, 5th edn. Miller NR, New man NJ (Eds). William and Wilkins. Baltimore 1998;36570-3723.
11. Nagppan N. Headache: A clinical approach in neuro-ophthalmology. Natchiar G (Eds). Arvind Eyc Hospital Maduri, 1501-15.
12. O'connor PS. Headache in neuro-ophthalmology, 5th edn. Kline L and Bajandas FJ (Eds). Jaypee Brothers Medical Publishers, New Delhi 2004;195-99.
13. Olesen J. Headache classification committee of internal headache society 1988;8:1-96.
14. Rang NP, Dala MM, Ritter 3 M, Moore PK. Migraine and antimigraine drugs in pharmacology, 5th edn. Chruchill-livingtone, New York 2003;190-93.
15. Raskin HS. Headache second edition. Churchill Livingstone New York 1988.
16. Rothner AD. Headache in pediatric neurology. Vol 1, 2nd edn. Swaiman KF (Ed). Mosby, St Louis 1994;219-26.
17. Samba Sivam M. Migraine in Neuro-ophthalmology. Natchiar G (Ed). Arvind Eye hospital, Maduri, 16.01-16.08.
18. Stewart WF, Shecter A, Rasmussen BK. Migraine prevalence: A review of population based studies. Neurology 1994;44:17-23.
19. Troost BT. Migraine in neuro-ophthalmology. 5th edn. Glaser JS (Ed). Harper and Row. London 1978;297-315.
20. Walsh JD, O'Doherty DS. A possible explanation of the mechanism of ophthalmoplegic migraine. Neurology 10:1079-1960.
21. Zwaan J. Headache in decision-making to ophthalmology. 2nd edn, van Heuven, Zwaan J (Eds). Mosby, St Louis 2000;28-29.

16 Nystagmus

Nystagmus is not a disease, it is manifestation of diseases involving either the eyes or extraocular neural structures with predominant ocular signs. **It is a clinical neuro-ophthalmic puzzle with about forty classifications**, none of which is very accurate.

Nystagmus is a disturbance of ocular posture.

Nystagmus is defined as repetitive, rhythmic oscillation of one or both eyes in any or all fields of gaze.

Exact mode of development of nystagmus is not well understood. During steady fixation the eyes are motionless, without any to and fro movement, that is brought about by **afferent path**, **efferent path** and **intra cerebral components**. Defect in any of them results in involuntary movements of the eyes, i.e. nystagmus. Ninety percent of nystagmus are brought about by afferent defect. Rests are efferent in nature.

The afferent nystagmus are due to defective vision. Defective vision in early infancy is more likely to cause nystagmus. The common conditions associated with nystagmus are—**Congenital cataract, albinism, aniridia, hypoplasia of optic nerve, achromatopsia,** and **optic atrophy**.

The efferent nystagmus are due to ocular motor disturbance

Nystagmus can be congenital or acquired.

Congenital nystagmus is always pathological.

Nystagmus is described clinically under following heads:

1. Morphology
2. Plane
3. Amplitude
4. Frequency
5. Degree

1. Morphology
   i. **Pendular nystagmus**—It has oscillation of **equal speed** and **amplitude** on each direction like a pendulum of a wall clock generally in primary position. They can be **horizontal, vertical** or **rotatory**. The **horizontal pendular nystagmus** is the **commonest type** of all nystagmus. The most probable etiology is sensory deprivation caused due to diminished central vision

The physiological nystagmus

They are to be elicited to be demonstrable. They last only during the presence of stimuli and do not have any neurological component. Some of then are diagnostic.

The physiological nystagmus are:

1. Optokinetic nystagmus and rail road nystagmus
2. End point nystagmus
3. Evoked vestibular nystagmus
4. Voluntary nystagmus

1. **Optokinetic (Opticokinetic) nystagmus**
   This is artificially produced jerk nystagmus that is elicited when the **eyes look at moving repetitive stimuli** through the visual field. Being a jerk nystagmus it has a slow and a fast phase. The first is **pursuit movement** while the second is **saccadic movements** in the opposite direction. The movements are controlled by **parieto-occipital path**.
   The example of this is **railroad nystagmus** or **train nystagmus** when a person sitting in a running train looks at successive passing scenario. The person picks up a part of floating scenario and follows it involuntary till it disappears from the field of gaze and then gives up to fix next object of interest. The fixing movement is towards the direction of the train. **The person is not aware of nystagmus.** A person sitting opposite him can observe the nystagmus. The nystagmus slows down with slowing of the train and disappear when the train stops.
   The same can be produced in office by rotating opto kinetic drum in front of the eye. The test is used to see if:
   i. If the person has vision or not
   ii. To diagnose:
      a. Defect in opticomesencephalic and fronto mesencephalic pathway.
      b. Malingering.

To produce horizontal nystagmus the drum is kept vertical. A horizontally placed drum when rotated produces vertical nystagmus.

The opto kinetic nystagmus is abnormal when it is asymmetric.

2. **End point nystagmus**—This is an **ill sustained** jerk nystagmus developing in normal persons in extreme horizontal gaze, more marked in abduction, it does not develop in down gaze. It is very faint in up gaze. The nystagmus consists of ten to fifteen beats on the side of the gaze. It has no localizing value.
3. **Evoked vestibular**—This is also a **jerk nystagmus** that can be produced by
   i. Displacement of endo lymph in semicircular canal.
   ii. Accelerations and de-acceleration of the body.

4. **Voluntary nystagmus**— Some people can produce **pendular nystagmus** at will for a brief period mostly during convergence. Children learn to produce voluntary nystagmus sooner than adults. The ability may be seen in many members of the same family.

Caloric test for vestibular nystagmus

If the labyrinth is stimulated in a normal person, the person develops nystagmus and vertigo. For diagnostic purpose the labyrinth stimulus is brought about by **cold** or **warm water** applied to the **tympanic membrane**. When cold water is applied to the right ear a nystagmus develops in the left side and when warm water is applied in the right ear, a right-sided nystagmus develops. This is remembered by mnemonic **COWS** where **C** stands for cold, **O** for opposite **W** for warm and **S** for same.

Rotational test for vestibular nystagmus

Rotation, acceleration of head movement causes a movement of the endolymph in the semicircular canal resulting in jerk nystagmus when the head is rotated the eye deviates in the direction of movement. The quick phase of nystagmus is towards the opposite side.

Latency in nystagmus

Nystagmus is said to:

1. **Manifest**—It is present with **both eyes open** and the frequency and amplitude does not increase when any of the eyes is covered. It is **bilateral**, **mostly horizontal**, may be **pendular or jerk nystagmus**. Sometimes there may be a combination of the two. The nystagmus disappears **during sleep** and is **reduced on convergence**. This is to generally **associated with abnormal head posture to keep the eyes in null zone.**
2. **Latent nystagmus**— This is a **congenital nystagmus**. It is generally **jerk nystagmus** and **bilateral**, may be pendular or torsional. **There is no nystagmus when both eyes are uncovered and straight.** As soon as any of the eyes is covered both the eyes develop jerk nystagmus towards the uncovered eye. The vision in the uncovered eye diminishes due to nystagmus but improves when both eyes are uncovered. The condition is mostly seen in **congenital esotropia**, less commonly in **hypertropia**. It is frequently associated with **dissociated vertical deviation**.
3. **Manifest latent nystagmus**— This is a manifest nystagmus that behaves like latent nystagmus when one eye is covered. If the dominant eye is covered, the manifest nystagmus becomes more severe.
4. **Nystagmus blockage syndrome**— This is seen in children with **infantile esotropia**. It is either **manifest nystagmus** or **manifest latent nystagmus**. The nystagmus is reduced on adduction with improvement of vision. The nystagmus in primary gaze is horizontal. The child may cross fix. The child turns the eye

towards the direction of convergence. The nystagmus is revealed when the esotropia has been corrected surgically.

Spasmus nutans

*This is a **transient syndrome** consisting triad of **nystagmus, head, nodding** and **torticolis** seen in **children**. The exact cause is not known. It is a **benign** condition, does not denote any specific disease. It generally **develops in first 18 month, lasts for a few years and passes off without any untoward affect**. The nystagmus is fine, horizontal, pendular and rapid. The nystagmus varies in different gazes. The nystagmus is asymmetric.*

*The **head nodding** is irregular and nonuniform, may be horizontal or vertical. The **torticolis** begins with nystagmus and disappears with it. The condition does not require any treatment. However, sometimes it may be associated with anterior visual pathway lesions that requires MRI to diagnose and needs specific treatment.*

PATHOLOGICAL NYSTAGMUS

Congenital nystagmus

All the types of nystagmus termed congenital nystagmus are **not really present at birth**, only a few may be present at birth, rest develop in **infancy** or **childhood** before development of visual fixation. It is more appropriate to call them as **infantile nystagmus**. Like all nystagmus they too have been classified variously.

The best classification is to divide them in

1. **Afferent nystagmus**
2. **Efferent nystagmus.**

The former is also called **congenital sensory nystagmus** and the latter is called **congenital motor nystagmus**.

Afferent congenital nystagmus accounts for 90% of all cases of congenital nystagmus. The condition is seen in cases of **bilateral, central, visual deprivation** developing in infancy, i.e. before 2 months of age. There is a long list of condition that cause afferent congenital nystagmus. The disorders may be congenital in origin or acquired in infancy. Most of them are **ocular**, a few may be in the anterior visual path.

The common conditions are— Hypoplasia of macula, albinism, aniridia, macular scar due to congenital toxoplasmosis, congenital cataract, congenital or infantile corneal opacity, congenital glaucoma, Lebers congenital amaurosis, retinopathy of prematurety, hypoplasia of optic nerve.

The efferent congenital nystagmus is more commonly referred to as congenital motor nystagmus or idiopathic infantile nystagmus.

Characteristics of congenital nystagmus are:

1. Have varied hereditary trait, may be sporadic, autosomal dominant or autosomal recessive.
2. May be present at birth or before two months of age.

3. The nystagmus is mostly **horizontal** and pendular, rarely may be jerk. The morphology can be vertical or circular. The nystagmus is **binocular, conjugate**. **Amplitude** is same in both eyes. The **plane** does not change with change of gaze. It is abolished during **sleep**. The nystagmus is **less in convergence**. It increases with fixation effort.
4. The nystagmus is frequently associated with head oscillation but **Oscillopsia is absent**. Latent nystagmus may be superimposed.
5. Children have poor distant vision but unexpectedly well near vision.
6. High error of refraction is common. **Astigmatism** is commonest error of retraction.
7. May be associated with squint.
8. In rare instances the nystagmus may be associated with neurological defects.

Congenital idiopathic nystagmus

This is a **hereditary disorder**. The nystagmus is mostly **latent**, **horizontal**, **pendular** and **coarse**. There may be **compensatory head posture** to dampen the nystagmus. The nystagmus may be so fine as to require magnification to be appreciated; a direct ophthalmoscope serves the purpose. It is always associated with **diminished central vision** with good near vision. The diminished vision is thought to be result of nystagmus and not the effect of nystagmus. The condition is **nonprogressive**, **lasting life long**. There are no other ocular or systemic diseases that can be corelated to it.

Management of congenital nystagmus consists of:

1. Improvement of vision by optical correction with contact lens.
2. Prisms to induce convergence.
3. Simultaneous recession of lateral rectus and injection of Botox in the muscles are also used to increase convergence.
4. Medical treatment consists of administration of Baclofen. This reduces the amplitude and frequency of nystagmus.

Acquired nystagmus

The list of acquired disorders that produce nystagmus is long. Some congenital anomalies may cause nystagmus later.

All acquired nystagmus are pathological

Broadly nystagmus can be divided into (Flow chart 16.1):

1. Those due to peripheral lesions.
2. Those due to central lesions.

Flow chart 16.1: Topographical classification of nystagmus

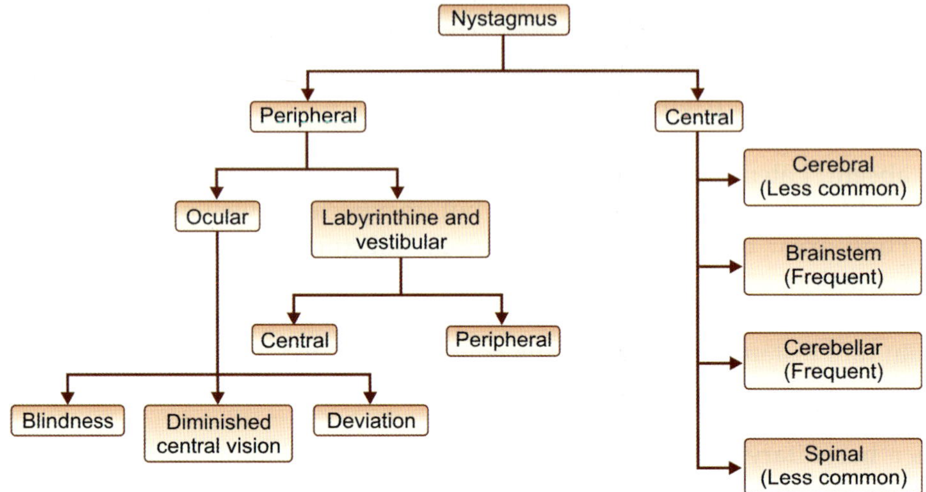

Difference between brainstem and cerebellar nystagmus

Brainstem	*Cerebellar*
1. Gaze nystagmus	Fixation nystagmus
2. Unidirectional	Multi directional
3. Horizontal	Horizontal
4. Vertical on up gaze	Up beat, down beat
5. Jerk, slow component towards the primary position, quick towards periphery.	Jerk, slow component towards the primary position, quick towards periphery.
Cause: Vascular, tumor, encephalitis, disseminated sclerosis, syrengio bulbia, vascular malformation.	Causes: Hereditary, ataxia, thrombosis of posterior cerebral artery, inferior cerebellar tumors

Acquired ocular nystagmus

1. **Nystagmus due to blindness** generally develops in persons who have been blind for some years, may be seen in newborn. It may either be present all the time or is precipitated when attention is required. It may be pendular or jerk nystagmus. The excursion is generally large and irregular. The rhythm may be variable and is bilateral.
2. **Nystagmus due to diminished central vision**— It is mostly seen when the central vision is developing, i.e. **in children of few months**. It is thought to be an attempt to overcome central scotoma. The nystagmus is pendular. It may be

lessened in primary position in later life. The eye when moved laterally may develop jerk nystagmus. The nystagmus may disappear on convergence. The common causes are **opacities developing in media** in infancy, or **hypoplasia of macula**. It is common is **albinism** and **achromatopsia**.

3. **Nystagmus in deviated eye**— Normally deviated eyes do not develop nystagmus unless the eyes are in extreme position of gaze. It is best observed in lateral gaze, such nystagmus is jerk nystagmus. It is seen more commonly **when a paralytic muscle is improving** in function or in early stages of partially developed paralysis of extraocular muscle. It is common following too much of tenotomy.

Acquired labyrinthine and vestibular nystagmus

The vestibular system consists of:

- Labyrinth
- The vestibular nucleus
- The vestibular nerve and its central connection.

In normal persons some degree of nystagmus develops when the labyrinth is stimulated with warm or cold water applied to the tympanic membrane. The direction of rapid phase of nystagmus thus created is remembered by the mnemonic COWS (cold opposite, warm same). The nystagmus is associated with **vertigo** and the eyes are involuntarily closed. There is a past pointing **without stretched arms**. **Romberg's sign** is present. The past pointing and **Romberg's fall** are on the side of slow phase.

The vestibular nystagmus results from disease of any part of the vestibular system. The causes may be **trauma, infection, inflammation, vascular or neoplasm**.

The nystagmus is jerk, generally horizontal, less commonly rotatory and sometimes vertical. It is fine and rapid. In mild nondestructive lesion the nystagmus is on the affected side, in destructive lesion the nystagmus develops on the opposite side. It is a subcortical phenomenon.

The labyrinthine nystagmus is divided into two broad groups each with characteristic features

1. Peripheral lesion
2. Central lesion

Characteristics of nystagmus caused by peripheral lesions:

1. The nystagmus is jerk nystagmus.
2. It is usually horizontal.
3. Most of the time it has a torsional part.
4. Nystagmus is accentuated when the gaze is directed towards the fast component.
5. It is uniplane.
6. It is self-limiting, resolves within days or weeks.
7. Noises may induce nystagmus.
8. Visual fixation reduces nystagmus and vertigo.
9. Direction of Romberg's fall is towards slow phase.

10. Tinitus and deafness are often present.
11. The common etiological factors are:
    i. Infection—Labyrinthitis, neuritis
    ii. Inflammation—Mieniere's disease
    iii. Toxic and drug induced
    iv. Vascular
    v. Trauma

Characteristics of nystagmus caused by central (nuclear) lesion:

1. It is a jerk nystagmus.
2. It is unidirectional.
3. Mostly vertical.
4. Pure horizontal or rotary nystagmus is less common.
5. Direction of nystagmus is variable, may change with convergence or change in direction of gaze.
6. Not influenced by removal of fixation.
7. Vertigo, tinitus and deafness are milder.
8. Romberg's direction of fall is not influenced by change in head position.
9. It is mostly chronic in nature.
10. Common etiological factors are:
    i. Demyelination
    ii. Tumor
    iii. Trauma
    iv. Vascular (stroke)
11. The lesions are generally bilateral.

Acquired central nystagmus (Brain)

Acquired nystagmus can result from lesions of various parts of brain and their connection, i.e. **cerebrum, cerebellum, brainstem** and some lesions of **spinal cord** even. **The central nystagmus are pathological.** Some of the physiological nystagmus, i.e. the optokinetic nystagmus and caloric nystagmus are used as diagnostic procedure in central nystagmus. There is overlap in clinical features of nystagmus of different origin.

Some of the common central nystagmus are generally dissociated and disconjugate nystagmus.

They are:

1. Upbeat nystagmus.
2. Down beat nystagmus.
3. See saw nystagmus.
4. Convergence retraction nystagmus.
5. Periodic alternate nystagmus.
6. Rebound nystagmus.
7. Gaze evoked nystagmus.
8. Gaze paretic nystagmus.

Upbeat nystagmus

This type of nystagmus is always present in **primary position**. It may be **congenital** or **acquired**. The latter is more common. There are **two types** of acquired variety, i.e. with **large amplitude** and with **small amplitude**. The fast phase is in primary position. Upbeat nystagmus is sometimes present in lateral gaze. This is a **jerk nystagmus**. The common causes are— **Multiple sclerosis**, hemorrhage in brain stem, encephalitis involving brain stem, posteriorfossa tumor, Wernicke's encephalopathy, cerebellar degeneration and drug induced. The pathological lesions are present either in brain stem or cerebellar vermis.

Downbeat nystagmus

Like upbeat nystagmus this is also present in **primary position**. It is a **jerk nystagmus**. The nystagmus does not follow the Alexander's law that states jerk nystagmus usually increases in amplitude with gaze in the direction of the fast phase. It is sometimes associated with **ocular dysmetria**, **rebound nystagmus** or **periodic alternating nystagmus**. It may be associated with vertical diplopia.

It is mostly due to **congenital malformation at the level of cranio cervical junction** in the brainstem in the form of **Arnold Chiari malformation**. Other conditions responsible are— Head injury, increased intracerebral pressure, hydrocephalus, Paget's disease, platybasia, hemorrhage in the brain stem, multiple sclerosis, cerebellar degeneration. **Many drugs** and deficiencies also cause the disorder. They are— Magnesium deficiency, B_{12} deficiency, Wernicke's encephalopathy, anticonvulsants, lithium toxicity.

The diagnosis of congenital malformation is confirmed by MRI, which may be helpful to plan surgical correction of the malformation.

See saw nystagmus

The disorder can either be **congenital** or **acquired**. The nystagmus is **pendular**, conjugate, disjunctive, vertical with torsional movement of both the eyes.

The condition is characterized by:

1. Elevation of one eye with depression of the contra lateral eye.
2. The rising eye intorts, the fellow eye extorts.
3. In congenital form the torsional movements are reversed.

The condition is commonly associated with **bitemporal hemianopia** and **diminished vision**.

The common causes are—Suprasellar growth, multiple sclerosis, Arnold Chiari malformation, trauma, mid brain hemorrhage.

Rare association are—Optic nerve hypoplasia, albinism and retinitis pigmentosa.

Convergence retraction nystagmus

It is a **rare** type of nystagmus. The nystagmus is **jerk**. It is associated with retraction of globe during convergence or an **attempted up gaze**. The retraction may be deep enough to be observed through closed lids as well. The convergence retraction nystagmus is best demonstrated by OKN target going downwards.

The common etiologies are—Congenital aqueduct stenosis, head injury, vascular malformation in brain stem, multiple sclerosis, basilar artery insufficiency. Some authors consider this as an ocular oscillation and not true nystagmus.

Periodic alternate nystagmus (PAN)

This is a **cyclic nystagmus** where the fast component changes direction in a regular cycle. It is a continuous process where the fast component reverses direction after every two minutes. The duration of the phenomenon may range from 1 minute to 6 minutes. The commonest duration being 4 minutes with a pause of few second between the change of direction. It can be **congenital** or **acquired**.

The nystagmus is **jerk** and remains horizontal even in **up gaze**. It may be associated with **head rotation**. Though it is designated as **central nystagmus**, it has been observed in severe bilateral visual loss due to optic atrophy, vitreous hemorrhage or even cataract. Correction of visual loss when possible abolishes nystagmus.

Other causes are— Anticonvulsants, Arnold Chiari malformation, multiple sclerosis, brain stem hemorrhage.

Rebound nystagmus

This **rare** from of jerk nystagmus is associated with **ataxia** and **cerebellar disorders**. It may be mistaken as PAN.

The nystagmus may be precipitated:

1. Following prolonged eccentric gaze with reversal of fast phase.
2. When the eye returns to primary position following prolonged eccentric gaze.

Gaze evoked nystagmus

This is said to be the **commonest** form of **acquired pathological nystagmus**. It is absent in primary position. It develops only during various gazes. It is presence does not have any localizing significance. It is a jerk nystagmus. It may be left or right beating.

It is commonly caused due to **drugs** and **toxins**. The common drugs that are associated with the disease are— Alcohol, tranquillisers and anticonvulsants. The next group consists of posterior fossa disorders that may be demyelination, infarction, injury, growth or cerebellopontine tumor. It has been reported in myasthenia gravis, dysthyroid oculopathy and cranial nerve palsy.

Gaze paretic nystagmus

This type of **jerk nystagmus** develops in **patients recovering from gaze palsy**. It has a slow frequency and large amplitude.

Ocular oscillations simulating nystagmus

There are some conditions that present as ocular oscillation without being nystagmus. They are involuntary, rapid to and fro, irregular without rhythm. Some of them may herald nystagmus and lesions of central nervous system. They may be subjective as in oscillopsia, i.e. that cannot be demonstrated clinically or objectively.

The common conditions are:

1. Oscillopsia
2. Opsoclonus
3. Ocular myoclonus (lightening eye movement)
4. Superior oblique myokymia
5. Ocular bobbing
6. Ocular flutter
7. Ocular dysmetria
8. Square wave jerks
9. Oculogyric crisis

1. Oscillopsia

This is an illusionary feeling of movement of environment usually due to **acquired nystagmus**. It could be **unilateral** or **bilateral**. It may be associated with other ocular oscillation like **opsoclonus**, **ocular flutter**, **myokymia**. Patient with intermittent exotropia may complain of oscillopsia. The condition is mostly seen in **internuclear ophthalmoplegia** due to involvement of **medial longitudinal fasciculus**. It may be horizontal or vertical. Vertical oscillopsia is seen in **superior oblique myokymia** and **downbeat nystagmus**. It can be caused by barbiturates as well.

2. Opsoclonus (Saccadomania, dancing eyes)

The movements are **saccades**. Other features of which are— Involuntary, chaotic, repetitive, conjugate in multiple direction, persist during sleep and coma. Patients recovering from opsoclonus may pass into ocular flutter. It may be seen in all ages. **The exact mechanism is not well understood.** Cerebellar dysfunction seems to be the common factor. The cause of cerebellar dysfunction differs at various age groups from viral infections to malignancies.

In infants, the most common causes is **neuroblastoma**. Other cause is **encephalitis** due to autoimmune reaction that responds to immunoglobulin and steroid. **In young adults** it is due to viral infection. In adults the common causes are metastatic neoplasm in brain stem from distant organs, vertebrobacillar insufficiency and multiple sclerosis.

3. Ocular myoclonus (lightening eye movement)

The condition though discussed under nystagmus is **not a true nystagmus** but has clinical similarity to nystagmus. The movements are bilateral, vertical, pendular in nature that persists in **sleep**. The rate of oscillation is 2 per second. The most characteristic features are **rhythmic movements** of some **nonocular muscles** as well. The frequently involved muscles are— soft palate, tongue, larynx, pharynx, facial muscles. The palate is most commonly involved. Involvement of diaphragm is also seen. Sometimes the extremities may show jerky movement especially in infants.

The condition is most probably due to bilateral pseudo hypertrophy of the inferior olivary nucleus in medulla. The condition lasts for the whole life. The GABA agonists are claimed to reduce the movement.

4. Superior oblique myokymia

This is observed as a benign condition sometimes in normal persons who complain of vertical oscillopsia and vertical torsional diplopia that causes blurring of images. The symptoms are aggravated if the person is asked to look in the direction of action of superior oblique. It is a **monocular feature**. The movements are so fine that they are appreciated only during ophthalmoscopy or slit lamp examination. The movements are **vertical** and **torsional**. They are **fast,** i.e. 15-20/seconds in proxyms.

It may follow **fourth nerve palsy** either due to trauma or neurological cause. It is also seen in **multiple sclerosis** and **cerebellar tumors**.

The condition is self limiting, treated by assurance that it is benign. Otherwise Carbamazepine (tegretol) propranol or gabapentine may be tried in consultation with neuro physician. Sometime surgical treatment be required, i.e. superior oblique tenotomy and recession of inferior oblique on the same side.

5. Ocular bobbing

It is seen in **comatose** patients with widespread **pontine hemorrhage or neoplasm**. It is also seen in obstructive hydrocephalus or metabolic encephalopathy. The movements are fast, conjugate, and downward followed by slow upward drift to the primary position.

The other types of ocular bobbing are:

a. **Reverse ocular bobbing**— A fast conjugate upward movements with slow downward drift to primary position.
b. **Inverse ocular bobbing**— Slow conjugate drift down with quick upwards movement with a gap in between.
c. **Converse bobbing**— Slow upwards movement followed by fast return to primary position.

6. Ocular flutter

This is a horizontal saccade. Patient recovering from opsoclonus go through ocular flutter. It is almost always associated with **ocular dysmetria**. It is intermittent group of several fine oscillations, develops in primary gaze.

7. Ocular dysmetria

This is either **over shoot** or **under shoot** movement of the eye during change of gaze, mostly seen in **cerebellar disorders** along with **nystagmus**. It is a conjugate movement. It is commonly associated with **intention tremors**.

8. Square wave jerks

These oscillations have rectangular appearance on eye movement recording, are seen in **Parkinson's disease, multiple sclerosis** and **progressive supra nuclear palsy**. They are nonrhythmic with small amplitude. They first obstruct fixation and then there is a foveal fixation. They are saccades.

9. Oculogyric crisis

This is **involuntary spasmodic deviation of both the eyes upwards** that may last for few minutes to few hours. It is caused by many drugs, commonly seen in Parksonism, encephalitis, neurosyphilis, trauma, multiple sclerosis.

Acoustic neuroma is unilateral growth that involves the vestibular nerve. It is slow enough to develop adaptive mechanism that dampen the vestibular features hence, **vertigo is less common**. **Nystagmus is common** that is **peripheral type**. The nystagmus is away from the lesion in early stage. As the tumor increase in size it presses the **brainstem**. The patient develops ipsilateral, slow, large amplitude nystagmus, hearing defect, lateral rectus palsy, diplopia and corneal anesthesia.

Uniocular nystagmus

This is a **rare** form of nystagmus. It can either be **central** or **peripheral** in origin when peripheral it is ocular. **It may be familial**. It could be horizontal or vertical. The **horizontal nystagmus** is jerk and due to lesions of medial longitudinal fasciculus. When vertical it is pendular and due to lesion of tegmentum. It should be differentiated from latent nystagmus which is a binocular feature but observed when one eye in covered.

The systemic causes are— Multiple sclerosis, meningitis, congenital syphilis, tumours of mid brain, spasmus nutans, ataxia.

The ocular causes are— Superior oblique myokimia, myokymia of lower lid, amblyopia, high errors of refraction, lesion of anterior visual pathway.

Positional nystagmus

Nystagmus is precipitated by sudden change of head position. The nystagmus may change in form or intensity with change in head position. It may be present in normal persons as well. It is **vestibular** in origin. It is also seen in **tumors of posterior fossa**. It is commonly due to **drugs** and **toxins**. Others cause are— Head injury, inner ear pathology, meningitis, syphilis, arteriosclerosis.

Management of nystagmus

Lack of precise knowledge about nystagmus makes it's management difficult.

The management may be broadly divided into two parts:

1. Directed towards the systemic causes that results in nystagmus, i.e. infection, inflammation, trauma, neoplasm etc. These are outside the domain of ophthalmologist. They are best treated by neuro physician or neuro surgeon.
2. Directed towards the ocular manifests. Which is managed by ophthalmologist. The aim of which are:
    - i. Improve vision
    - ii. Correct physical appearance by way of:
        - a. Minimize nystagmus
        - b. Correct head posture
        - c. Manage squint and amblyopia.

The above goals are achieved by a combination of:

a. Medical treatment
b. Optical correction
c. surgery:

a. The medical management consists of:
   i. GABA agonist, anti convulsants, sedatives and tranquillisers. They are Gaba pentin, baclofen, clonazepam, valproate, carbamazipine.
   ii. Retro bulbar injection or infiltration of spastic extraocular muscle with botulin toxin type A (Botox).
   The therapeutic agents are best administered under supervision of physician.
b. Optical correction consists of salvaging the best correctable vision by:
   i. Spectacles
   ii. Contact lenses
   iii. Uniocular telescope for distance
c. Squint is managed by:
   i. Optical correction
   ii. Prisms— they are used to dampen the action of stronger muscles and place the eyes in position of least nystagmus.
   iii. Surgery to correct squint and to move the eyes into null zone. This is claimed to correct abnormal head posture. The commonest procedure is known as Kestenbaum— Anderson procedure.

BIBLIOGRAPHY

1. Averbuch-Heller, Tussa RJ. Fuhry L. A double blind study of gabapentine and baclofen in treatment of or acquired nystagmus. Ann Neural 1997;41:818-25.
2. Averbuch-Heller-L, Leish RJ. Medical treatment for abnormal eye movements. Pharmacological, optical and immunological strategies. Ast Nz Jraph 1997;25:7-13.
3. Daroff RB, Troost RW. Upbeat nystagmus, JAMA 1973;225:312.
4. Deborah Pavan Langston. Extraocular muscles. Strabismus and nystagmus in manual of ocular diagnosis and therapy. 3rd edn, Little Brown, 1981;323-35.
5. Dell'osso LF, Daroff RB. Nystagmus and saccadic intrusion and oscillation in neuro-ophthalmology, 3rd edn, Glasser JS, Lippincott-Williams and Wilkins (Eds), Philadelphia, 369-401.
6. Duke Elders. Uniocular nystagmus in system of ophthalmology, Vol XII. Duke Elders, and Scott-I (Eds), Henry Kimpton, London 1971;882.
7. Gami NK. Examination of a case of nystagmus in bedside approach to clinical neurology. Current books international, Calcutta 1983;56-59.
8. Gitt Inger JW. Downbeat nystagmus in manual of clinical problems in ophthalmology. 1st edn, Gittinger JW and Asdourian GK (Eds). Little Brown and company, Boston 1988; 182-84.
9. Helveston AM, Ell is FD, Plager DA. Large recession of horizontal rectus for treatment of nystagmus, Oph 1991;98:1302-05.
10. Kanski JJ. Nystagmus in clinical ophthalmology, 2nd edn, Butterworth, London 1889;475-77.

11. Kline LB, Bajandas FJ. Nystagmus and related ocular oscillations in neuro-ophthalmology, 5th edn, Jaypee Brothers Medical Publishers, New Delhi 2004;75-86.
12. Lyle TK, Wybar KC. Nystagmus in Lyle and Jacson's practical orthoptoic. 1st edn, Jaypee Brothers Medical Publishers, New Delhi 1994;592-600.
13. Martyn LJ. Nystagmus in paediatric ophthalmology. Vol 2, 2nd edn. Harley RD (Eds), WB Sanders company, Philadelphia 1980;800-07.
14. Mason S. Swash M. The cranial nerves in Hutchison's clinical methods, 17th edn, ELBS, London 1982;291.
15. Mukherjee PK. Nystagmus in Paediatric ophthalmology, 1st edn, New Age International, New Delhi 2005;628-35.
16. Natchiar G. Subhuram supranuclear disorders of the eye movement and visual integration in modern ophthalmology, Vol 2, 2nd edn, Jaypee Brothers Medical Publishers, New Delhi 2000;921-922.
17. Roy FH. Oscillopsia in ocular differential diagnosis, 1st edn, Jaypee Brothers Medical Publishers, New Delhi 1985;450.
18. Sharma P. Nystagmus in strabismus simplified, 1st edn, Modern Publishers, New Delhi 1999;155-63.
19. Wheller DI. Nystagmus in current ocular therapy, 5th edn, Fraunfelder FT, Roy FH (Eds), WB Saunders Company, Philadelphia 2000;407-10.